TEXTBOOK OF PSYCHOLOGY
FOR HOMEOPATHIC STUDENTS

Recommended for various Universities for Degree and Post-graduate Courses

Dr. Bichitra Bhusan Misra

B.II.M.S. (Bam. University), MD (Hom.) Utk. University,
Homeopathic Medical Officer (Govt. of Orissa)
I/C, H.O.D., Dept. of Repertory,
Previously teaching S.P.M. and Currently teaching Repertory:
Theory, Clinical and computer Repertorization,
Therapeutics and Psychology at Biju Pattanaik Homoeopathic
Medical College and Hospital, Brahmapur - 76 00 01

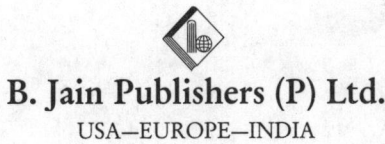

B. Jain Publishers (P) Ltd.
USA—EUROPE—INDIA

TEXTBOOK OF PSYCHOLOGY FOR HOMEOPATHIC STUDENTS

First Edition: 2010
3rd Impression: 2017

No part of this book may be reproduced, stored in a retrieval system or transmitted, in any form or by any means, mechanical, photocopying, recording or otherwise, without any prior written permission of the author.

© with the author

Published by Kuldeep Jain for
B. JAIN PUBLISHERS (P) LTD.
D-157, Sector-63, NOIDA-201307, U.P. (INDIA)
Tel.: +91-120-4933333 • *Email:* info@bjain.com
Website: **www.bjain.com**
Registered office: 1921/10, Chuna Mandi, Pahargani, New Delhi-110 055 (India)

Printed in India by
J.J. OFFSET PRINTERS

ISBN : 978-81-319-0542-5

Dedicated to
Loving Memories
of My Beloved Younger Brother

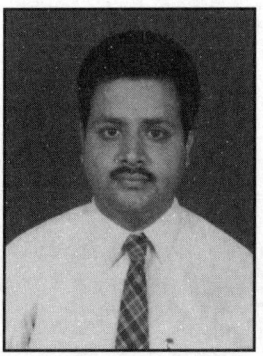

Late Shree Rabi Narayan Misra
(4.01.74-21.11.06)

ACKNOWLEDGEMENT

Neither the Taj nor Rome was built by a single person, although the credit goes to the Emperor. Similarly, this book is the outcome of several persons, who have been in the background and I must express my gratitude to all of them.

First, I express my sincere gratitude to my father **Sri Krishna Chandra Misra,** who infused in me English grammar and the art of writing and my mother **Smt. Sushila Misra,** who handed over the art of imagination and creativity in writing to me.

Next, I put across my indebtedness to **Sri Upendra Sahu,** my beloved teacher, who taught me English grammar during high school, which played a great role in bringing about this book.

Again, My deepest and biggest thanks are also due to **Sri Premananda Rath**, my eldest brother-in-law and **Swarnanjali,** my younger sister, who enthusiastically supported this gracious foundation with all their potential perspectives and without their support, this digest might not have come through.

I also acknowledge my deep gratitude to B.Jain family:

- **Late Shree P.N. Jain,** who had promised to give me a breakthrough as an another, and his word has come true at last
- **Shree Kuldeep Jain,** who took so much interest in publishing the book
- **Dr. Rohit Jain and Shree Manish Jain** who on the very first look of the rudimentary manuscript, gave a positive response for its publication
- **Dr. (Ms.) Taru Bhagat**, for her superb editing, **Dr. (Ms.) Geeta Rani Arora,** for her excellent coordination **and Dr. Harpreet Kaur** for her pains taking follow-up and without their team effort of tough grinding, this book might have lost all its beauty and nicety.

I also express my thanks to **Mr. Shantanu Kumar Sahu,** Proprietor, Gananath Homoeo Hall, Berhampur for his constant encouragement while the book was in progress.

Last but not the least, I acknowledge my thanks to **Osho Sambit,** my eight years old son, whose sweet smile and antics always wipe away my agonies and worries.

FOREWORD

I have known Dr. Misra since the last twenty five years. He was a colleague of mine for a few years. He has always regarded me as his mentor and guide, and I take great pride in it. He is silent, yet dynamic. He is disciplined, yet aggressive. He is obedient, yet hard working and meticulous. This book is the outcome of his pen. It is my grand privilege to forward the book to the homeopathic world.

I am sure this book will meet the long-felt need of our profession. Although Psychology was introduced in our curriculum thirty years back, until date this subject has not gained its due attention. Rather, this subject has been grossly neglected due to the non-availability of a standard book. Dr. Misra's attempt in this respect is praiseworthy. I have gone through the book and have found total coverage of the subject in a lucid and simple style with dozens of illustrations. This book, the first to be written in India on Psychology for homeopathic students (as per the course prescribed by the Central Council of Homoeopathy) will be welcomed by homeopathic teachers and students alike. Now, graduates as well as postgraduate students will no more run from pular to post to understand this subject. This single book will cater to all their needs to understand Psychology. Moreover, the book highlights the clinical application of Psychology in the realm of homeopathy.

In conclusion, the book is a welcome addendum and in a way a trendsetter in the field of behavioral science as applicable to homeopathy. I hope this book will be a success in its mission to trigger advance attempts in the trail.

Prof. (Dr.) Niranjana Mohanty
Advisor, Indian Institute of Homeopathy Former Physician
—Dean of Homeopathic faculty (Utkal University)
—Principal-cum-Superintendent/H.O.D., P.G./ Dept of Repertory,
Dr. A. C. Homeopathic Medical College and Hospital, Bhubaneswar
—National President I.I.H.P.
—Member, C.C.H. (New Delhi)

PREFACE

I trust in totality. I am absolutely against ritualism. I trust in totality in the sense that either you should do something in totality with a full effort or not do anything at all. Hence, it is obvious on my part to subscribe the view that no learning is better than ill learning. Similarly, I also subscribe that no teaching is better than ill teaching. It is unfortunate that the education imparted in psychology in our institutions has just become a ritual. In our curriculum, the main endeavor of teaching psychology is just fixed to the completion of the course by hook or by crook within a stipulated period without taking into account its practical benefits in the realm of homeopathic treatment, education, research and administration. It is felt that this arrangement cannot cater to the present need of our profession. Hence, it is felt that the subject has been grossly neglected in our curriculum. In many homeopathic institutions, teachers are hired from general colleges or from private sources who are entrusted the teaching of psychology to homeopathic students. They teach psychology to the students in their own style, manner and whim without realizing its relevance to homeopathy. Surprisingly, no guidelines are issued to them for teaching psychology in homeopathic institutions. Hence, they fail to correlate the prescribed lessons to the students of homeopathy. Also, interestingly, some homeopathic teachers attribute Hahnemann's views in a distorted form in relation to psychology. No doubt, our immortal Master has given sufficient instructions to deal with a patient from a psychological point of view but his views should not be wrongly interpreted. In a truer sense, the development of the science of psychology belongs to the post-Hahnemannian era.

I have tried my level best to give a solution to the plight and predicament delineated above. Reading psychology has been a passion and pleasure for me since the last two to three decades. The present work is the outcome of 18 months of rigorous study and hard work. I have carefully evaluated the course that has been prescribed by The Central Council of Homoeopathy, New Delhi, to give the real spirit of psychology that is needed to our profession. I have consulted more than SIX dozen books, out of which most of the material has been incorporated from the category of foreign authors, as a substantial contribution comes from their side. My attempt in this venture is to:

a. Offer an introductory course in psychology.
b. Present the profession the complex concepts of psychology in a lucid and simplified manner.
c. Bring forth the clinical relevance of the subject.
d. Cover the syllabi of psychology as prescribed by C.C.H. Thus, it will help the students to understand the various principles and utility of psychology.
e. Present authenticity of the subject matter.
f. Present the faculty of Organon of Medicine, homeopathic Psychology as a handbook in imparting education to the students.
g. Present various topics in a sequential arrangement so that the book will become useful as a ready reference.

I sincerely hope that the book will prove beneficial to all for whom it has been written. If this book helps you even as little as a candle in the dark, I will feel that my entire effort has been successful. Anyhow, you being a part of this mission are at liberty to write to me with your views for improvement of the book, which will be acknowledged in the next edition of the same.

—**Dr. Bichitra Bhusan Misra**
Tulasi Nagar,
Brahmapur – 760001
Orissa
17 Nov., 2007

PUBLISHER'S NOTE

B.B. Misra's 'Textbook of Psychology for Homeopathic Students' is a valuable acknowledgement of the realization that many of the era's diseases spring from the mind, or are psychological in origin, and some could, given proper guidance encouragement and motivation, be cured by timely psychological intervention. Many develop unwholesome cravings from sweetmeats, many turn to substance dependence or abuse as an escape from frustration or monotony and very few know about psychological ideas of personality improvement, the value of a regular life, of regular habits and so it is hoped that tomorrow's homeopathic doctors will enlighten their patients and illumine their lives, possibly saving them from frustration and poverty.

Kuldeep Jain
C.E.O., B. Jain Publishers (P) Ltd.

CONTENTS

Dedication .... *iii*
Acknowledgement .... *v*
Foreword .... *vii*
Preface .... *ix*
Publisher's Note .... *xi*

Chapters

1. Psychology: An Introduction 1
2. Psychology: Its Relation to Other Sciences 21
3. Schools of Psychology 29
4. Psychology of Cognition: Sensation 41
5. Psychology of Cognition: Perception 69
6. Learning (Scientific Study of Behavior: Pavlov, Skinner and Watson) 93
7. Freud and Psychoanalysis 117
8. Neo-Freudian Psychodynamics 147
9. Psycho-somatic Manifestation of Dreams 169
10. Emotion 187
11. Remembering and Forgetting (Memory) 209
12. Intelligence 229
13. Thinking 265
14. Personality 279
15. Motivation 305
16. Aptitude 323
17. Attention and Distraction 331
18. Psychology of Anxiety and Anxiety Disorders 345
19. Conflict 367
20. Frustration 375
21. Dimensions of Developmental Psychology 387
22. Developmental Psychology 411
23. Model Questions 437

Bibliography *447*

Chapter 1

PSYCHOLOGY : AN INTRODUCTION

When we think of psychology, generally we think of it as a mysterious subject. We believe that by reading psychology, we,

1. can read somebody's mind.
2. can predict the future course of action of the concerned person.
3. feel that we can understand the nature and character of the man too by doing so.
4. can obtain fascinating information about ourselves.
5. can solve various personal and allied problems of our life, etc.

Though we are not absolutely wrong about such associations, yet we must remember that psychology belongs to science and science never believes in anything. Science is not mystery. It is also not black magic. A magician might have shown the action of a breezy fan or so-called aeroplane to Asoka or Akbar, and people around him. The people of that time might have observed it with awe and wonder. Probably, people of those days had taken it as a mystery or personal effect. Now the scenario has changed. Aeroplanes, TV's, computers, etc. have become child's play due to the phenomenal progress of science. Yes, we can predict a lot of animal, as well as human behavior by reading psychology. But those efforts must be looked through a scientific method instead of a mystery or black magic. Psychology should not be categorized under "mysticism" or "occultism". Psychology is one of the youngest, yet rapidly growing science. It has entered almost all the fields of human concern like health, medicine, education, warfare, economics, industry, etc. Study of psychology has a tremendous impact on homeopathy. Psychology is needed by us from drug proving to inducing euthanasia for a dying patient of cancer. Without the study of psychology, our science will become sterile in many ways. Today, psychology concerns one and all. Although Hahnemann has left us glimpses of psychology in his scattered literature, yet a serious effort for its exploration in relation to homeopathy has not been undertaken. Today we need a serious and relevant study of psychology from a homeopathic point of view, which is the call of the day. You will be happy to know that the first scientific laboratory was started in Leipzig in the year 1879, a few years after the departure of the immortal soul of our Master Hahnemann. Anyhow, psychology has now become very important for homeopathic education, treatment, research and administration.

Our age belongs to science and its off-shoots; information and technology, popularly known as IT. After its advent, dramatic concepts were developed and phenomenal achievements were accomplished in the field of homeopathy. We have absorbed IT in toto in homeopathy. Now there comes the turn of psychology. Psychology has already played a wonderful role in every walk of life. Today we need it for further fortification of our science. The subject of psychology has two aspects:

1. Pure.
2. Applied.

Pure psychology formulates broad principles, brings theories and recommends technique for the study of human behavior.

In *applied psychology*, the theoretical teaching finds its practical shape in applied aspects: Clinical psychology, Criminal psychology, Industrial psychology, Educational psychology and now, Homeopathic psychology.

Psychology has become a part of us since its very inception, although we are not actively aware of it. Hahnemann, Boenninghausen, Kent, Boger and even Murphy, the messiah of homeopathy have talked a lot about psychology directly or indirectly in their literature. Now it is high time for us to explore and use psychology for the purpose our research, treatment and education. Moreover, homeopathy has also a lot to contribute to psychology. To cite an example, the people of psychology are not aware of Hahnemann's miasmatic theory. Approaches like Hypnotism, Psycho-analysis and even Catharsis have only been able to palliate many cases instead of curing them. When these approaches are utilized judiciously with homeopathy, humanity can get a new light. In fact, our future belongs to genetics, homeopathy, psychology and yoga. Today we can safely accept and further develop homeopathic psychology as a branch of homeopathy. Homeopathic psychology is an attempt to apply the knowledge of pure psychology to the field of homeopathy.

DEFINITION OF PSYCHOLOGY

The word psychology takes its origin more than two thousand years ago. But the credit goes to Rudolf Goeckle (1547-1628), who coined the word "Psychology." This word is derived from two Greek words "*Psyche*", means soul (it differs from Indian terminology of Soul. You should go through Patanjali Yoga Pradeep or alike Indian literature to perceive the real essence of the soul) and "*Logos*" meaning "discursive knowledge" or "a rational course of studies". Psychology is a relatively new subject, but it has a long history, as long as human beings who have tried to understand themselves and the environment around them. The subject of psychology is becoming increasingly popular day by day.

Is Psychology the Study of the Soul?

It has already been mentioned that psychology is the science of soul. This concept has been described in ancient Greek literature. Accordingly, soul was termed as an inner flame, which is responsible for the function of bodily processes. It is also mentioned that the soul leaves the body after death or in other words death occurs when the soul departs from the body. Moreover, it was believed that women and servants have no soul. The ancient Greek philosophers (as earlier, psychology was a branch of philosophy) also held that the soul has no physical existence. It can neither be seen nor touched. Moreover, it cannot be destroyed after death. They sternly believed that death can occur to a body and never to the soul.

Criticism

The above definition somehow seems to be mystical and does not cater to the needs of qualifying for a scientific certification. The definition was rejected on the following grounds:

1. Soul cannot be observed.
2. It coincides with religion.
3. The term 'soul' appears to be philosophical.
4. A scientific study cannot be carried out for the soul. Science cannot exist for something that does not exist.

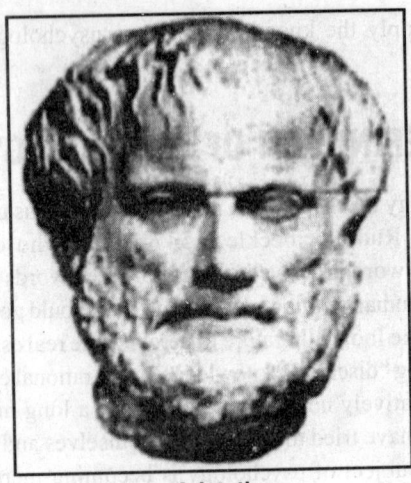

Aristotle
(384 B.C. - 322)

Is Psychology the Study of Mind?

After rejection of psychology as the science of soul as mentioned above, some Greek philosophers like Aristotle defined psychology as the study of mind.

Criticism

The word "mind" has to suffer almost equally to that of soul. Of course mind is less vague and less mysterious in comparison to the soul, still it was rejected on the following grounds:

1. What is mind? Who is there to answer?
2. How can the mind be studied?
3. Mind involves a mental process but it does not have a separate existence.
4. Mind lacks unanimous agreement amongst psychologists regarding its nature.
5. Studying the mind of animals or humans is difficult and confusing because mind is related to subjective experience. Moreover, there rises a question, "How to study the mind of an animal?"

Is Psychology the Study of Consciousness?

After the rejection of psychology as the science of "soul" and "mind", it was defined as the "science of consciousness" by Wilhelm Wundt, who gave psychology a scientific status by opening the first psychological laboratory in Leipzig in the year 1879.

Criticism

Wundt's definition was again rejected like the above for reasons described below:

1. There is a diverse opinion about consciousness. Some psychologist do not accept it even as a process.
2. The behavior of man and animal do not come under purview consciousness, being subjective in nature.
3. Such a definition of psychology constricts its scope for expansion.
4. Psychology also studies unconscious and sub-conscious levels.
5. This definition restricts itself to only human beings and restrains us from studying the consciousness of an animal.

Naturally this definition cannot be accepted.

Psychology: What is it?

In fact, psychology is the product of philosophy and physiology. It has to traverse a long way from its very inception. Anyhow, William McDougall, a British psychologist was the first person to give a practical definition to psychology. He defined psychology as the science of behavior. This definition was accepted by almost all the psychologists. This definition sets up the most comprehensive definition of psychology. In other words, psychology may be defined as the positive science of conduct of living creatures. It fulfils all the criteria that have been criticized above. Anyhow, in recent times we find a better definition given by Robert A. Baron in his book *"Psychology"*. According to him, psychology is the **"science of behavior and cognitive process"**. Two parts of this definition deserve further comment.

First, note that psychologists view their field as basically scientific in nature.

Second, this definition suggests that psychologists view their field broad in scope; indeed they perceive it as being concerned with virtually everything we do, feel, think or experience.

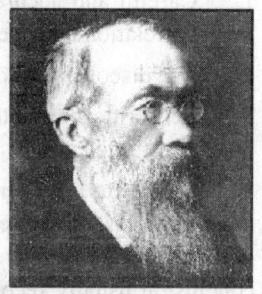

**Wundt
(1832-1920)**

The term behavior denotes observable action or reaction of a living organism – everything we see or do through subtle changes in the electrical activity occurring deep inside our brains. If it can be observed and measured, then it fits within the boundary of psychology. Similarly by cognitive process, the psychologist means every aspect of our mental life – our thoughts, memories, reasoning, decision making and so on – in short, all aspects of mind.

Psychology: Is it Science or Not?

Wilhelm Wundt was the first psychologist who tried to give a scientific status to psychology. His novel venture gave a new turn to psychology and the real scientific spirit was instilled in psychology.

Now Let Us Study What Science is?

The simplest definition for science is "accumulation of systematic knowledge". Systematic means the method that is used in reaching the goal, whereas knowledge refers to the goal of science. We must know that it is not however the subject matter of a study that makes it a science, but its methods. It is the method of science that distinguishes itself from art and philosophy or religion. Thus, we must have a basic understanding about the scientific methods.

SCIENTIFIC METHODS

Definition

Karl Parson in his book "*Grammar of Science*" states "the scientific method" is marked by the following features:

1. Careful and accurate classification of facts and observation of their correlation and sequence.
2. The discovery of scientific laws with the aid of creative imagination.
3. Self-criticism and the final touch stone of equal validity for all normally constituted minds.

George L. Lundberg in his book "*Social Research*" quotes, "Scientific method consists of systematic observation, classification and interpretation of data. The main difference between our day to day generalization and the conclusion usually recognized as scientific method, lies in the degree of formality, rigorness, verifiability and general validity of the latter.

L.L. Bernard in his book *"The Field and Method of Sociology"* asserts that science may be defined in terms of six major processes that take place within. These processes are:

1. Testing
2. Verification
3. Definition
4. Classification
5. Organization
6. Orientation

(These also include prediction and application.)

Steps in Scientific Method

1. Observation

The first step in scientific methods is observation. A casual and random observation may give a clue, it may even reveal a fact or phenomenal truth or reality, but this must be properly observed. The study must be made very carefully and closely. The observations usually need various equipment, apparatus and instruments. These equipments must give precision in measurement so that an objective end may be achieved.

2. Recording

Next to observation there comes the role of recording. Recording is needed, because through it we can establish a relation between facts. The recording must be accurate and should be done very carefully. The experimenter must be free from prejudiced convictions and personal emotions with a knack of detached objectivity.

3. Classification

Relevant data is collected from the given field and then classified or grouped as per the facts. The scattered data usually fails to express the relevant facts and may put one in a state of confusion. In census, we record in the multiple of 5 because without such classification we cannot conclude to something relevant. If we record the individual age of everybody then we cannot evaluate steps of solving the problems. Hence, classification is a part and parcel of scientific methodology. The classification should be realistic and should be done in such way that a relationship can be evolved. By classification we reach generalization from particularization. A scattered pattern of particulars generally does not convey anything useful, whereas generalization gives a practical utility. Classification should be an organized representation of particular patterns so that a plausible, realistic strategy of generalization can be developed.

4. Generalization

Next step is generalization. By generalization the scientific laws are derived for general application.

5. Verification

Simply propounding a law is not sufficient for qualifying it as a scientific method. The law must be verified from time to time depending upon the conditions.

From the above study we can safely term a subject scientific, if it:

a. does not support on hearsay, superstition or personal belief, having no objective verification.
b. sets up a cause and effect relationship.
c. takes up the method of objective investigation on systematic and controlled observation with a scientific approach.
d. stands for generalization, verifiability of observed results or inferred phenomena.
e. predicts for future application.
f. has an applied or practical aspect.
g. involves scientific method.
h. bears factuality.
i. has universal application, under any given condition.
j. testifies the veracity.

Let us review psychology in the light of the above mentioned norms:

a. Almost all the methods used in psychology are more or less scientific in nature.
Psychology uses scientific methods to collect data about individuals and groups to analyze and predict their behavior. The experimental

methods used in psychology are exact. In experimental methods, dependant and independent variables are used precisely. Even laboratory instruments like chronoscope (a highly sensitive clock) are used to determine the interval down to the thousandth part of a second. Psychologists deal with observable behavior and establish fact by objective evidence. Hence psychology should be called as science.

b. Psychology as science helps us to understand, control and predict behavior through experimental methods in a given condition.

c. Psychological findings are applicable for future verification, researches and new findings for a practical and fruitful life.

d. Psychology studies the facts of behavior and is hence factual.

e. Psychology follows all the foot steps of scientific methods like testing, verifying, defining, classifying, organizing, etc. and establishes laws of psychology which are universal. Under given conditions, they can be verified from time to time.

f. Psychological laws can be verified and reverified. For example, it has been found that behind every mental abnormality there is a history (rather a cause) of frustration. This fact has been verified very frequently.

g. Psychology discovers cause and effect relationship in human behavior. For example, psychology has discovered why and under which circumstance a child becomes a delinquent. These findings have immense value in the treatment, as these findings are scientific. Thus, psychology discovers the "how" of behavior together with its "what".

h. Psychology predicts human behavior. It has already been mentioned earlier that psychology discovers the cause and effect relationship. This helps in predicting human behavior.

Finally, we can bind the present mission as follow:

"Psychology as a behavioral science which aims to study the behavior in groups. Human beings are by nature social. They live in social situations form birth to death. Their personality is shaped by interaction with the external social environment. It is beyond imagination to think that a human being can develop harmoniously without social interaction in isolation. In modern psychology, we study how society influences the behavior of an individual and vice versa. How an individual learns in a group? The behavior of an individual originates in social milieu. We know that the behavior of an individual is studied in terms of social interaction. Psychology as a science studies scientifically cultural and social problems of society. Psychology has successfully collected an enormous data on problems of minority groups, group dynamics, etc. and has devised measures to solve social problems. Thus, we see *psychology as a behavioral science"*

(Chauhan, 1991)

Limits of Accuracy in Psychology

A science is a systematic body of knowledge gathered by careful observation and measurement of events. The things and objects are systematized and classified into various categories, followed by formulation of general laws and principles. Later, these formulations and generalizations are established. They describe and predict the events as evidently as possible. A science is engaged in discovering those conditions and factors that determine the cause of the occurrence of a particular event using scientific method of experimentation and observation. Science seeks to explain the phenomena within its scope.

Branches of Psychology

Psychology has extended its tentacles in all aspects of human life extending from infant to old, from normal to abnormal, crime to military and many more. Following divisions are recognized by various psychological associations of the world including Association of American Psychologists, who are in the forefront.

1. General psychology
2. Abnormal psychology
3. Social psychology
4. Experimental psychology
5. Para-psychology
6. Geo-psychology
7. Developmental psychology
8. Educational psychology
9. Clinical psychology
10. Physiological psychology
11. Comparative psychology
12. Dynamic psychology

13. Occupational psychology
14. Industrial psychology
15. Legal psychology
16. Military psychology
17. Political psychology
18. Engineering psychology
19. Child psychology
20. Folk psychology
21. Consumers psychology
22. Individual psychology
23. Evaluation and measurement psychology
24. Personality and social psychology
25. Consulting psychology
26. Rehabilitation psychology
27. Philosophical psychology
28. History of psychology
29. Community psychology
30. Psycho-pharmacology
31. Humanistic psychology
32. Population psychology
33. Psychology of women
34. Psychometric psychology and many other divisions.
    And now,
35. Homeopathic psychology

We will discuss a few of the various branches of psychology under two headings:

    A. Pure

    B. Applied

A. Pure Psychology

Important branches of pure psychology have been highlighted below:

1. General Psychology

It deals with the fundamental principles of all psychology. It specially deals with normal human adults, leaving other subjects to specialized fields. It studies topics of human behavior of greater importance like sensation, perception, emotion, learning, motivation, thinking, memory, personality, etc.

2. Abnormal Psychology

Psychology studies both normal and abnormal behavior. Psychoses, neuroses and other abnormalities come under its purview. Psychology studies all these abnormal conditions, tries to find out its causes and remedial measures. For example, psycho-analysis, founded by Freud plays a significant role in treatment of various abnormal behaviors.

3. Social Psychology

Social psychology is the science of behavior of the individual in society. Social psychology is a bridge between psychology and sociology. This has been already accepted as a major branch of psychology. It is concerned with behavior and experience of an individual in a group, in a community and in society. It also studies the behavior of a group; its formation, interaction, its influence over the society, etc. Sociology deals with its other aspects like socialization of personality, social motives, behavior, aggression, conflicts, leadership, propaganda, etc. Social psychology also studies how rumors are spread, how beliefs and attitudes develop. In recent days it has attached itself with mass communication, cognitive dissonance, population research, etc. Its need has grown to a greater extent in the field of community medicine.

The great difference between social psychology and sociology is its approach to the problem. Social psychology explains society through the study of an individual whereas, sociology explains individuals through the study of society and its forces. The main subjects of sociology are family, group dynamics, mob, crowd, opinions, propaganda, rumor, leadership, social tensions, conflicts, fashion, culture and process of socialization.

4. Experimental Psychology

The most important method of contemporary psychology is the experimental method. It includes specializations in child, educational, social, developmental, physiological, comparative psychology, etc. This is one of the most valuable branches of psychology in the sense that it uses scientific methods in its study. Its scope is gradually enlarging and amplifying with the modern equipment and gadgets.

5. Para-psychology

Para-psychology is that branch of psychology which attempts to study various mental phenomena, such as E.S.P. (i.e., Extra Sensory Perception), Psycho-kinesics, Bio-location, etc., which suggest that the mind can secure knowledge by means other than the usual perceptual process. Now this branch has specially engaged itself in exploring telepathy, rebirth and allied phenomena.

Herewith some para-psychological phenomena are given in a nutshell:

i. *Telepathy:* The apparent communication of thoughts between one person's mind to another's, which cannot be done with the normal range of senses.

ii. *Clairvoyance:* The supposed ability to see into the future, or know things without making use of any of the five senses.

iii. *Precognition:* To foresee events of the future without the use of any of the five senses.

iv. *Psychokinesis:* This is also known as P.K. and Telekinesis or 'Mind Over Matter'. P.K. is thought to be influenced by a person's 'willing'. In P.K., exercising of power over objects outside of human physical reach is done, by which an object of physical character can be moved with the act of mind. A person gifted with P.K. can move a dice in space or manipulate the falling of cards as per his desire. Levitation of floating in space without any physical help is another example of P.K.

v. *Bi-location:* Appearance of an individual can be seen at two places simultaneously.

vi. *Psychometry:* An individual gifted with this ability can gather information about a person. The individual just touches an object that belongs to the person and reveals the past, present or future of the concerned person.

vii. *Dowsing:* An individual's ability to sense the presence of underground water, ores, lost articles, etc.

viii. *Psychic Healing:* An individual can heal a sufferer through transmission of his psychic powers, which cannot be explained by normal means.

6. Folk Psychology

This is the branch of psychology that studies superstitions, mythologies, along with culture, music, art, religion, etc. in a given context.

7. Geo-psychology

This branch of psychology explains the relation of physical environment in relation to weather, climate, soil, etc. with behavior.

8. Developmental Psychology

Psychology studies man as a dynamic being. Growth and development is a part and parcel of this dynamic activity. Developmental psychology studies the various stages of development of man in relation to the behavior of an individual from birth to old age. It attempts to find the abnormality of development and tries to solve it through its unique way (see last two chapters of this book).

B. Applied Psychology

It has already been mentioned that psychology is not only a theoretical study. It conversely, helps to find a solution to various problems concerning various aspects of human behavior. Applied psychology has the following important branches:

1. Educational Psychology

Educational psychology involves the understanding of children at home as well as in the classroom. The main purpose behind this is to examine and evaluate their learning along with emotional and motivational problems. The educational psychologist mainly studies the process of teaching and learning in the educational set up. Educational psychology deals with the problems of guiding and training the individual in various ways to learn new concepts and activities. Educational psychology is needed to understand child's abilities, activities, interest and limitations for better educational guidance. The study of educational psychology trains an individual what to teach and what not to teach, when to teach and when not to teach, how to teach, where to teach and why to teach. It also helps the educational system to bring about utmost development in the field of education. Today's education, may it be general or medical or homeopathic cannot run without educational psychology.

2. Clinical Psychology

Clinical psychology concerns itself with diagnosis, treatment of severe adjustment problems such as those found in psychotic, neurotic and delinquent behavior. A clinical psychologist chiefly:

a. Facilitates diagnosis by administering psychological tests.
b. Interprets the findings.
c. Carries out psychotherapy.
d. Conducts researches on problems of clinical nature.

A clinical psychologist also concerns himself for the followings:

a. Counselling psychology.
b. Industrial psychology.
c. Engineering psychology.
d. Consumer psychology.
e. Legal psychology.

The scope of clinical psychology has widened in India in recent days. It is estimated that clinical psychology employs almost $1/3^{rd}$ of all psychologists in clinical set up. In recent days, worries, anxieties, frustrations, etc. have become a part of our life. Such traumatic experiences lead us to various behavioral disorders like anxiety neurosis, psychoses, sexual deviants, anti-social personalities, etc. Hence clinical psychology now occupys a lions share in the field of psychology. Now, we the homeopaths should bring forth the importance of miasmatic and constitutional treatment of a mentally aberrant individual with due documentation in our clinic.

3. Physiological Psychology

Physiological psychology is the study of the physiological basis of behavior. Physiological psychology is primarily concerned with the relationship between psychological processes and the underlying physiological events with special focus of emphasis on the study of the nervous system and endocrine glands. It also encompasses the study of sensation and perception, thinking, learning, etc. including motivated behavior, emotion, learning, memory, cognition, etc. In recent days, special foci has been put in the study of heredity, metabolism, drug addiction and diet.

4. Comparative Psychology

It is the comparative study of animal species in relation to processes of psychology, neurology and biochemical activities. The animals often studied are rats, dogs, monkeys, pigeons, etc.

This branch emerged from the evolution concept by Darwin, who highlighted psychological evolution also. His work highlights the characteristics of the mental and emotional life of animals and people, which are transmitted from generation to generation like morphological characteristics.

5. Differential Psychology

It studies the individual difference through measurement and assessment of mental abilities by various tests.

6. Dynamic Psychology

Dynamic psychology mainly studies normal motivation including both conscious and unconscious aspects.

7. Occupational Psychology

It is an application of the differential psychology in occupation. It deals with selection of people in a particular job. Various mental and aptitude tests are carried out to evaluate interest, temperament and other personality variables for the recruitment of suitable candidates.

8. Industrial Psychology

Industrial psychology is related to human factors in industry such as personal problems, safety management, prevention of accidents, morale of employees, rehabilitation, etc. along with factors like bargaining, labor unrest and their welfare, processing grievances, commercial advertisement, effective leadership, production, etc. Its main objectives are increasing productivity in a cost effective way, using the principles of scientific management with those of comprehensive understanding of human problems in the industry.

9. Legal Psychology

Legal psychology is concerned with finding the cause behind the crimes. It also deals with the methods and techniques required for the detection of crimes along with suggesting remedial measures for its control or cure.

10. Military Psychology

This division of psychology is concerned with making use of psychological principles and techniques in the domain of military activities. Military psychology is also utilized for recruitment of better personnel for the armed force. It involves in making strategies against enemy camp, boosting the morale of soldiers and people or the nation during wartime.

11. Political Psychology

This branch of psychology is concerned with the psychological principles and techniques in the field of politics. It includes study of mass behavior, public opinion, leadership abilities along with diplomatic manipulation of mass psychology, etc.

12. Engineering Psychology

This owes its origin to the period of Second World War. Engineering psychology is involved in designing and operating machines and equipment. This psychology is gaining a new height in recent days where an engineer and a psychologist walk hand in hand. The design or the model is conceptualized by an engineer. The psychologist also contributes in relation to perception, learning, etc.

13. Developmental Psychology

Developmental psychology studies the physical and mental development of the human organism from womb to tomb.

14. Child Psychology

Child psychology is a branch of developmental psychology. It includes the study of sensory and motor development of the child, his specific ability including growth and development of various milestones, perception, intelligence, thinking, reasoning abilities, etc. Child psychology also studies the behavior of gifted, normal and below normal children.

Homeopathic Psychology

It is the latest entrant in the realm of psychology. Homeopathic psychology concerns itself the various behaviors that evolve with homeopathic education, treatment, research and administration.

Homeopathic psychology pertains to both pure and applied aspects.

In pure aspect we study behavior of various diseases and in applied aspects we go for case taking, evaluating symptoms, repertorisation, etc.

As far as the pure aspect of homeopathic psychology is concerned, various processes of behavior have been explained in detail in *Organon of Medicine* and *Chronic Diseases* by Hahnemann. Stalwarts like Boenninghausen, Kent, Boger, Roberts, etc., have immensely contributed in relation to various behavior patterns of the patient and the drug in their literature.

Homeopathic psychology will help us in formulating homeopathic education also. We should study the behavior of the patient, students, public, etc. so that we can evolve a better psychological approach to our education in homeopathy.

We can also study the behavior of various medicines in relation to proving, clinical observations and patients so that our prescription will become more precise and time saving.

Homeopathic psychology can also be utilised for various research purposes. It will enable us better understanding of various behaviors related to incurable diseases with their variables. This can help us in fixing various parameters and measurements. Aspects like building hypothesis, formulating research design, analysis of data, statistical utility, etc. can be better understood and hence can be applied with the help of homeopathic psychology.

Goals of Psychology

Till now we have come across the major branches of psychology that exist today including homeopathic psychology. Naturally, you may ask what is there in common that ties them up together under the single crown "psychology"? The answer is that psychologists, regardless of their branches or areas of interest, share common goals and methods, like scientists, who seek to describe, explain, predict and control what they study. Hence, let us go for a discussion under the following headings to appreciate the goals of psychology:

1. Description
2. Explanation
3. Predication
4. Control

1. Description

Let us take a question: Whether there are gender differences in aggressive behavior? Many people deem that males are more aggressive than females. Some people may not subscribe to this, argue that this may be only stereotype and it is not true always. When this problem appears before psychologists, first they try to find out: Do men and women essentially differ in aggressive behavior? A number of research reports reveal the fact that males do behave more aggressively than females, at least as far as physical aggression is concerned. Now the psychologists do describe that gender differences in aggression do exist. Next, they will go for explanations about the description.

2. Explanation

The above description may be taken up by related branches of psychology for explanation.

If this is taken up by a physiological psychologist, he may explain the above phenomena on the basis of anatomy or body chemistry. He may even attribute possession of a greater amount testosterone as the cause of aggression in males.

The above theory may be carried out by a developmental psychologist. He may explain it on the basis of early training of the child; the way he was trained to behave like a boy or girl.

Similarly a social psychologist may explain the differences on the basis of community oriented constraints against aggressive behavior.

3. Prediction

Simply giving explanations like above are not sufficient to reach a goal. The explanations must be tested and found true. If any of the explanations are found to be correct then it should be permissible for prediction.

If gender differences in aggression are attributed to testosterone because males posses a larger amount it, then the psychologist will predict that reducing testosterone would reduce aggressive behavior in males.

Similarly, if the psychologists' explanation about early training is considered, they would predict that there would be fewer sex differences in families where the parents did not stress on gender difference in behavior.

Again, if sex differences in aggressive behavior are due to community oriented constraints, the psychologist will predict that removing or lessening the constraints will result in a higher level of aggressive behavior in females.

4. Control

If any or all of these explanations for sex differences in aggressiveness are found to be true; that is to say, if predictions are supported by research we can easily control aggressive behavior of an individual to a greater degree. Each of the predictions could be tested through research and the results can be used to indicate which of the explanations is the most successful to control aggressive behavior.

Chapter 2

PSYCHOLOGY : ITS RELATIONSHIP AND DIFFERENCES FROM OTHER SCIENCES

OVERVIEW

We can divide all the sciences under two categories:

1. **The Positive Science**

    This category incorporates:

    a. Physical sciences like physics, chemistry, etc. and,

    b. Life sciences like botany, zoology, etc.

    Positive science studies facts as they are and in no way concerns itself in enquiring what ought to be. It simply reveals obvious truths.

2. **The Normative Science**

    This category includes sciences like logic, philosophy, ethics, etc.

    This science teaches us what one should be, without bothering about its feasibility of application.

    Psychology belongs to the category of positive science. Of course, we may not equate it with other positive sciences like physics, chemistry, etc., still it has a relationship with both the types of science. Let us explore it further.

Philosophy

Earlier, psychology was a branch of philosophy. Various philosophical and psychological phenomena have been well described by Aristotle (384 BC-322

AD) and Rene Descartes (1596-1650), the Father of Modern Philosophy. Now psychology is completely an independent science with its distinctive methodology and perspective, although it has its origin from philosophy.

Philosophy comes from the Greek via the Latin word '*philosophia*' which means "love of wisdom". It is the study of nature, meaning of the universe and of human life. Philosophy examines facts and values as a systemic whole. Don't we often exhort to our friends not to be philosophical. Philosophical attitude implies to look into the matter as a whole, even in the context of the entire world or universe. Hence, psychology falls under the purviews of philosophy. Moreover, the philosophical truths must be centred on psychological facts. Epistemology is the branch of philosophy, which is centred on psychology. Thus, psychology bears a marked resemblance to philosophy. Still psychology diverges from philosophy under the following grounds:

a. First, psychology is a positive science and very concerned or related to science, whereas philosophy is normative science and less concerned with science or scientific methodology.

b. Secondly, psychology seeks objective evidences whereas philosophy is generally concerned with subjective conditions. Hence, psychology resorts to scientific experiments, observations, etc., whereas philosophy adheres to logic, intuition, meditation, etc.

c. Third, psychology is concerned with behavior whereas philosophy is concerned with philosophical outlook.

d. Last but not the least, the major differentiating point lies in respect to their perspective. The perspective of philosophy is synthetic whereas the perspective of psychology is analytical.

Logic

The word logic comes from 14th century French word, "*logique*" via Greek "*logikç*" which means 'art of reasoning.' Logic deals with the theory of deductive and inductive arguments and aims at discriminating good and bad reasoning. It involves sensible arguments and thoughts keeping emotions and whims apart.

In logic, the rules and criteria in association with concepts, judgements and inferences are discussed. Psychology also studies conception, judgements inferences, etc. from a psychological point of view. In this aspect, psychology seems to be in close relation with logic. Hence, it is better that logic be based on psychological findings and psychology must be based on logic before arriving at any principle. Despite such close resemblance, there exist differences between the two.

Firstly the nature of both psychology and logic differ. We must know that logic is a normative science whereas psychology is a pure science. Secondly, psychology is concerned with the process of thinking whereas logic tells how to think. Thirdly, the field of psychology is wider and embodies anything under the sun, whereas logic is concerned only with thought. Logic is less concerned with affective and conative processes. Finally, the standpoint also differs between these two. The stand point of logic is normative whereas the standpoint of psychology is factual.

Ethics

Ethics is a system of moral principles. Ethics is the science of ultimate good. It teaches us what one should do and not do. It examines the right and wrong of our action from ultimate truth. Ethics observes what is right or wrong in a given context.

Psychology is a positive science of behavior which is concerned with factuality. It does not bother what is right or wrong. Ethics is interested in evolving 'what ought to be' whereas psychology is concerned with 'what it is'. Ethics takes the help of psychology to know the psychological basis of moral decisions. An ideal ethic can be built only on true psychology. Ethics place high goals for human beings. Many a times a common man finds himself incapable or helpless to follow the norms erected by ethics. He loses moral judgment. But it is the psychology that facilitates the path to follow in actual life.

Moreover, the field of ethics is very limited whereas anything under the sun can be attributed to the scope of psychology. Ethics studies psychological principles from an ethical point of view whereas, psychology studies moral principles only as mental phenomena. Again, ethics is concerned with volition whereas psychology is involved in cognition, conation and affection.

Sociology

We know that sociology is related to society. Sociology is the scientific study of nature, development of society and social behavior. It attempts to understand the social system in order to arrive at a causal explanation of its course and effects i.e., study the social relationship within every institution. It tries to find an explanation for the nature of social order and social disorder which characterize the social life of man. Both psychology and sociology are closely related to each other in the following way:

a. Both belong to positive science.
b. Both are factual.
c. Both use scientific methods.
d. Both have limited predictive value.

Despite the above similarities, both differ from each other in many ways, some of which are described below:

One of the important points of difference between psychology and sociology lies in its approach towards an individual. Psychology teaches that every action of an individual has some psychological basis and studies a human being as an individual in a given environment. Sociology emphasises on society more than an individual. Hence, the basis of social behavior of man is his inclination to live in a group or society. Naturally, the standpoint of psychology is individual whereas the standpoint of sociology is society, mass, group, etc.

Psychology studies the individual apart from his caste, creed, religion or geographical distribution, whereas sociology studies man in context of society and as part of it.

The method envisaged for study by psychology and sociology also differs.

A Note on Social Psychology

We must remember that society is composed of individuals. Hence, an individual cannot appreciate the human values, activities, inter-relationships, etc. without understanding human psychology. Hence psychology and sociology are interdependent. Both are supplementary and complementary to each other. Social psychology is the science of behavior for the individual in society. Social psychology is a bridge between psychology and sociology.

Anthropology

Anthropology studies each and every aspect of human life ranging from the biology and evolutionary history of Homo sapiens to the future of society and culture. It also studies the enviornment and the various cultures that staunchly differentiate them from other animal species. It looks into the aspect of humanity like:

a. How the people live?
b. What they think?
c. How the people interact with their environments?

It also tries to comprehend the entire series of human diversity and what all people share in common. Here anthropology must take the help of psychology to enrich itself.

Anthropologists also quest for some basic questions like:

a. When did humans evolve?
b. Where did humans evolve?
c. How did humans evolve?
d. How do people adapt to diverse surroundings?
e. How have societies developed and changed from the ancient past to the present?

Naturally, anthropologists answer the above questions which help us understand what it means to be human. Here psychology must take the help of anthropology to enrich itself.

Obviously, psychologists and anthropologist help us to learn ways to meet the present-day needs of people all over the world. It also suggests of living for today and tomorrow. Hence, both are interdependent and naturally follow each other well.

Biology

Psychology is a positive science of behavior. The term behavior is taken in totality. Behavior has an extensive and comprehensive meaning. It includes all activities of life: External as well as internal processes including cognition. Psychology studies the origin of man including his biological developments. It describes the racial, sexual, physical, social and individual characteristics of a man and the principles of his adjustments to the environment. Hence, biological principles became a part of understanding the human behavior. For example, a person suffering from gastritis or asthma may become sluggish. Moreover, a specific hormone produces a specific action on a human being. Hence, the behavior of an individual is decided by hypo, normal or hyper-secretion of hormones. Behavior cannot be fully grasped without the knowledge of various biological principles. Despite such close resemblance, there exists essential differences between psychology and biology which can be assessed by the following lines:

a. Biology is the scientific study of natural processes of living things. It encompasses the study of the body and cells of living things. Thus, the discipline of biology covers all the physical and biological activities. On the other hand, psychology concerns itself with behavior and limits itself to study the observed behavior.

b. Biology studies man only as a living being whereas psychology studies man as an individual in relation to his environment.

From above, it is clear that biology and psychology are independent and interdependent discussions. Of course, both can be manipulated for the betterment of humanity.

Physiology

Psychology is the positive science of behavior. It has originated from dual sources of physiology (positive science) and philosophy (normative science). Yet it has its own individuality and speciality.

Physiology is the science of functioning of living organisms. It involves itself with the study of physiological activities in a living organism like circulation, respiration, digestion, etc. All these have a concern with health which guides the subsequent behavior of a person. For example, a person suffering from an acute episode of gastritis or asthma may not greet you cheerfully. His behavior may not be up to the mark or expectation.

Moreover, we cannot deny the relationship of psychology with physiology. The study of physiological processes helps us in understanding the mental behavior of an individual.

The field of psychology and physiology are separate and different. Physiology, as told above, is related to physical activities while psychology is related to the behavior of an individual including mental activities. Again, physiology concerns itself with different physical activity, whereas psychology is interested in the study of reaction of the physical organism as a whole towards external stimuli.

Anyhow, now-a-days another approach called physiological psychology is becoming more popular, which studies the physical activities connected with mental processes, having a special focus on endocrinology.

Medicine

Medicine includes the following features:

1. A drug is a substance used as a therapeutic agent to treat sick individuals.
2. It implies the science and art of healing of sickness including clinical specialists like, medicine, surgery, pediatrics, etc.
3. It attempts to study both health and disease. It studies man in disease and disease in man. It aims to:
    a. promote positive health of the individual,
    b. provide him specific protection against various diseases,
    c. diagnose a case as early as possible,
    d. provide early treatment to diseases,
    e. minimise the disability in the patient and,
    f. rehabilitate him in a due place in case he becomes physically or mentally handicapped.
4. Finally, the medicine is used for community approach which includes the total study of man in health and disease in clinic, hospital, laboratory including family setting, community or society with an aim to prevent, cure, palliate or rehabilitate as per the nature of disease with the current trend available in the health world.

Medicine and psychology are interrelated and interdependent as both are interested to heal the sick and promote positive health.

A doctor is supposed to have knowledge about human psychology and behavioral patterns. Similarly, a psychologist must have basic knowledge about the agent, host and environment that cause diseases. It is also hoped that the psychologist must have basic knowledge about anatomy, physiology, pathology along with medicine. As a homeopathic physician, we need to know psychology better because we treat the patient as a whole. Our holistic approach consists of taking the case along with considering the constitution of the patient and adopting the technique of analysis and synthesis in prescribing. Hence knowledge of psychology is a must for us. Similarly, psychologists and psychiatrists should have homeopathic knowledge in relation to vital force, miasms, etc. so that several illness that comes to them can be referred to a homeopathic physician for treatment. Psychological approaches like psychoanalysis, free associations, dream analysis, catharsis, etc. have given marvellous results in various psycho-somatic illnesses. But there are many types of cases which are not amenable to these approaches. Conducting session after session of such therapies has proved futile. Hence, if the chronic nature of diseases is perceived accurately by the psychologist, then the patient can be treated in a better way by the judicious approach of both, the psychologist and homeopathic physician. Hence, let the psychologist and homeopath start conjointly a new era with interaction and research, so that the entire humanity can be given super succour. In coming days, the disease is shifting from the physical to the mental plane due to the development of better preventive medicines and comprehensive healthcare provided by the government and other allied agencies for physical diseases. Moreover, the exposure of an individual into the world of pornography and crime in TVs, computers (pre-recorded), internet and other associated agencies has induced sickness on the mental plane. The author is of stern apprehension that in future the building of asylums will be overtaking that of hospitals. It may so happen that most of the hospitals which are existing today will be converted into asylums. So we need homeopathy, psychology and yoga in an appreciable proportion to curb this menace.

Chapter 3
SCHOOLS OF PSYCHOLOGY

Initially, psychology had no separate existence and it was a branch of philosophy. In olden days it was full of conjectures and it was ever believed that women and servants have no souls, and at night the soul left the body. It was Wilhelm Wundt (1832-1920), a German professor who was trained in medicine and physiology who initiated a psychological laboratory at Leipzig in 1879. His task was to study the mind in a laboratory. He was the first person to give psychology a scientific status. His school is designated as structuralism. Later there occurred development of other schools. Woodworth sarcastically comments, "First psychology lost its soul, then the mind, then it lost its consciousness; it is still a behavior of sort". In fact this is the whole journey of psychology. Now let us go through important evolutions of psychology.

1. Structuralism

As mentioned above, it was William Wundt, who initiated this school of structuralism. It was the first attempt of Wundt to expose psychology into an arena of science. Hence William Wundt is credited as the first scientist of the psychological world. He focused his experiment on conscious experience of mind. He endorsed thoughts, feelings, sensations, perceptions, ideas, etc. as the structure of mind. Hence his school is called the *school of structuralism*. He carried out various experiments with these elements of mind. Wundt and his followers conducted experiments taking a subject—a human being. The subject (sometimes the psychologist himself also) is exposed to various stimuli like light, colors, etc. to get the feel of it. Then he is asked to note down or narrate his feelings. This art of such experience is called *introspection*. Introspection means being reflective, looking inward: An examination of one's own thoughts and feelings. Although subjective feelings have no role to play in science, yet the attempt of experimentation in itself was a part of scientific study, which paved the path for the following generations to promote psychology towards a scientific status.

The Leipzig laboratory became fruitful and ultimately brought colors to its establishment. It produced most of the leading psychologists of the world. Among those renowned psychologists, the name of Edward Bradford Titchener (1867-1927) deserves a special mention. Titchener was an English born psychologist. He took training in Germany and was later established in America. He became the champion of structural psychology. He also became the professor of psychology at Cornell University. His primary goal was to establish psychology as a science as firmly as physics and chemistry. To attain this purpose he set up a special laboratory at Cornell with various equipment. He tried to redefine psychology as the science of consciousness. Though it looks somehow unnatural because science seeks clarity and objectivity, and consciousness does not qualify to be science, yet the use of the word science was important as this stage may be taken as a transitional period. Titchener avowed that psychology is the study of experience. He broke consciousness (or experience) into the following three basic elements:

1. Physical sensation.
2. Feelings.
3. Images like memory and dreams.

Let us take an example to highlight the concept of Titchener. When we are asked for a report on perception of a rose (flower), we combine the visual sensation (that we see) with feelings of smell and with images (from past experience). Through such experimentation, Titchener concluded that the structure of the human mind was made up of more than 30,000 separate sensations, feelings and images.

Wundt and Titchener are called the structuralists who explored systematic study of mind through the structure by identifying.

Plus Points of Structuralism

Structuralism ushered a new era in the realm of psychology. This was in the transitional phase and was moving towards the scientific world. Structuralism cut itself off from the domain of philosophy and metaphysics, and marched towards scientific psychology. The concept of

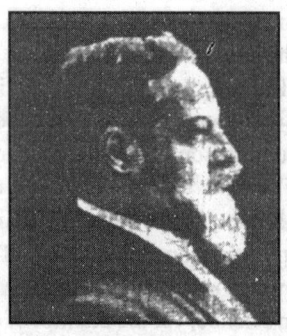

Titchener
(1867-1927)

soul and mind was totally rejected and later psychologists engaged themselves in scientific psychology.

For the first time "introspection" was introduced in the school of structuralism. This was a sort of experimentation, a part of scientific goal. Even today, despite its limitations, it forms a method in psychology.

Structuralism is credited with establishing the first psychological laboratory, which paved the way for systematic observation of the activities of the mind. This school ultimately inspired the future psychologists for carrying out scientific studies and experimentations.

Minus Points of Structuralism

Structuralism is regarded as a very limited system which cannot cater to all needs of human behavior.

The worst drawback of this school is in its interpretation of structure of the mind. The word structure is related to anatomy. We do not find structure of mind in anatomy. The so-called structures are in real sense processes. Hence they are more related in the terms of physiology and anatomy.

Introspection too is related to personal or subjective experience, which may vary from person to person—truly or falsely. We cannot accept somebody's experience as absolute and similarly we cannot categorically reject somebody else's claims of experience. Moreover, a real consensus cannot be reached for scientific enquiry. Again, it lacks objectivity and measurement whereas science is based on objectivity and measurement. Hence, the very conception of introspection seems to be non-scientific.

The method of introspection belongs to private and personal aspect; and we have to remember that science does not accept private, mysterious or personal views.

2. Functionalism

Functionalism was started by William James. He was of a rare genius, who was well versed with the diversity of various subjects like science, art, philosophy as well as religion. He is called the 'Father of Psychology' in U.S.A. He was born on January 11, 1842 in New York and he died on August 26, 1910, in Chocorua, N.H. He was the leader of the philosophical movement of pragmatism and the psychological movement of functionalism. He was highly influenced by Emanuel Swedenborg, which reflects in his literature. At the age of 18,

James learned art under the tutelage of William M. Hunt, an American painter of religious subjects. Later, he took a course in chemistry and anatomy at Lawrence Scientific School. He also studied medicine at Harvard Medical School. He was deeply interested in religion and philosophy. His all round approach of study ultimately reflected in his future works. He heavily broke over-structuralism and severely criticized their work and established his own school called '*Functionalism*'.

In 1872, James was appointed as an instructor in physiology at Harvard College where he worked till 1876. He adopted a biological approach to the study of mind (i.e., physiological and psychological) which was revolutionary in its approach. James had to face a lot of challenges from students who felt that psychology was imbibed with the theological aspect of mind. He also had to face opposition from structuralism. The school of structuralism had already produced superstars like Wundt and Titchener. Anyhow, his marriage in 1878 with the charming and inspiring Alice H. Gibbenes of Cambridge brought a new lease of life for him. With her cooperation and assistance, he published the world famous book "*The Principles of Psychology*" by 1890, which brought name, fame and laurels for him. This book was a great breakthrough into the then existing world of psychology.

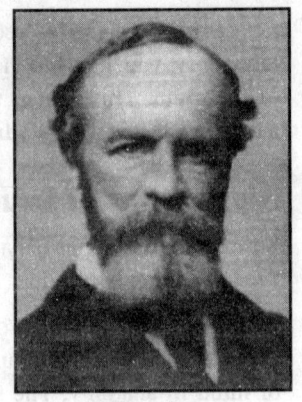

William James (1842-1910)

William, as mentioned above was an all rounder and he was well aware of religion, science, art, philosophy, etc. Hence, his approach to life was holistic and perhaps his exposure to the above branches of human learning made him reject structuralism and criticized it under the following grounds:

1. Consciousness or experience cannot be divided into elements. According to William James, it is sheer nonsense to separate ideas, thoughts, sensations, perceptions, etc.
2. Structure does not divulge about what the mind actually does or how it goes about doing.
3. He stressed that knowing the function of mind which is lacking in structuralism is more important.

William James was a knowledgeable person in the subject of anatomy. He utilized this knowledge along with the inspiring work of Darwin, propounded his doctrine of functionalism and advocated the theory of mental life and behavior.

1. According to James, consciousness or mental life is a continuous, flow of unity, a stream that carries the organism in its adaptation to the environment.
2. James also supported Darwinian theory and stated that the mind is a recent development of the evolutionary process and its function was to help man adjust to the environment.

According to James, habits are nothing but a function of the nervous system. When we repeat an activity, time to time, our nervous system is put into a pattern so that in subsequent episodes, the act is carried out like a machine. He also accepts that the mind forges association, revises experience, starts and stops, and even reverts back and forth in time for the development functional ability to adjust with the environment.

The main exponents of this schools are John Dewey, James Rowland Angell (1869-1949), J.M. Cattel, Edward Thorndike, R.S. Woodworth (1869-1962), etc.

3. Behaviorism

John B. Watson (1878-1958) was the founder of this school. He brought a new revolution in the field of psychology. He presented a novel doctrine to the world of psychology which was quite different from the contemporary theories of structuralism and functionalism. He was inspired by Ivan Pavlov, who had promulgated the theory of classical conditioning (see Chapter VI). Interestingly his doctrine of behaviorism fits into the tradition of scientific materialism, beginning from evolutionary biologist Jacques Leob, the famous author of *"The Mechanistic Conception of Life"* and concept of Russian psychologist (rather reflexologists) I.M. Seehenov and Vladimir Bekheterve.

Watson freed psychology from the contemporary and controversial mental approach. He gave the world a totally new objective psychology. He entirely rejected the idea of consciousness because it could not be proved scientifically. Consciousness lacks objective evidence, which is a part of scientific method.

Watson applied Pavlov's approach in the field of human behavior. In his famous experiment with an 11 months old infant, named Albert, he conditioned the baby's behavior to the fear of a rat (in reality those white rats were inoffensive by nature) by substituting the rat with a sudden loud noise. He affirmed that consciousness cannot be touched, seen or demonstrated by any scientific test. He also criticised its subjective experience, which may be a matter of confusion and contradiction, and varies from person to person. He also categorically rejected the older concept of psychology in relation to soul, mind, etc. He asserted that if you intend to make psychology a science, then it should have observable and measurable behavior. He also rejected the above method of psychology and tried to project human beings as complex machines which respond in a particular fashion to a particular kind of stimulus. He supposed that the behavior of an individual is controlled by the environment. We should remember that Watson was an extreme environmentalist. He proposed that environment is more important than heredity. He strongly believed in conditioning. One of his quotes are frequently found in many books on psychology, that deserves special attention:

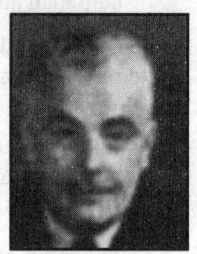

Watson
(1878-1958)

"Give me a dozen healthy infants, well informed and my own specified work to bring them up in and I will guarantee to take any one at random and train him to become any type specialist I might select – doctor, lawyer, artist, merchant, navy chief and yes, even beggar-man and thief, regardless of his talents, penchants, tendencies, abilities, vocations and race of his ancestors."

This attempt of Watson's brought psychology nearer to physical sciences like chemistry and physics.

Plus Points of Behaviorism

1. Watson ushered in a new era in the field of psychology by propounding behaviorism. It freed psychology from the clutches of controversial mentalistic approach of human behavior.
2. His sound concept is extremely useful in learning. His work is adhered by many nations and institutions as programmed learning.
3. His work contributed a lot in the field of learning, motivation, emotion, developmental psychology, etc.
4. His methods are used to help maladjusted children.
5. Behaviorism advocated the use of theory of reinforcement. For example, one child may be rewarded for a good work and punished for a bad work. This helps in the acquisition of desirable behavior and for giving up the behavior that is not desired.

Minus Points of Behaviorism

Despite the above mentioned plus points, behaviorism suffers from the following shortcomings:

1. The mechanistic approach to behavior advocated through S-R (stimulus-response) is too simple.
2. No doubt S-R has a role to play in relation to behavior, but it is too narrow. Later, psychologists belonging to Gestalt school suggested that this is a part of the whole. According to them, an individual perceives the thing as a whole and not as a mere collection of its constituents or elements.
3. It has also been asserted that the whole may differ from the sum of its parts.
4. Behaviorists failed to explain complex human behavior, such as our use of language, in terms of stimuli and responses, that is, without reference to mental activity.

4. Gestalt Psychology

This school was developed in Germany around 1912 under the leadership of Max Wertheimer (1880-1943), Kurt Koffka (1886-1941), Wolfgang Kohler and Kurt Lewin (1890-1947). Later all of them went to United States of America to expand their work, Kohler being their chief spokesman.

The German word "*Gestalt*" means configuration or in a simpler term means totality with a meaningful expression. This approach is synthetic rather than analytical and hence was the outcome as a reaction to contemporary psychology: Structuralism, functionalism and behaviorism. It opposes the atomic and molecular approach to behavior. Accordingly, an individual perceives an object as a whole and not merely as a collection of its constituents or elements. It rejects the very idea of mechanistic approach to behavior through a simple 'Stimulus-Response' connection. The school asserts that an individual perceives as per the whole or total situation and a perception always involves a problem or organization. It emphasizes that a sort of organization definitely exists between 'Stimulus–Response' which ultimately helps in forming an organization. Let us take the example

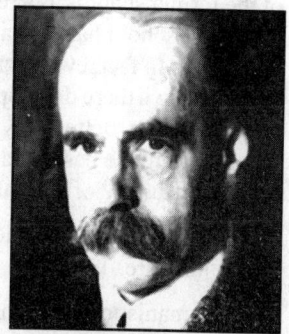

Max Wertheimer
(1880-1943)

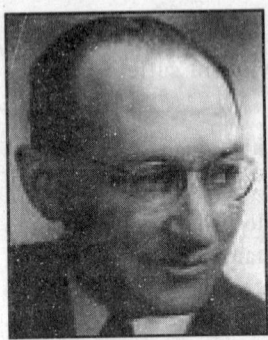 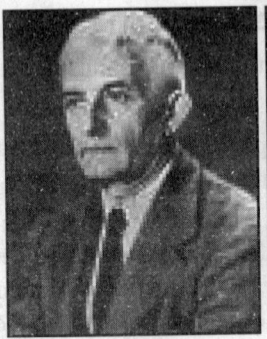 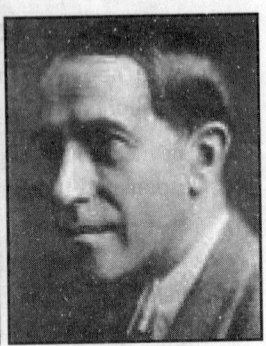

Kurt Lewin (1890-1947)   Wolfgang Kohler (1887-1967)   Kurt Koffka (1886-1941)

of a rose. When we look at a rose, we perceive it as a pattern or we perceive in it a conceptual image, which is called Gestalt. The Gestalt includes color, form or pattern and even its fragrance. The Gestalists go further deep and claim that when the component of a thing is brought together by the mind, something new, which may be very valuable and comprehensive may come up than the component originally found.

5. Psycho-Analytical School
(See Freud and Psychoanalysis, Chapter VII)

RECENT TRENDS IN CONTEMPORARY PSYCHOLOGY

Till now we have observed that developments of later schools are the outcome of the former schools as a reactionary measure. It has also been observed that the newer school had to waste a lot of energy to prove their superiority over the former. In fact, every school has some plus points and some minus points. In recent days there developed an eclectic approach so that mankind could be benefited in a better way. Hence, recent psychology has developed by incorporating the best of each school. Anyhow, much benefit is derived from schools of behaviorism and psychoanalysis.

In recent days there developed three approaches, that deserve a mention at this juncture. They are:

1. Humanistic psychology.
2. Transpersonal psychology.
3. Cognitive psychology.

1. Humanistic Psychology

Humanistic psychology is based on humanism in psychology. The chief exponents of this school are Abraham Harold Maslow, Carl Rogers and Gordon Allport. Their view closely corroborates with what our Master Hahnemann had said long before. They preached that human beings are not mere complicated and refined machines but every human being has a purpose of living. They also did not accept that human beings are not the victim of conflict of ego and Id (Freud). They advocated that each human being has a full potential to develop a purposeful living, is competent of adopting himself to his environment for a positive and purposeful destiny. They also assert that these goals are simple and lead to attaining self- realization.

Abraham Harold Maslow (1908-70) was an American psychologist and one of the champions of the humanistic school in psychology. He proposed that an individual has some basic needs like food and sex. After satisfying these basic needs, the individual proceeds to the highest need for what he called self-actualization (or the fulfillment). Accordingly, he views that self-actualization could only be attained once basic needs had been fulfilled.

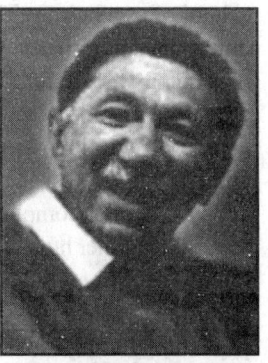

Maslow (1908-1970)

Carl Rogers (1902-87) was also an American psychologist who developed a client-centred psychotherapy, "client" meaning "patient". This method stresses the relationship between therapist and client and the client's use of this relationship to guide the course of therapy. This approach emphasizes that each person has the capacity for self-understanding and self-healing. The therapist tries to demonstrate empathy and genuine caring for clients, allowing freedom to them to reveal their true feelings without the fear of being judged.

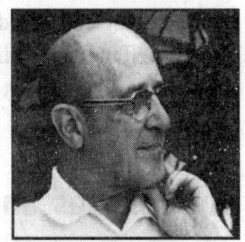

Carl Rogers (1902-1987)

2. Transpersonal Psychology

In contemporary psychology, transpersonal psychology has a distinct place. This school has been established on the work of Abraham Maslow's self-actualization. Accordingly, it emphasizes the study of personal experience that seems to transcend ordinary existence. Transpersonal psychology studies what we think and how we feel in our changed state of awareness. The changes of awareness can be induced and studied during sleep, deep concentration, through specific drugs and transdental meditation.

3. Cognitive Psychology

This school was developed as an extension of cognitive outlook of Gestalt school of psychology. This school does not accept the molecular approach of human behavior. It accepts an individual's higher cognitive abilities. Cognitive psychology focuses on various cognitive activities like – perception, language, attention, memory, knowledge, reasoning, problem solving abilities and the effects of emotion. It recognises an individual's intelligence, capacity and adaptability to a given situation. It accepts an individual as an able problem solver in various complicated activities. By this, cognitive psychology attempts to explore higher human mental activities like insight, creativity, etc. The main theme of this new school is cognitive revolution (sometimes called 'White Box Theory' in contrast to behaviorism as 'Black Box Theory'). Cognitive psychology categorically rejects the S-R (i.e., Stimulus-Response) approach of behaviorists. They advocate that the human mind does not accept information from its environment in exactly the form and style it is conveyed to them. The conveyed information is compared with the information already consigned in the mind. Then it is scrutinized and often metamorphosed into a new shape. Finally, it is comprehended, preserved and operated as per the need.

Approaches and Methods of Cognitive Psychology

Within cognitive psychology there are three main approaches:

I. *Experimental cognitive psychology:* The traditional experimental approach.
II. *Cognitive neuro-psychology*: The study of brain-damaged subjects.
III. *Cognitive science*: Computational modelling.

Experimental cognitive psychologists apply the traditional methods of psychology. They observe the behavior of subjects who are put into one or more time bound tasks followed by recording their responses.

They investigate cognition and test hypotheses under controlled laboratory conditions. Experiments are carried out to test word memory, accuracy, speed, problem solving, object recognition and reaction times without the individual's conscious awareness. Here, we must remember that it is not a sweeping restitution to introspection. Immediate report treated in a prudent and solicitous way can supply useful information and evidences about the cognitive abilities.

Cognitive neuro-psychologists study the impaired abilities of brain-damaged subjects. Their primary methodology is to look for dissociation: Comparing normal performance and impaired performance.

Very often brain damage affects many cognition processes. Hence, it is not possible for psychologists to carry out study on a selective basis. Moreover, it has also been found that cognitive processes are inter-related and affect one another even in brain damage. The most difficult task is that there occurs a compensatory mechanism so that a confirmatory study cannot be evolved easily. Hence it is a challenge for the researchers to reach a genuine and feasible conclusion.

Anyhow, neuro-psychological findings are used to develop and test theories of normal cognition.

Cognitive scientists within cognitive psychology concentrate in constructing and testing computational models. The computational model was thought as an alternative to test the theories suggested by cognitive psychologists. The theory forwarded by cognitive psychologists tended to be obscure and hard to test. It is felt that the computational model be an alternative with a view to obtain precision.

Computational modelling has become a more acceptable method as it simulates human behavior. Usually a digital computer is programmed to display artificial intelligence. Cognitive psychologists consider that we owe our cognitive abilities to the information-processing potential of the brain. They also assert that the brain comprises of specialized interacting components which process and store information received by our senses in a structural form. Then the information is mobilized to exhibit intelligent behavior. Hence, psychologists assert that similar behavioral study is possible from a computational model.

Now-a-days, cognitive psychology is gaining new heights and is becoming very popular. Edward Tolman, a U.S. psychologist, one of the founder psychologists and   Jean Piaget, a Swiss psychologist have made notable contribution in the field of cognitive psychology.

■

Chapter 4

PSYCHOLOGY OF COGNITION : SENSATION

Everything we know comes through the process of sensation or sensory experience. Sensation is the first response of the organism to a stimulus. Without sensory experience, an individual cannot enhance his knowledge and experience new things, new events, new situations, etc. It is the first step towards the direction of perception. Hence precedence of sensation is a must for later perception of the object or stimuli. One cannot think of perception without sensation. However, it is difficult to discriminate between the two. Strictly speaking, sensation and perception are not different entities, rather they exist like two sides of a coin. Pure sensation is a myth from a psychological point of view. However, conceptually, both the terms can be comprehended separately.

Titchener defined sensation as "An elementary process which constitutes atleast four attributes — quality, intensity, clearness and duration." Quality is the most important attribute which permits us to distinguish one elementary process from another, hot, cold, red, blue, etc. Intensity refers to brightness or brilliance of color, loudness of sound, magnitude of pain, etc. Intensity enables us to compare the sensory experience within one area of experience. Clearness in sensation is explained in terms of figure and ground perceptions. That which is in the figure is clearly conscious; that which in the fringe is partly in the consciousness. Duration defines the temporal course of sensation. A sustained tone creates a different sensation compared to a short click—even though they have the same intensity and pitch. Some sensations also produce the attribute of extensity. Tones; of course do not have extensity, but they have volume.

Introspective psychology was most successful in the area of sensory psychology. Functionalists did consider sensation in terms of its role on adaptation but failed to emphasize it in their system. Watson studied sensory processes in animals to provide a comparative picture in relation to sensory processes in human beings. It is important because of the methodology it provided for the study of sensory processes. The Gestalt psychologists and psycho-analysts did not contribute anything new to the understanding of sensory psychology. Contemporary research and interest in sensation is primarily along the neuro-physiological lines.

Elementary Processes of Sensation

E.B. Titchener defines sensation as an elementary process which constitutes atleast 4 attributes, which are as follows:

1. Quality

Different sensations have different qualities. The sensation of brightness of color cannot be compared to that of listening to music. Hence, each sensation differs in quality from the other. Moreover, we find difference in quality of the same sense. The music of pop songs differs from that of jazz or Indian classical music. Colors like red, green, blue, etc. differ from one another.

2. Intensity

A sensation of the same quality may differ in intensity. Every stimulus has its own intensity in a given circumstance to reach the threshold and produce a sensation. A color may be deep (say maroon or black) or light (say lemon-yellow or white). Similarly, the sound may be loud or mild under a given circumstance. We all know that greater the intensity, stronger the sensation.

3. Clarity

A stimulus appears more clear when it remains in the centre instead of in the fringe or ground. Observe the following figure, which is popularly known as "Figure Ground Phenomena" in psychology.

Now, from this figure, the central or figure part of the picture seems to be clear. This phenomenon is called figure-ground phenomenon. Here the part that remains noticeably separated from the rest of the visual

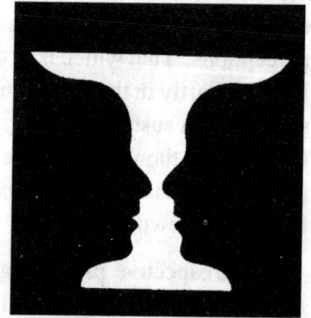

Figure Ground

field is called the 'Figure' and the background against which it is watched is called the ground.

Hence, the clearer the stimulus, the better the sensation of the object.

4. Duration

Each stimulus has a duration to produce a sensation. The longer the duration, stronger is the sensation. The sensation differs in relation to duration.

Along with the above 4 points, the following attribute may also be added:

5. Extensiveness

A sensation occupying a larger area produces different sensations to that of a smaller area. During election time, political leaders display a larger portrait of themselves, which possess a different sensation to their counterparts who display a smaller portrait. An example from filmland may be seen. In film "NH", two superstars were cast. In those days "R" was the superstar and on the top. His portrait was displayed in a bigger form. Some years later "R's" popularity was on the decline while "A" was the reigning superstar. Then the display on the poster was opposite to lure the audience for a second visit.

Types of Sensations

Psychologists claim that there exist as many organs as sensations, the study of which is neither feasible nor desirable. Anyhow, we can carry out our studies on sensations under three heads:

a. Organic sensations.
b. Motor senses.
c. Specific senses.

a. Organic Sensations

Organic sensation is related to internal organs. They do not belong to a specific sensation.

Sensation of well being or restlessness can be of a wide range. They are spread all over the body and no particular part can be allocated to it.

Specific sensations like cutting or burning are usually of confined nature and its locality is fixed.

Sensations like hunger or thirst or pain cannot be attributed to any of the above. Their locality is yet to be confirmed.

These sensations are connected to some fundamental biological needs of the body. The organic senses help in maintaining homeostasis.

b. Motor Sensations

These sensations are concerned with motion. Sensations like pulling, contraction, tension, etc. are attributed to motor sensations. They are caused by muscles, tendons, joints, etc. When the embedded nerves of the muscles, joints or tendons are affected by the action or movement of other muscles, tendons or joints, then motor sensations are produced. Motor sensation gives us the knowledge of primary qualities of objects like, distance, direction, position, etc. Generally motor sensations are not noticed by us. In case they come to our notice, then we should suspect the existence of some pathological state.

In psychology, the motor sensations are divided under the following 3 heads :

i. Sensation of Position

We can feel this type of sensation keeping both of our hands stretched laterally while standing in a motionless state.

ii. Sensation of Free Movement

This type of sensation generally occurs when we move our arms in all the directions.

iii. Sensation of Restricted Movement

Such type of sensation can be perceived by lifting a heavy object.

c. Specific Senses

Specific sensations are related to specific sense organs like – eye, ear, tongue, nose, skin, etc. We know there exist 5 sense organs viz.

i. **Eye** : Vision pertains to sight (visual sensations).
ii. **Ear** : Auditory pertains to hearing (auditory sensations).
iii. **Tongue** : Gustatory pertains to taste (taste sensations).

iv. **Nose :** Olfactory pertains to smell (olfactory sensations).
v. **Skin :** Tactile pertains touch (tactile sensations).

THE EYE AND SENSE OF SIGHT

Eyes are the sensory organs meant for vision. These organs are situated in a quadrilateral, pyramid shaped, bony cavity called orbit on both sides of root of the nose. Now it will be convenient for us to study this organ of special sense under two heads:

I. Accessory structures of the eye.
II. Eyeballs.

Let us explore first, the accessory structures of the eye, that surrounds the eyeball.

I. Accessory Structures of Eye

1. **Eyebrows:** These are the two curves of thick skin over the eyes with thick hair. Eyebrows prevent sweat entering the eyes, by soaking it.

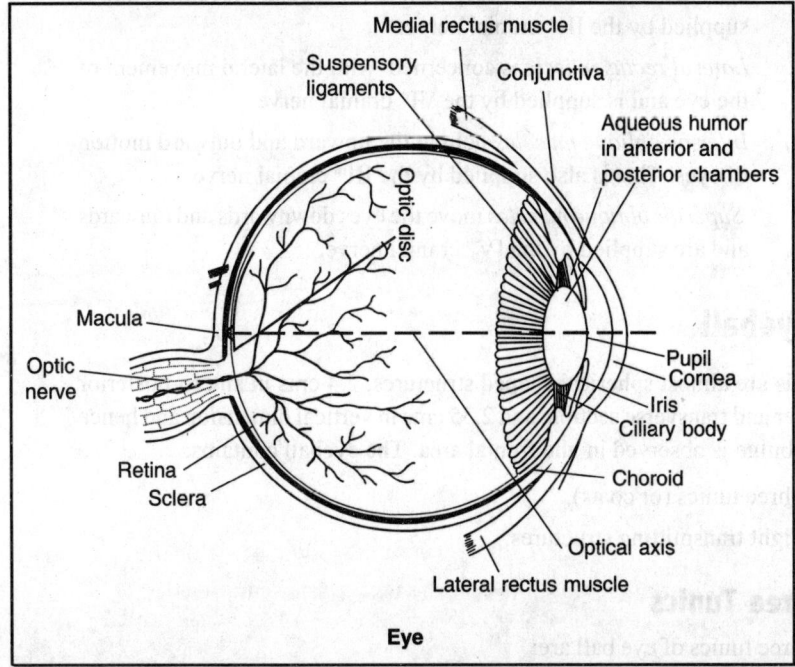

Eye

2. **Eyelids:** There are two eyelids – upper and lower. Eyelids give protection against various inimical agents that can enter the eyes. Both the eyelids are lined internally by the conjunctiva and covered externally by the skin. The upper eyelid is larger and more flexible in comparison to the lower eyelids.
3. **Lacrimal Apparatus:** This part of the eye is involved in the production of tears and it consists of :
    a. A lacrimal gland situated in the lateral end of the upper eyelid.
    b. Lacrimal duct, lacrimal sac and naso-lacrimal duct through which the tears are carried to the nasal cavity.
4. **Extrinsic Muscles of Eye:** The eyeball has six extrinsic muscles, each performing a special type of function. These muscles originate from the posterior bony wall of the orbit and ultimately insert into the sclera.
    a. *Superior rectus muscle* is involved in the movement of the eyes upwards and inwards. This is supplied by the IIIrd cranial nerve.
    b. *Inferior rectus muscle* is helpful in the movement of the eyes downwards and inwards. This is also supplied by the IIIrd cranial nerve.
    c. *Medial rectus muscle* is responsible for medial movement and is supplied by the IIIrd cranial nerve.
    d. *Lateral rectus muscle* is concerned with the lateral movement of the eye and is supplied by the VIth cranial nerve.
    e. *Inferior oblique muscles* help in the upward and outward motion of eyes. This is also supplied by the IIIrd cranial nerve.
    f. *Superior oblique muscles* move the eyes downwards and outwards and are supplied by the IVth cranial nerve.

II. Eyeball

Eyeballs are almost spherical shaped structures, 2.4 cms in antero-posterior diameter and transverse section, and 2.35 cms in vertical dimension and hence a little bulge is observed in the frontal area. The eyeball contains:

A. Three tunics (or coats).
B. Light transmitting structures.

A. Three Tunics

The Three tunics of eye ball are:

a. *The outer fibrous tunic comprises of two parts:*
  i. The anterior one-sixth transparent part called *cornea*.
  ii. The remainder five-sixth opaque part called *sclera*.
b. *Middle vascular tunic, contains:*
  i. Choroid.
  ii. Ciliary body.
  iii. Iris.
c. Inner nervous coat containing the retina.

B. Light Transmitting Structures

The light transmitting structures are:
i. Aqueous humor.
ii. Lens.
iii. Vitreous humor.

Now let us go ahead and explore the above one after another.

Three Tunics

a. Outer Fibrous Coat

  i. **Cornea:** It forms the anterior one-sixth of the outer coat. It is transparent and has a convex anterior surface. It is richly supplied by sensory nerves. The cornea is hard, transparent and a curved part. It is situated in front of the eye. It is convex in shape. The gap between the cornea and lens is know as anterior chamber, which is filled with a fluid called aqueous humor. Aqueous humor supplies nutrition to the cornea and crystallized lens.
  ii. **Sclera**: It is the posterior five-sixths of the outer coat. It forms the white of the eye and is continuous with the cornea in front. Sclera safeguards the internal structures and upholds the shape of the eyeball. The optic nerve passes through the posterior aspect of sclera and reaches the retina.

Cornea allows light to enter the eye. It does not get blood supply. If the cornea had blood vessels they would interfere with the entry of light waves into the eye. Because blood is the source of defence against foreign substances, the absence of blood vessels in the cornea makes it one of the few tissues in the body that can be transplanted from one person to another with little chance of antibody rejection. Its nutrition is supplied by lymphs. The covering over the cornea forms the conjunctiva. Conjunctiva is a modified epidermis of cornea. It is the inner layer of eyelid projection. Cornea has the following main layers from within outward:

- Layer of optic nerve fibres
- Layer of ganglion cells
- Inner plexiform layer
- Inner nuclear layer
- Outer plexiform layer
- Outer nuclear layer
- Rods and cones layer
- Pigment cell layer

b. Middle Vascular Coat

i. *Choroid:* It is a thin, darkly pigmented and highly vascular membrane. It lines the posterior compartment of the eye and lies between the inner surface of sclera and retina. Choroid has two basic functions:

- To support the blood vessels that supply fuel to the retina.
- To absorb light waves that have scattered after corneal refraction. If the choroid does not prevent these scattered rays from striking the retina, the image would be blurred.

ii. *Ciliary Body:* It is the anterior continuation of the choroid and it lies between the choroid and iris. The ciliary body contains ciliary muscles. The suspensory ligament of the lens is attached to the ciliary muscle.

iii. *Iris:* It is the anterior continuation of the ciliary body. Iris is a pigmented membrane and the color of eye is dependent on its pigments. Iris has a central opening called pupil. Following two sets of iris muscles control the pupil:

- Circular muscles which reduce the pupillary size
- Radial muscles which increase the pupillary size

c. Inner Nervous Coat

Retina: It is the innermost nervous coat of the eyeball and lies immediately inside the choroid. The retina contains :

i. Nerve cells and nerve fibres present on the inner surface (facing the chamber of eye)
ii. Some special structures called 'rods and cones' which are on the outer or choroidal surface of retina. These rods and cones receive the light and set up impulses which are transmitted through the optic nerve.
iii. Optic disc is the point where the optic nerve leaves the eyeball. This point is not lined by the retina and is hence, insensitive to light. So this point is also called the *blind spot*.
iv. Macula is a small area on the retina which is situated just lateral to the entrance of the optic nerve. It is exactly opposite the centre of pupil. Direct or near vision is focused on the macula.

As light passes through the cornea and the aqueous humor, it comes across the iris, a colored membrane. Iris consists of a group of muscles. There exists a small opening in the centre of the iris called the pupil, which controls the amount of light that enters the back of the eye. The pupil can open to about five-sixteenths of an inch in diameter at its widest and one-sixteenth of an inch in diameter at its narrowest.

The widening and narrowing of the pupil are governed by two sets of smooth muscles under the control of the autonomic nervous system. In periods of stress, the sympathetic system stimulates the pupils to dilate and during relaxation, the parasympathetic system stimulates the pupil to contract.

It has various functions. It controls the opening of the pupil. Since it is pigmented, no light passes through it and we perceive a clear picture.

Light Transmitting Structures

i. *Aqueous Humor*: It is a fluid present in the both the anterior and posterior chambers of the eye.
   The space between cornea and anterior surface of lens is called anterior chamber.
   The narrow space between iris, lens and ciliary body is called posterior chamber.
ii. *Lens*: Lens is the transparent, biconvex structure that lies immediately behind the iris and pupil. The lens is a spherical structure located behind the pupils. It is attached to the ciliary body by means of suspensory ligaments. The thickness of the lens is checked by ciliary muscles through the suspensory ligament. Aqueous humor supplies nutrition to the lens.

iii. *Vitreous Humor*: It is a jelly-like fluid which fills the space between the lens and retina. It maintains the shape of the eye. It gives shape and firmness to retina and it keeps the retina in contact with the choroid and sclera.

Principle of Accommodation

Light must pass through the lens and vitreous humor, which has the same basic nutritive function as the aqueous humor, before it reaches the retina.

The pupil dilates when there is either intense light or near vision and the lens becomes convex in shape. At this time its power increases. When there is dim light or distant vision the lens became more spherical, and its power decreases.

This adjustment of the lens to light and distance is known as the principle of accommodation.

Mechanism of Vision

When light falls upon the retina, two phenomenon happen:
1. Photochemical changes.
2. Electrical changes.

Photochemical change takes place in rods and cones of the retina. Rhodopsin is a chemical substance that is found in rods. Light breaks the rod pigment into retinene, which is an aldehyde form of vitamin A. When rhodopsin comes in contact with light it is activated and it breaks down into retinal retinene and opsin. If the intensity of light is very strong, the retinol is further converted to vitamin A. Interestingly, the whole process is reversible i.e., vitamin A can again be converted to retinol and retinol into rhodopsin. This photochemical reaction starts the visual response and induces changes in electrical potential which are transmitted through the bipolar cells to the ganglion cells and then along with fibres of the optic nerve to the brain. (Note: Retinene is also called retinol)

The electrical changes adjust itself in frequency to intensity of light, which can be recorded by an Electro-retinogram (E.R.G.).

Cornea receives the light like a window, which is further regulated by the iris and pupil. Now the image is focused on the retina through the lens. The pigmented choroid darkens the interior of the eye, which prevents scattering and reflection of light. The image then arouses the receptors present

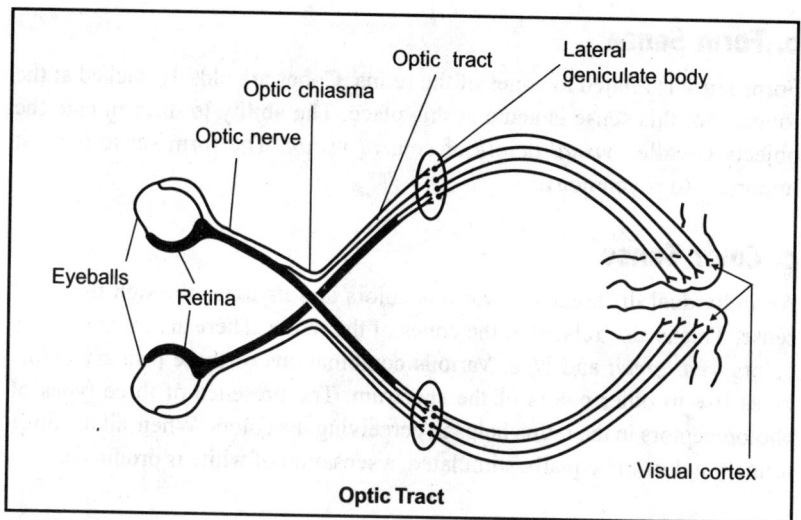

Optic Tract

in the rods and cones of the retina producing impulses. These impulses are then carried through the optic nerve i.e., 2nd cranial nerve, which arises from the ganglion cells present in the retina. The nerve passes posteriorly and medially through the cranial cavity, via the optic canal. Then it passes through the optic chiasma. Here the fibres of the optic nerve split in two halfs. The fibres converge and move to the opposite sides of the optic tract while the other half continues in the same tract. By the crossing over of fibres, each optic nerve is connected to both the sides of the brain. The visual centre lies in the cortex of the occipital lobe of the brain.

The stimulation of the retina with light yields three types of sensations:

a. Light Sense

An individual perceives light of all degrees of intensities through light sense.

The minimum amount of light energy through which the visual sensation is generated is called minimum light. After determining the minimum light, if the intensity of light is gradually increased, one can appreciate a difference in the amount of illumination, called light difference. The least perceptible difference of illumination bears a constant relation to the total illumination and is known as *Weber's Law*. The light difference is also influenced by the adaptation of the eye. This difference may be affected by various disorders of the optic nerve.

b. Form Sense

Form sense is related to cones of the retina. Cones are closely packed at the fovea. So, this sense is acute at this place. The ability to discriminate the objects is called *visual acuity* or *central vision*. The form sense is most important to psychology.

c. Color Sense

An individual differentiates various colors and its tones through the color sense. This is also related to the cones of the retina. There are three primary colors, *red, green* and *blue*. Various combinations of these primary colors gives rise to other colors of the spectrum. The presence of three types of photoreceptors in the retina helps in perceiving the colors. When all the three primary colors are equally stimulated, a sensation of white is produced.

Diseases of the Eye that Interfere in the Sensation of Vision

1. Emmetropia

It is normal refractory function of the eye.

2. Ametropia

It is deviation from the normal refractive state of the eye.

3. Myopia (Short sightedness)

In this condition, the patient can see the near objects without any difficulty but he cannot see distant objects clearly. This occurs due to an increase in the antero-posterior diameter of the eyeball, by which the image is formed in front of the retina. This condition can be corrected by using concave lenses.

4. Hypermetropia (Long Sightedness)

This state is the opposite of myopia. In this condition, the patient cannot see near objects clearly. The decrease of antero-posterior diameter of the eyeball is responsible for causing this condition. The image occurs behind the retina. This condition, generally occurring in old age, is also called *presbyopia* in which there are defects in accommodation due to sclerosis of the lens. Both the conditions can be corrected by using convex lenses.

5. Astigmatism

Astigmatism may be associated with either myopia or hypermetropia. This causes blurring of vision. The error can be corrected by using cylindrical lenses.

6. Night Blindness (Nyctalopia)

It is the incapability of a patient to see in dim light or at night. This occurs due to deficiency of vitamin A and hence a supply of this vitamin will correct the condition.

7. Color Blindness

It is a defect of the retina in which the patient cannot see one or all colors.

8. Glaucoma

It is an increase in the intraocular tension produced due to excessive collection of aqueous humor (in the anterior chamber). This may lead to blindness due to retinal damage. Hence the case must be properly treated.

9. Cataract

Opacity of the lens is termed as cataract. It is caused by degenerative changes in the cells of the lens. Homeopathic medicines like *Silicea*, *Fluoricum acidum*, *Causticum* may give good results especially in early stage. *Cineraria lotion* is also found to be very effective in cataract. However, very often such conditions need surgical intervention.

THE EAR, SENSATION OF HEARING (AND EQUILIBRIUM)

The human ear is an amazingly delicate organ, no less interesting or intriguing in structure then the eye. It is concerned with the functions of hearing and equilibrium. It is divided into the following three parts:

1. External ear.
2. Middle ear.
3. Internal ear.

The first two parts are concerned with collection of sound waves while the third one is basically the organ of hearing. The outer ear collects sound waves, the middle ear amplifies it, and the inner ear transduces it.

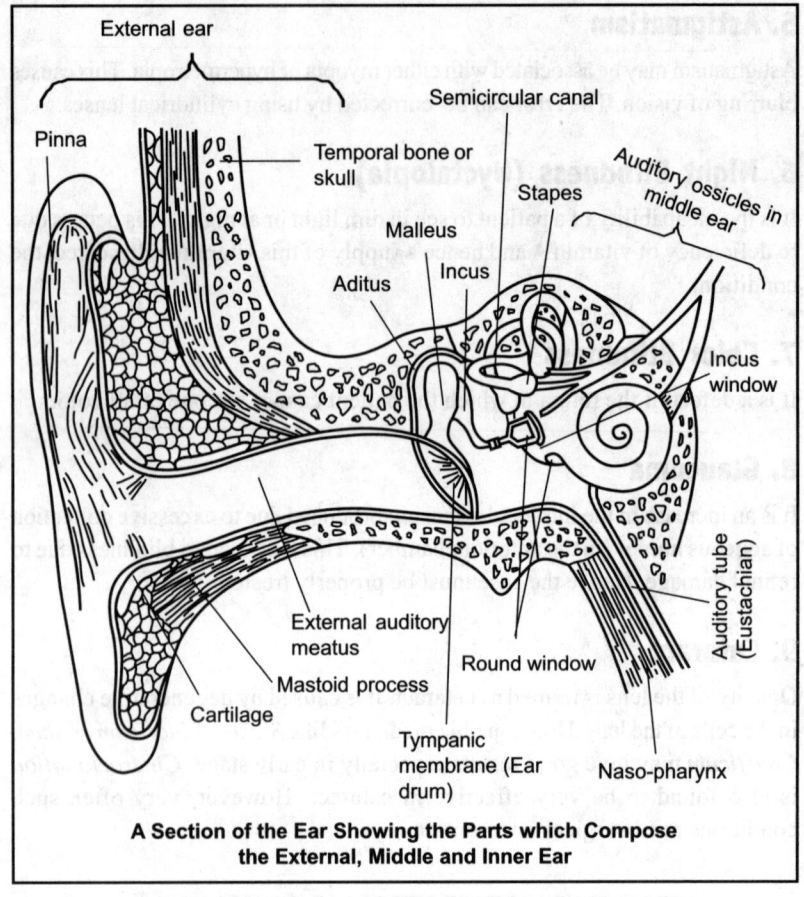

A Section of the Ear Showing the Parts which Compose the External, Middle and Inner Ear

Parts of the Ear

1. External Ear

It is the only part which remains outside the skull. It embraces the following structures:

a. Pinna or Auricle

It is a funnel shaped organ made of elastic fibro-cartilage and striated muscles. Its main function is to collect the sound waves. Without the pinna, we would have less amount of sound. It aids in channelizing the sound waves. It also helps us to recognize the direction from where the sound is coming.

b. External Auditory Meatus

i. External auditory meatus is a small canal, 2.5 cms in length. It joins the tympanic membrane. It contains wax secreting glands and transmits the vibrations of sound to the tympanic membrane.

2. Middle Ear (Tympanic Cavity)

Beyond the eardrum, there exists an air-filled cavity called the middle ear or tympanic cavity. Tympanic membrane or ear drum forms the lateral wall of the ear. It is elastic in nature. It can move back and forth. This matches the incoming sound in frequency and amplitude. The inner surface of the tympanic membrane is lined by ciliated columnar epithelium while the outer concave surface is lined with stratified squamous epithelium.

It has the following structures :

a. Two *foramina* that exist in the medial (inner) wall called:
   i. *Fenestra ovalis* or oval window (synonym: Fenestra vestibule).
   ii. *Fenestra rotundum* or round window (synonym called Fenestra tympani).
b. *Eustachian tube* through which the middle ear is connected anteriorly to the naso-pharynx.

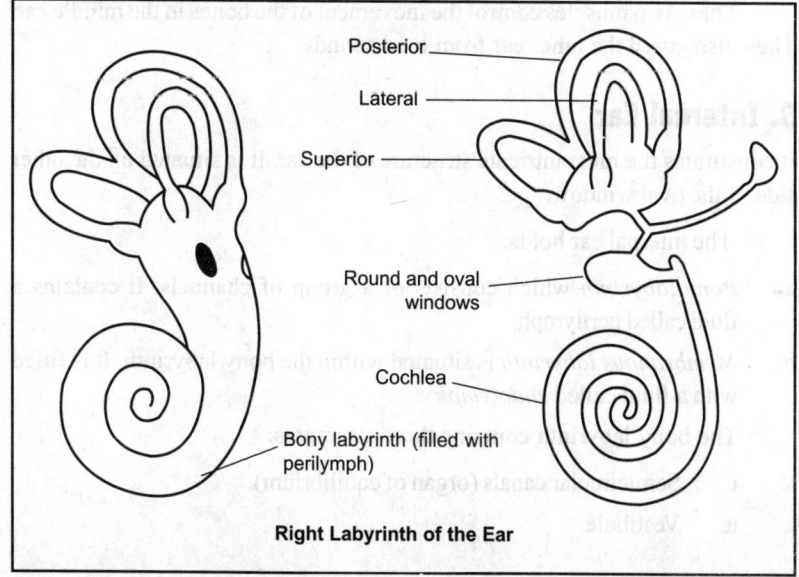

Right Labyrinth of the Ear

c. *Auditus,* a narrow passage that connects the middle ear posteriorly with mastoid antrum.

d. Three *auditory ossicles* which are situated across the middle ear. The three ossicles are:

   i. *Malleus* (roughly resembles a hammer).
   ii. *Incus* (roughly resembles an anvil).
   iii. *Stapes* (roughly resembles a stirrup).

The handle of malleus is attached to the middle of the tympanic membrane or ear drum. The head of malleus is connected to incus by ligaments, so that whenever the malleus moves, the incus moves with it. The opposite end of the incus in turn articulates with the stem of stapes, while the faceplate of the stapes is positioned against fenestra ovalis, where sound waves are transmitted into the cochlea.

The hammer launches the process, proceeding the anvil into movement which, in turn, pushes the stirrup into the oval window. The vibrations are maintained equally in the three bones.

It has two muscles, namely:

   i. Tensor tympani, supplied by the Vth cranial nerve.
   ii. Stapedius, supplied by the VIIth cranial nerve.

These two muscles control the movement of the bones in the middle ear. They also guard the inner ear from loud sounds.

3. Internal Ear

It constitutes the most intricate structure of the ear. It is situated on the other side of the oval window.

The internal ear holds:

a. *Bony labyrinth* which consists of a group of channels. It contains a fluid called perilymph.

b. *Membranous labyrinth* is situated within the bony labyrinth. It is filled with a fluid called *endolymph.*

The bony labyrinth contains three structures:

   i. Semicircular canals (organ of equilibrium).
   ii. Vestibule.

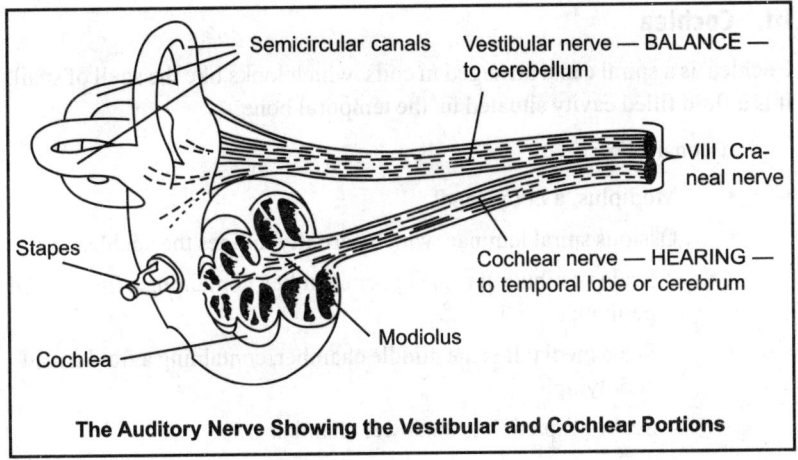

The Auditory Nerve Showing the Vestibular and Cochlear Portions

    iii.   Cochlea (the organ of hearing).

The semicircular canals and vestibular sacs, form the upper portion of the internal ear whereas, the cochlea forms the lower portion.

i. Semicircular Canals

Each ear has three semicircular canals lying at right angles to each other. They are called posterior, superior and lateral semicircular canals. Each semicircular canal has a distended end called *ampula*. The nerve endings of vestibular nerve are inserted in the ampula. The ampula also contains some hair – like projections, which are not involved in hearing. These are basically concerned with body balance and posture. The semicircular canals are mainly related to head movements, and their damage impairs the ability of an individual to maintain an equilibrium.

ii. Vestibule

It is the middle part that is situated between the cochlea (anteriorly) and semicircular canals (posteriorly). The vestibular sacs are sensitive to the head position and movement. Vestibule contains hair-like receptor cells submerged in fluid. When the posture is changed, the head moves and in its succession, movement also takes place in the fluid. This movement stimulates the receptors in the vestibule. Sensory impulses stirred up by these stimulations are carried to the cerebellum. These specific receptors control forward, backward and linear movement. In this way it maintains the body posture.

iii. Cochlea

Cochlea is a spiral canal arranged in coils, which looks like the shell of snail. It is a fluid filled cavity situated in the temporal bone.

It consists of:

- Modiolus, a bony canal
- Ossious spiral laminae, which partially divides the cochlea into:
  - Scala vestibuli: It is the upper chamber, containing a fluid called perilymph
  - Scala media: It is the middle chamber, containing a fluid called endolymph
  - Scala tympani: It is the lower chamber

  The scalae communicate through the helicotrema

The membrane between scala vestibuli and scala media is called Reissner's membrane.

The membrane between scale media and scala tympani is called as basilar membrane. The basilar membrane is also called auditory strings. It has different sections with different lengths. The strings generate different sounds at different places.

Organ of corti is the auditory receptor which rests on the basilar membrane.

Mechanism of Hearing

Sound waves in air enter the external ears through the pinna. From here the waves travel to the tympanic membrane via the external auditory meatus. These sound waves cause vibration in the middle ear i.e., at the tympanic membrane. Then these vibrations are transmitted by malleus, incus and stapes to the fenestra ovalis. From fenestra ovalis, the vibrations enter the organ of corti passing through perilymph and endolymph. From the organ of corti, the impulses produced by vibrations are carried to the brain stem via the cochlear portion of VIIIth cranial nerve. Here a phenomena called spatial summation of impulses occurs. This means transmission occurs through many nerve fibres rather than a few. The fibres are then carried to the auditory center of brain which is present in the temporal lobe of the opposite side.

Loudness is determined by three ways:

1. When the sound becomes louder, the amplitude of vibration of the basilar membrane and hair cells also increase, so that the hair cells stimulate the nerve endings at more rapid rates.
2. As the amplitude of vibration increases, it causes more and more of the hair cells on the outer edge of the resonating portion of the basilar membrane to become stimulated; transmission occurs through nerve fibres.
3. The outer hair cells do not become stimulated significantly until the vibrations of the basilar membrane reaches high intensity

Theories of Hearing

There exists some theoretical explanation about hearing, out of which the following two are important:

1. Helmholtz's place or Resonance theory.
2. Rutherford's frequency or Telephone theory.

1. Helmholtz's Place or Resonance Theory

Helmholtz formulated this theory in 1864. According to him, the basilar membrane of the cochlea with its hair cells acts as a tune resonator and the fibres of the basilar membrane can be compared to the strings of a piano. He also clarified that the narrow end or the base of the cochlea is tuned to high pitches (i.e, frequencies) while the wider upper end of cochlea, is tuned to low pitches. In other words, different parts of the basilar membrane are related to different pitches. Each part is assigned a pitch and different pitches go to different parts of the temporal lobe. Pitch of sound is controlled by the area and intensity of the activated place. Hence, if an external stimulus aroused more area of basilar membrane with great intensity, then there will generate a high pitch. Recent electro-physiological studies of the ear have unfolded the veracity of this theory.

2. Rutherford's Frequency or Telephone Theory

Rutherford in 1866 propounded the frequency theory of hearing. According to this theory, cortex is the location where sound is analysed. Cochlea simply acts as a passive instrument like a telephone to transmit the sounds from the external ear. It also propounds that the bacillary membrane is supposed to vibrate as a whole and not in parts. The intensity of sound is determined by the number of active nerve fibres involved in it. Although it is the advanced theory to the former one, it still failed to explain loudness of sound.

Mechanism of Equilibrium

The endolymph present in the semicircular canals is activated by the movement of head. Consecutively, endolymph stimulates the nerve endings in the ampullae. The impulses are conveyed to the brain through the vestibular portion of the VIIIth cranial nerve. These impulses produce sensations which make an individual conscious of the position of the head. Thus there occurs adjustment and maintenance of balance and equilibrium.

SMELL AND TASTE

Smell and taste are separate senses. Still psychologists (like Robert A. Baron and Michael J. Kaisher) and physiologists (like Arthur C. Guyton and John E. Hall) prefer to discuss them under one head for two reasons:

1. Both respond to agents in solutions; stuffs that have been dissolved in fluid or gas.
2. Both senses are strongly tied to primitive emotional and behavioral functions of our nervous system and hence, are intimately interrelated.

Sensation of Smell (Olfaction)

Nose is the organ of smell. The sensory nerves of smell are olfactory nerves (first cranial nerve).

Smell is the least understood of our senses mainly because this subject belongs to subjective evidences, which cannot be collected from lower animal experiments. Another reason attributed for it is that the sense of smell is poorly developed in human beings in comparison to that of some lower animals. Human beings possess about 50 million olfactory receptors which is almost one fourth or 25 percent in contrast to that of a dog.

The stimulus for sensation of smell consists of molecules of different substances or odorants that exist in the air. These molecules enter the nasal passage, where they dissipate in the nasal tissues, which are soggy in nature resulting in their coming in contact with receptor cells of the olfactory epithelium. Our olfactory senses are limited in terms of range of stimuli to which they are receptive. Human olfactory receptors can detect only substances with molecular weight between 15 and 300. That is the reason why

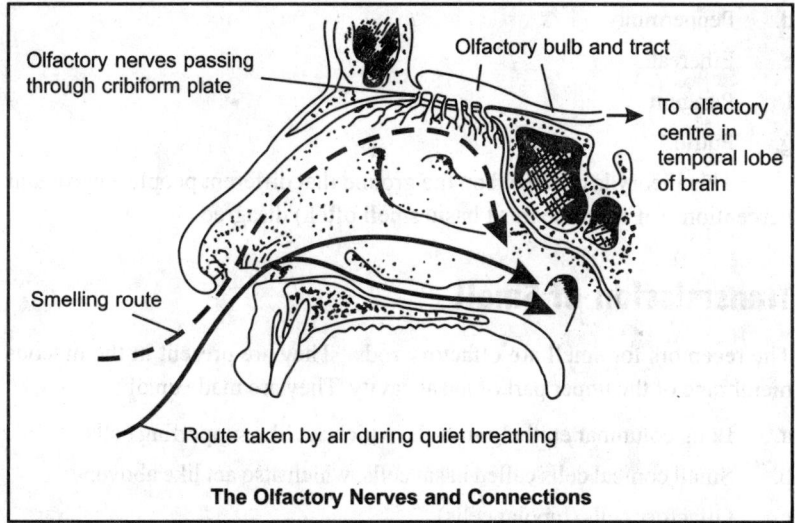
The Olfactory Nerves and Connections

we are able to detect the smell of alcohol and not table sugar in a mixed drink. The molecular weight of former is 46 and 342 respectively.

Theories of Smell

Stereo-chemi'cal Theory

This theory states that substances differ in smell because they have different molecular shapes

This theory is being criticized for the following reasons:

1. Nearly identical molecular shapes can have extremely different fragrances.
2. Substance with different chemical structures can produce very similar odors.

Theory of Primary Odors

This theory suggests that there exist basic or primary odors, similar to primary colors in color vision. Primary odors are:

a. Camphoraceous.
b. Musky.
c. Floral.

d. Pepperminty.
e. Ethereal.
f. Pungent.
g. Putrid.

This theory is criticized on the ground that different people's particular perceptions (of even the most basic smell often) disagree.

Transmission of Smell

The receptors for smell are olfactory rods. They are present in the mucous membrane of the upper part of nasal cavity. They are made up of :

a. Long columnar epithelium cells, which act like supporting cells.
b. Small conical cells called basal cells, which also act like above.
c. Olfactory cells (bipolar cells).

The olfactory receptors send impulses to olfactory cells (bipolar cells) that form the first order of neurons. The axons of these neurons form the olfactory nerve i.e., 1st cranial nerve. This nerve passes through the cribriform plate of ethmoid bone (i.e., root of nose) and terminates in the olfactory bulb. Cribriform plate separates the brain cavity from the upper reaches of the nasal cavity. The cribriform plate has numerous tiny holes through which an equal number of small nerves pass upward from the olfactory membrane in the nasal cavity to enter the olfactory bulb in the cranial cavity. The olfactory bulb has short axons that terminate in the multiple globular structures within the olfactory bulb called glomeruli. Olfactory bulb has mitral and tufted cells, which along with the above mentioned axons form the second order of neurons. From the olfactory bulb, the sensations are carried through the olfactory tract to transmit the sensation of smell to the central nervous system.

Anosmia means loss of smell.

Hyperosmia is morbid sensitiveness to smell.

In *cacosmia* the patients complain of imaginary odors that do not exist.

SENSATION OF TASTE (GUSTATION)

Taste is related to tongue. Two types of special structures are seen on it:
1. Papillae.
2. Taste buds.

PSYCHOLOGY OF COGNITION : SENSATION

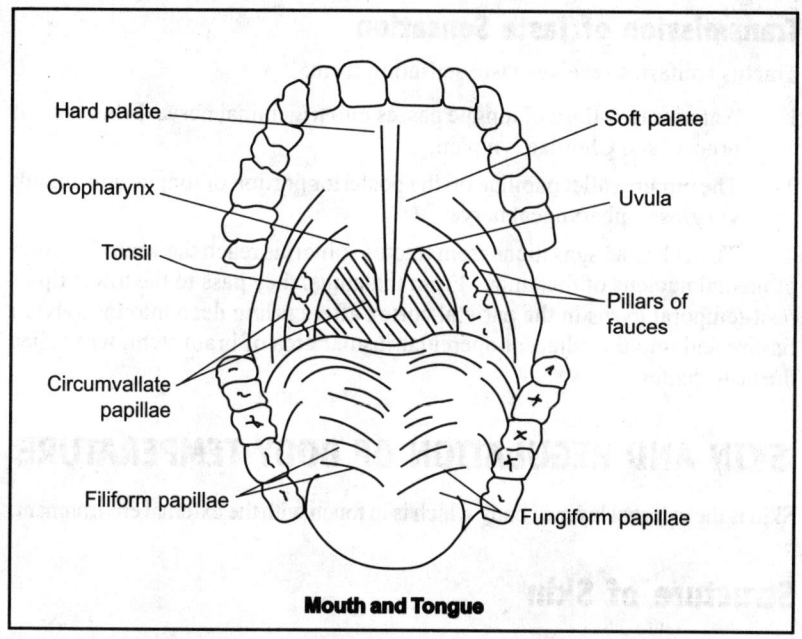

Mouth and Tongue

Each papillae is assigned to a cluster of buds. The taste buds are the sense organs of taste. Human beings possess 10,000 taste buds. Each taste bud contains several receptor cells. These buds are lined by stratified squamous epithelium and are flask-like with a wide bottom.

We can perceive literary hundreds of different tastes, But they are the combination or amalgamation of four primary tastes, which are as follows:

Sour: This taste is caused by various acids. The edges of the tongue are sensitive to it.

Salty: This taste is elicited by ionized salts. One can perceive this taste with the help of the tip and anterior part of tongue.

Sweet: This taste is caused by sugars, glycols, alcohols, aldehydes, ketones, esters, etc. Tip and anterior part of tongue are assigned with this taste.

Bitter: Quinine, caffeine, strychnine and nicotine. Posterior part of tongue is sensitive to this taste.

Transmission of Taste Sensation

Tractus solitarius receives taste sensation from:

1. Anterior two-third of tongue passes into trigeminal nerve. From there it proceeds to Chordae tympani.
2. The circumvallet papillae on the posterior portion of tongue and mouth via glosso-pharyngeal nerve.

Then all taste sensations from tractus solitarius reach the ventral portion of medial nucleus of thalamus. From thalamus, they pass to the lower tip of post-temporal gyrus in the parietal cortex after curling deep into the sylvian fissure and into the adjacent opercular insular area of brain stem, where lies the taste center.

SKIN AND REGULATION OF BODY TEMPERATURE

Skin is the external layer of body which is in touch with the external environment.

Structure of Skin

Skin consists of :

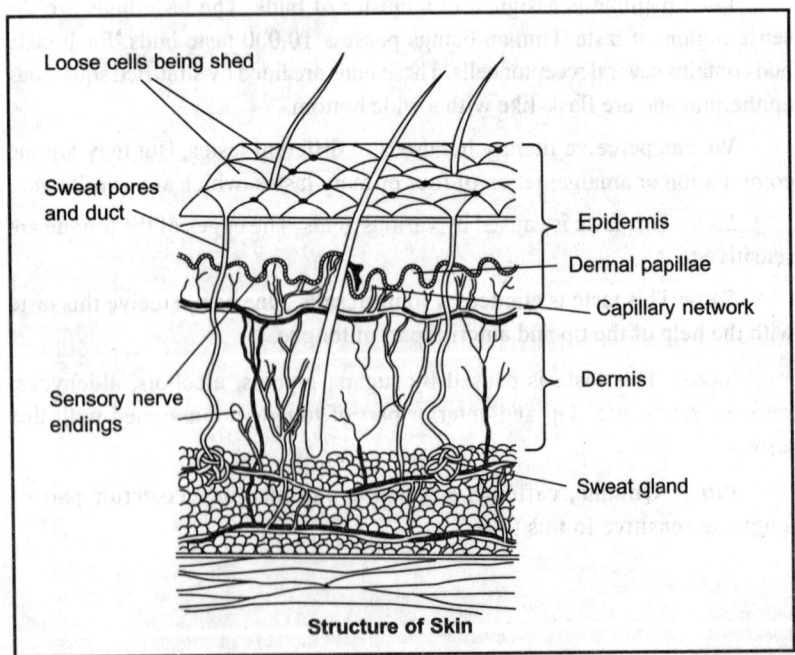

Structure of Skin

A. Epidermis, the outer layer.
B. Dermis, the inner layer.

A. Epidermis

It is made of stratified epithelium and contains the following layers:

1. *Stratum Corneum*: It is the most superficial layer of skin consisting of cell which are dead or desquamating. It has scale-like cells which are constantly being replaced. These cells have a protein called keratin which acts like a buffer and protects the skin from acids and alkalies of a mild nature.
2. *Stratum Lucidum*: This is the thin glistening or translucent layer made up of indistinct non-nucleated cells.
3. *Stratum Granulosum*: It is of two to three layers possessing spindle-shaped triangular or rhomboidal cells with granules in the cytoplasm. The granules change keratin in stratum lucidum.
4. *Stratum Germinativum*: It is also called Malpighian layer or the germinative layer of epidermis. It mainly contains prickle cells and melanocytes. This layer replenishes the horny cells of the superficial layer, which is regularly exfoliated. The layer is devoid of blood supply and the nutrition is supplied by lymph. Mitosis is intensified in this layer at night.

B. Dermis

It is the inner layer which forms the true skin. It comprises of connective tissues, blood vessels, lymph, nerve fibres, etc. It contains melanophore cells containing melanin pigment, sweat and sebaceous glands, hair roots and erector pili muscles, contraction of which produces straightening of the hair.

Secretions of Skin

The two secretions of skin are sweat and sebum.

1. Secretion of Sweat

Sweat is secreted by sweat glands that exist in the dermis. It is of two types:
   a. *Eccrine,* which are found throughout the body.
   b. *Epocrine,* which are found over the axillary skin, skin of mons pubis, scrotum, nipple, etc.

These glands are entwined tubular glands and their ducts open in the epidermis.

Sweat glands are more numerous in the palms of hands and soles of feet. The secretion of sweat is controlled by sympathetic nerves. Everyday an average of 500-1000 ml of sweat is produced in 24 hours inside our body. Sweat becomes insensible when the amount is 600-800 ml. However, when the amount reaches about 1-2 litres a day, it becomes noticeable. Sweat contains mainly water, some salts and traces of other waste products.

2. Secretion of Sebum

Sebum is a greasy secretion produced by the sebaceous glands. They are small, flask-shaped glands present in the dermis. They have a duct which opens into a hair follicle. The sebaceous glands are present in the skin of many parts except the palm of hands and soles of feet. Sebum keeps the skin oily and prevents it from drying.

Functions of Skin

1. It protects the underlying structures from injury.
2. The normal body temperature i.e., 98.4° F (37° C) is maintained by a balance between heat production and heat loss.

   Heat is produced by increased activity of liver and other glandular structures, metabolisms like oxidation of foods stuff and combustion of fat, severe exercise, etc.

   Loss of heat occurs, through the skin by conduction, convection, radiation and evaporation. Body temperature is controlled by a 'heat regulating centre' that exists in the hypothalamus.
3. Skin excretes salts like sodium chloride and metabolites like urea.
4. Skin provides sensation of awareness of environment.
5. Sebum and sweat are secreted by the skin.
6. Synthesis of vitamin D from ergosterol of skin is caused by the action of ultraviolet rays of sun.
7. Skin is concerned with beauty and attraction of an individual.
8. Melanin present in skin protects skin from ultraviolet rays.
9. Absorption of some oils, fat soluble substances, drugs, etc. occurs through the skin.

Cutaneous Pain

This can be caused by injury to skin, pathological states of skin, release of chemical substances that produces itching, etc.

There are chiefly four different types of tactual sensations: Warm, cold, pain, touch or pressure. We find differential distribution of touch sensation for different parts of the body. The lips and cheeks have hot spots. The cold spots are found just below the shoulder blade. The tip of nose is sensitive to pressure.

SENSATION OF SOME OTHER PAINS

Pain is experienced in all parts of the body. The pain can be caused by physical, mechanical, electrical and thermal stimuli. We have already discussed cutaneous pain. Let us discuss some other important pain sensations.

Visceral Pain

Visceral pain is generated as an expression of altered physiology of an internal organ like kidney, liver, pancreas, etc. Among various pains, the pancreatic pains are the most severe ones. Sometimes sensation of pain becomes migratory to nearby or distant areas and is designated as referred pain e.g., pain arising from the liver is felt at the inferior angle of right shoulder, which you might have read in *Chelidonium*.

Deep Pain

This type of pain is produced in the receptors of muscles, tendons, joints, etc. The pain is generated due to occlusion of blood supply resulting from the powerful contraction of a muscle. Sometimes, such pain may also be a referred pain like above.

Headache

A headache may occur due to a variety of conditions like anxiety, tension and pathological changes in intracranial blood vessels, visual defects, etc.

PATHWAY OF PAIN

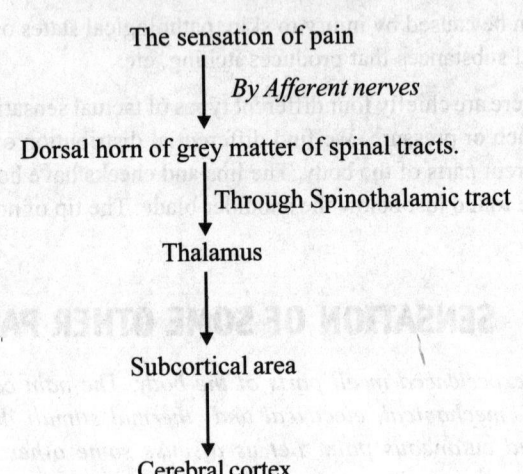

The sensation of pain
↓ *By Afferent nerves*
Dorsal horn of grey matter of spinal tracts.
↓ Through Spinothalamic tract
Thalamus
↓
Subcortical area
↓
Cerebral cortex

Chapter 5

PSYCHOLOGY OF COGNITION : PERCEPTION

We live in an environment. While interacting in the environment we have to interact with a variety of stimuli, and reception of such stimuli through our sense organs is called sensation. Sensation is the experience of raw materials whereas this sensation is learnt through perception. It is perception that gives meaning and awareness to a particular sensation. Perception adds a comprehensive understanding to the stimulus.

WHAT IS PERCEPTION?

What happens to us when we see a rose? We appreciate its color. We receive its fragrance. We also feel its tender, smooth and soft touch. We interpret this object as a rose flower recalling it from our past experience. We perceive the given object as a rose. Hence perception is the interpretation of the meaning of sensations. When we look at a rose, its various sensations of color, smell, touch, etc. are aroused inside us. Perception is a mental activity, which provides us awareness of the situation by giving us exact knowledge of it. Perception is not merely a mechanical association with an object alone; it adds knowledge about it too. Hence, sensation is regarded as a whole in perception. In our case, the mere pink color of a rose does not certify it as a rose or the sensation of color alone is not enough for the identification of rose. The real meaning of sensation is expressed in perception.

SENSATION AND PERCEPTION

Sensation and perception are like two sides of a coin and cannot be separated. The distinction between perception and sensation is similar to the one between a whole and its part. Sensations are the basic elements of perceptions. Perception of the external world depends on the sensation of form, heat, cold, color, sound, taste, smell, density, range, etc. Just as the whole cannot exist without its parts, in the same way, perception cannot exist in the absence of sensation. For example, the perception of a rose involves the experience of the sensations of color, smell, touch, etc. To express the same scientifically, the analysis of the perception of a rose yields three sensations. Sensations are the rudimentary and simple experiences. Sensations are the direct or primary responses while perceptions are secondary or reflective responses to the physical stimuli. Here we have to note that although we talk of first and second response, the gap between these two is not perceptible. We say so for understanding the relativity only.

VARIOUS PROCESSES IN PERCEPTION

The mechanism, by which an organism amends a sense impression to perception by adding knowledge and meaning to, is called the process of perception. Perception is a complex process and comprises of the following five steps:

1. Selection Process

Selection is the first step of our perception process. We are always exposed to various stimuli in the environment. Still it is neither desirable nor feasible to perceive all the stimuli at a given moment. Hence our perception is based on a selective process.

2. Receptor Process

The second process in perception is the receptor process. The rose, by virtue of its presence, stimulates three different receptor cells i.e., olfaction, visual and tactile. Now, let us assume that you receive two auditory stimuli at a time: Say a phone call from a friend and door bell being rung by a guest who is waiting at the entrance of your home. Here you receive both the auditory stimuli simultaneously. At this juncture, you decide to attend first to the telephone call and later to the door bell. Similarly, when you watch a favorite TV programme, very often the breaking news appears at the bottom of the screen. Here you alternately watch both the items with the help of receptor process.

3. Unification Process

This is the third step in the process of perception. For the perception of a rose, simply, the reception process of visual, tactile and olfaction separately does not give it a meaning. The process of meaningful unification of the different sensations is necessary for the process of perception.

4. Symbolic Process

This process is the fourth step in the process of perception. From our daily life, we know that most things have an experience attached to them. A rose reminds us of the friend, we love most. Thus, the rose becomes a symbol of our dearest friend. The rose will always be a rose but every time we perceive a rose, because of this symbolic process attached to the rose now has more meaning than a just being a flower.

5. Affective Process

This is the fifth process to perception. A rose may remind us of our beloved friend. The friend is not a lifeless object. He came to us and presented a rose, which left us with some happy memories. So the rose also reminds us of sweet memories. Of course, the affective process may also represent sad moments. For example, once the author had to depart with his beloved lecturer, who died in an accident. The author accompanied the dead body till the graveyard as a token of respect to the departed soul. During this journey, he was exposed to a particular type of fragrance of an incense stick. Although two decades have passed, he detests that particular brand of incense sticks because whenever he comes in contact with that fragrance, the sad moments of his beloved teacher's departure ensue.

Moreover, perception is a complex process where past experience plays a crucial role, which is obvious from above.

CHARACTERISTICS OF PERCEPTION

The main characteristics of perception are as follows:
1. Attention.
2. Unity and continuity.
3. Persistency with varied efforts.
4. Free adaptation to varying conditions.

5. Learning by experience.
6. Reproduction in perception.

1. Attention

Attention is the prime step of perception. Everyday you come to college. Can you exactly name the shops, automobiles, clinics, departmental stores, saloons, buildings, etc. you pass everyday? Can you tell the place where roses are sold. Most probably you cannot recall everything that has been asked. This happens because you do not pay attention to those shops, stores, etc. Hence, perception cannot occur without attention despite proximity of sense organs and objects.

2. Unity and Continuity

As mentioned above, scattered sensations cannot lead us to perception as that lacks meaning. The perception of a rose includes the unity and continuity in the sensations, which enables us to perceive a rose.

3. Persistency with Changing Efforts

Every stimulus to which we expose ourselves may not be static or constant. Hence the perceiver has to constantly change his efforts for complex perceptions. How do you react to an intruder in your campus? You put a sharp glance into him, listen and talk with him so that his personality and intention can be discovered. These varying perceptions have a unity and persistency.

4. Adjustment to Varying Circumstances

Under some circumstances, there are frequent changes in sensation and perception. In cricket, the batsman keeps an eye on the action and movement of the bowler. In this process, the batsman has to undergo various types of adjustments in sensation and perception. The batsman has to adapt himself every now and then to the changing behavior of the bowler.

5. Learning by Experience

It is a debatable question whether we enter the world with experience (i.e., born with some kind of ready knowledge) or we learn everything by experience. This has given rise to the controversy of nature versus nurture. Anyhow, we have to accept that both innate factors (the way a bee collects honey, which is not learned or taught) and experience are needed to provide a complete account of our perceptual abilities. But the major chunk of perception seems to be learnt.

6. Recollection of Past Experiences

The example of the rose which was discussed earlier justifies this aspect of perception. We can take an example from our clinic where past experience also counts much for perception. When a patient undergoes severe aggravation under so called homeopathic treatment (say for scabies), then the next time he will perceive the treatment of homeopathy in relation to the previous experience. A kindergarten student, whose mother is very affectionate, perceives her Miss (lady teacher) also as an affectionate teacher when she first comes in contact with her.

PERCEPTUAL GROUPING

When a child is riding a cycle he is not only riding a cycle alone. Simultaneously, he develops other perceptions of distance, accident, speed of cycle, etc. to adjust with the environment. This total approach is called the Gestalt approach.

Similarly, when you attend a phone call you perceive the picture of your friend, the place from where he is communicating with you, the time factor, etc. all while you are answering the phone call. This in totality is called Gestalt.

Similarly you cannot call the wheel of a chariot, a chariot. You also cannot call the banner of a chariot, a chariot. So also, the seat where the conqueror sits cannot be called the chariot. Chariot as a term, refers to a totality. This totality of perception is called Gestalt approach

The tune generated from the harmonium is very pleasant for listening, but if it is analyzed in its notes, the tune vanishes. This is called Gestalt.

In German, the word for it is 'Gestalton', while in English it is Gestalt. Gestalt is very important in perception. The Gestalt psychologists maintain the real form of the object is to be taken as a whole. They first introduced this theory on the subject of perception in psychology. In 1912, Wertheimer announced, on the basis of his experiments, that perception by the various sense organs, eyes, nose, ear, tongue, etc. takes place as a whole. A face is beautiful because of the effect of this Gestalt.

According to the Gestalt theory, perception is controlled by the physiological activities in the nervous system, which is a result of stimulation from physical objects. Whatever the person sees depends to a great extent on the sensations from the perceived object.

The orchestra in a film's music is very attractive because the sounds of many instruments are incorporated in it.

Just observe the following asterisk's cited below. You might have seen such asterisks in many books. You might have noticed that there are four divisions of arrangement. The arrangement of asterisks and the spatial relation depends not on the perceiver but the perceived objects too. These independent factors set up the explicit organization in the field of perception.

```
*  *        *  *        *  *        *  *
*  *        *  *        *  *        *  *
```

The psychologists belonging to Gestalt school have discovered some laws of organization which we will now study.

LAW OF PERCEPTUAL ORGANIZATION

In psychology, this perceptual organization is divided into:
A. Gestalt Factors in Organization
    I. External
        1. Law of Wholes
        2. Law of Figure and Back Ground
            a. Similarity
            b. Proximity
            c. Symmetry
            d. Homogeneity
    II. Central
        1. Law of Familiarity
        2. Law of Mental Set
    III. Reinforcing
        1. Law of Pragnaz
        2. Law of Good Figure
            a. Law of Continuity
            b. Law of Closure

B. Personal Factors in Organization
   I. Mental set
   II. Social milieu
   III. Past experience
   IV. Emotion
   V. Needs, drives and motivation.

A. Gestalt Factors in Organization

I. External Factors

1. Law of Wholes

This is the most important law of organization. The word Gestalton has been brought from German language. It means a form, structure, configuration, or pattern of physical, biological, or psychological phenomena so integrated as to constitute a functional unit with properties not derivable by mere summation of its parts. It emphasizes that in perception, the whole is perceived at a time. Accordingly, all the sensations converge in the mental faculty in an organized structure. In the given figure you perceived all the asterisks as a whole and asterisk as a solitary item.

  *   *   *   *   *   *   *   *

The Law of Wholes means that the whole is noticed first in perception. This is the reason why a person sometimes overlooks minor and insignificant defects in the picture.

Now let us look at the following figure.

The figure can be seen under two aspects.

First, you may discover the face of a young lady, provided you see one of her ears, her neck and the pupil of her eye.

Secondly, you may also see an old lady just altering the parts. The part, which was previously observed to be the young lady's neck, now becomes an old woman's mouth and chin.

Figure of a Lady

Hence different parts of a figure depend on the meaning attached to the whole. Their meaning is analyzed on the basis of the meaning of the whole from the particulars.

2. Law of Figure and Background

Psychologists belonging to Gestalt school also maintain that every perception of a sensation is always based on something in the background. This background has an effect on the perception of the object or figure. We have observed in various advertisements that every figure has been treated with a contrasting background so that it can have a better effect. This law of figure and background is not restricted to visual perception only but is also applied to tactile and auditory perceptions.

Factors Determining Figure and Background

a. SIMILARITY

When two parts become similar in any way e.g., color, figure, extension, etc.,, they tend to express in an organized form. Let us examine the following figure:

We see an organized framework of three vertical and five horizontal lines of stars. Similarly, if our attention is focused on the circles, we see an organized figure in the form of four perpendicular and two horizontal lines. In general, we do not notice the square that stands on the right. You might

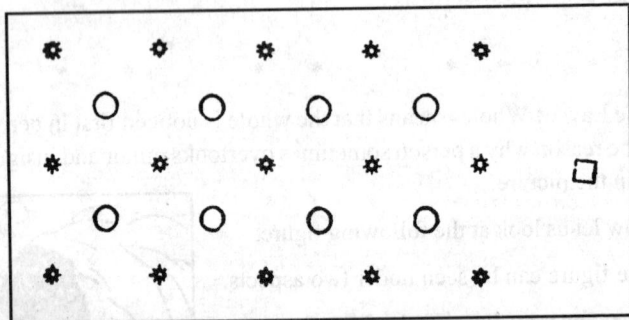

have taken it as a printing mistake as it neither forms a pattern with circles nor with the stars.

b. PROXIMITY

Objects in close proximity in time and space tend to express a perception as a whole. When we look at the night, we form the stars in groups or patterns and perceive them as a whole.

c. SYMMETRY

The various parts, when placed in an order or symmetry, tend to be organized into a whole.

d. HOMOGENEITY

Two parts of equal intensity or brightness are easily assimilated in a perception. Let us take the example of the following figure:

In the above figures, A and B, there are two concentric circles. In the case of A there are two concentric circles while in B the gap between the same circles has been darkened which gives the appearance of a ring, instead of two circles.

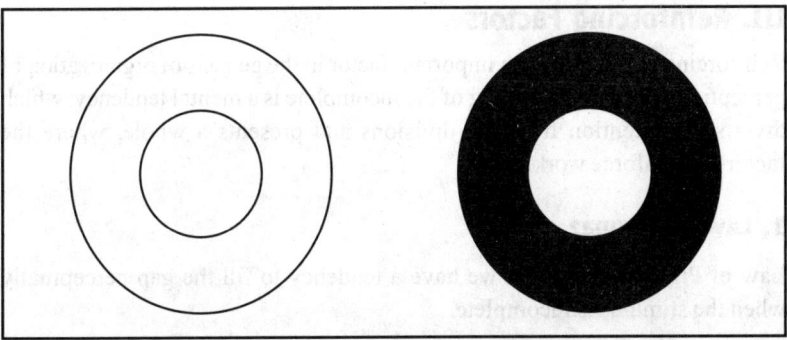

II. Central Factors

Gestalt psychologists suggest the following central factors for the organization of perception along with the factors mentioned above:

1. Familiarity

We have to understand three points in this respect:

a. An individual can perceive an organization if he is familiar with it. If he is familiar with a picture quiz he can immediately perceive it and can recall with clarity and alacrity.

b. If the same picture quiz is presented to some uninitiated person he will not be able to figure it out.

c. Again if the same picture is presented in part to the first person who is familiar with it, he will be not be capable of making it out, not withstanding his familiarity.

Therefore, the Gestalt psychologists offers the view that familiarity may or may not be related to perception.

2. Mental Set

Mental set plays a crucial role in the organization of perception. For example, a philosopher looks at the truths of the universe while a trader always looks at the world with profit and loss in mind a doctor looks at the world with diseases and treatment, a saint advises to renounce the world, etc. The difference in mental set is the cause of diverse perceptions of the same thing by different individuals in a given time or the same people at different times. This factor can also be attributed to personal factors.

III. Reinforcing Factors

Reinforcing factor is also an important factor in the genesis of organization of perception. The supplementing of the incomplete is a mental tendency, which diverts our attention from the divisions and presents a whole, where the factors of reinforce work.

1. Law of Pragnaz

Law of Pragnaz states that we have a tendency to fill the gap perceptually when the stimulus is incomplete.

2. Law of Good Figure

It has basically two principles:

a. Law of Continuity

It is also called the law of direction. Continuity also has an effect on organization. Through this principle we see a line straight or curved by perceptual groping.

b. Law of Closure

Closure too, when compared to continuity, has an effect on the organization of parts. This law refers to perceptual processes which organize action; we perceive a whole form, not just disjointed parts.

Let us observe the following figure:

On first seeing it, one observes a triangle, a circle, a square, another circle and a hexagon (from center to periphery).

Now look along the lines of each figure. Now, nothing will be visible.

These lines do not make any angle, as they do not meet.

A careful observation, similar to the preceding one, of the two circles, the square, the triangle and the hexagon will reveal that there is no such figure in the picture.

The illusion of figures in the first case was caused by closure, which did not allow the attention to dwell on the gaps, so that the figures appeared organized.

B. Personal Factors in Organization

I. Mental Set

(Already discussed.)

II. Social Milieu

Affairs, circumstances and people are perceived in consistent with the interest, attitude and values of the group to which the individual belongs. Effects of group predispositions are very strong and they modify our perceptions. Women perceive a social gathering differently from men, may be due to social training. The prevailing attitudes and beliefs in society also influence the selective nature of perception. Hindus perceive the cow, its dung, the river Ganges, etc. differently from hope of other religions. A man may go to church without covering his head but it is not so in a Gurudwara.

III. Past Experience

Experience also counts in perception. When a patient undergoes severe aggravation under so called homeopathic treatment, next time he will perceive the treatment of homeopathy in relation to his previous experience. A student, whose mother is very affectionate, perceives his Miss (lady teacher) also as an affectionate teacher when he first comes in contact with her.

IV. Emotion

The role of emotions cannot be overlooked. We observe from our day to day lives we excuse many faults of others when we happy. We know that a person in love looks at the world through rose – colored glasses. They perceive everything in a joyous state.

V. Needs, Drives and Motivation

Motivation and emotion also play an important role in the process of perception. For example, if you ask a hungry man to complete the word 'Me–, he may fill up with 'al' or 'at', which will give rise to the word 'Meal' or 'Meat', whereas other people who are not hungry may answer with Mean or Meet, etc.

It is said that a poet lost his way while passing a dense forest. He had to take rest on a tree for his survival. At night he became very hungry and perceived the moon as a 'Roti' or 'Chapati'. Hence perception is greatly modified with the need, drive and motivation.

Till now we talked about 5 senses and its related perceptions. There are many people who claim that there exists another sense called 6th sense and extra sensory perception, to which science has no sanction. Anyhow, let us have a bird eye view over their claim.

BEYOND NORMAL PERCEPTION - SOME NOTES

Psi Phenomena (Extra Sensory Perception and Psycho Kinesics)

The branch of psychology that deals with psi phenomena is called parapsychology. The term 'psi' was introduced by the British psychologists Drs. Robert Thouless and W.P. Weisner in the year 1946. You should not bother for the full form of this word as this is not an abbreviated form. The word 'psi' (y), is the twenty-third letter of the Greek alphabet which includes both the phenomena of ESP (related to mental aspect) and P.K. (related to physical aspect) because of their close relationship. **Psi phenomena** cannot be accounted for natural law or knowledge apparently acquired by other than usual sensory abilities.

ESP (*Extra Sensory Perception*)

The short form of extra sensory perception is ESP. Extra Sensory Perceptions are generally cognitive in nature. These occur beyond the use of the ordinary sensory channels (i.e. not related to visual sensation of eye, hearing sensation of ear, olfaction sensation of nose, taste sensation of tongue or tactile sensation of skin); hence the term extrasensory perception frequently used to assign these phenomena. Followings are the examples of ESPs.

a. *Clairvoyance;* supernormal awareness of objects or events, which are not known to others.
b. *Telepathy;* the thought transference of between persons.
c. *Precognition;* having knowledge of facts, of future events.

P.K. (*Psycho Kinesics*)

See chapter I under 'Branches of Psychology, no. 6'

The existence of Para psychological phenomena continues to be a subject of dispute, and a majority of conventional scientists categorically reject such findings as unscientific and hence it has remained inconclusive. Anyhow some associations and organizations are carrying out researches in PSI phenomena in the USA and UK. Among these; "Parapsychology Laboratory of North Carolina's Duke University" under the initiation of Joseph Rhine deserves a mention here.

ERRORS IN PERCEPTION

We look through eyes; listen through ears, smell through nose, etc., yet we cannot rely upon these senses always. Sometimes we perceive something for something else, which is not present there. Such conditions are called errors of perception. Errors of perception are very common in our day to day life. These errors depend upon one's physical and psychological conditions and environment under which the stimulus is interpreted. We will study errors of perception under:

I. Illusion
II. Hallucination
III. Delusion

I. Illusion

Perception is the correct interpretation of sensation whereas an illusion is a misinterpretation of the correct meaning of a perception. An illusion is a mistaken perception. An illusion always has an apparent stimulus of external nature. An illusion is not a dream. In an illusion, the perceived object is present whereas in a dream it is absent. It also differs from imagination as the object of perception is not a creation of the mind of the individual. In a state of illusion, a person may take a snake for a rope. In a normal condition also, a stick appears crooked when held partly under water. Illusion may be related to a sane as well as in an insane individual. A sane individual after close search or check will understand his error whereas an insane individual will persist with the erroneous interpretation, even after repeated demonstrations of his error.

Types of Illusion

In psychology, illusion has been classified under:
1. Personal
2. General

1. Personal Illusion

Personal illusion pertains to a person alone. It differs from person to person. In a dark night some people mistake a rope for a snake but a person unfamiliar with a snake cannot make this mistake. On the other hand, he is more likely to mistake a snake for a rope.

2. General Illusion

General illusions are of a universal kind and pertain to one and all. Examples of such illusions are:

    a. The illusion of merger of railway tracks at a distance.
    b. Seeing water in a sunny desert (or even on pitch road in summers).
    c. Geometrical illusions like Muller – Lyer illusion, Horizontal – Vertical illusion, etc.

Now let us discuss some important illusions.

1. **Illusion Caused by Stimulus Factor**

Let us examine above figure. The horizontal and vertical lines are of equal length, yet the vertical line seems to be longer than the horizontal line. This type of illusion is caused by the stimulus factor.

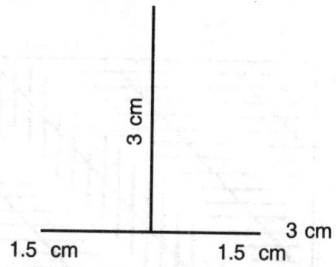

2. Muller-Lyer Illusion

Here exist two straight lines i.e., AB and CD. Both the lines are of equal length. But AB appears longer than CD because of movement of eye. The factor of eye movement seems to be a potent cause for this illusion. This illusion is called Muller – Lyer illusion.

AB is the feather headed line while CD is the arrow headed line. While comparing, we have to exert more eye movement in perceiving the feather headed line than in arrow headed lines. Therefore, the previous appears longer than the last.

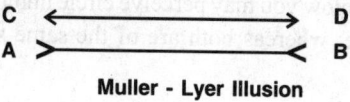

Muller - Lyer Illusion

3. Fan's Illusion

Observe the two horizontal lines in the figure below. The distance between the two parallel lines is equal all the way across the figure. But they appear unparallel. This illusion is also called Hering's illusion.

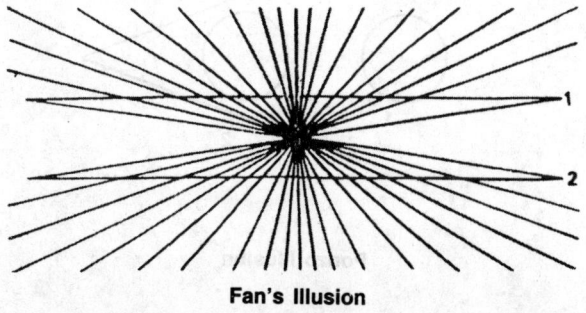

Fan's Illusion

4. Zollner Illusion

Observe the following figure.

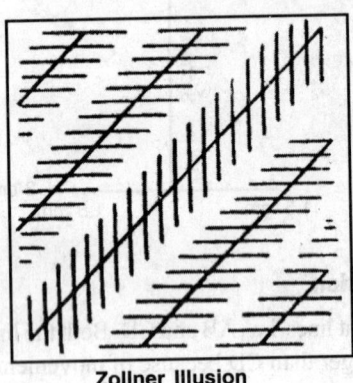
Zollner Illusion

All the lines in the figure are drawn parallel to each other but they look unparallel.

5. Ponzo Illusion

From the figure given below you may perceive circle number two to be bigger than circle number one; whereas both are of the same size. This is called Ponzo illusion.

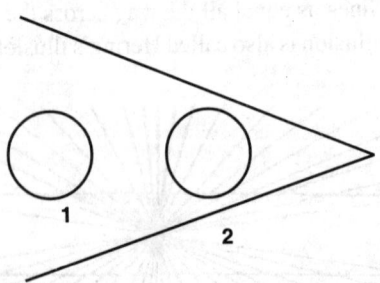
Ponzo Illusion

6. Jastrow Illusion

When you observe the following two crescents – one and two, crescent one seems to be bigger than number two. This is called Jastrow illusion.

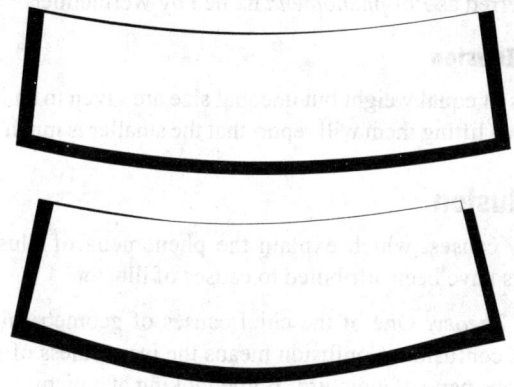

Jastrow Illusion

7. Contrast Illusion

Observe the following two rings—A and B. Both the rings are of equal diameter. But B appears smaller than A. This so because A is encircled by asterisks while B is encircled by circles. We tend to observe the whole picture with the result that the tendency towards wholes or a perception of good figures (see below) comes into play. This illusion is caused by eye movement, confusion, etc.

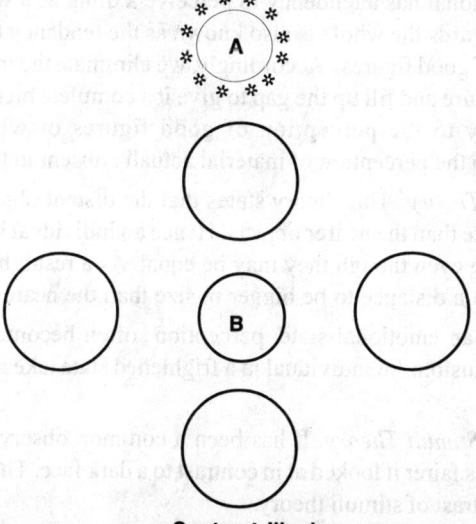

Contrast Illusion

8. Illusion of Movement

You might have seen a movie in a cinema hall. Here you perceive a moving picture which in fact does not move. This is called illusion of movement. This is very often referred as *Phi-phenomena* named by Wertheimer.

9. Size-Weight Illusion

When two boxes of equal weight but unequal size are given to an individual, then the individual lifting them will report that the smaller is much heavier.

Causes of Illusion

There are many causes, which explain the phenomena of illusions. The following factors have been attributed to causes of illusion:

1. *Confusion Theory:* One of the chief causes of geometrical and alike illusions is confusion. Confusion means the inexactness of perception of the various parts of a picture. While looking at a picture, the person becomes so engrossed in it that he does not notice the peculiarities of the parts or the merits and demerits of the picture. It has been found that if the Muller – Lyer illusion is examined by narrowing down the over range of vision, the illusion could have been greatly reduced.
2. *Eye Movement Theory*: The movement of the eyes has a lot to do with the creation of illusions. For example, the Muller – Lyer illusion justifies this.
3. *Good Figure Theory*: The Gestalt school of psychology postulated that an individual has a tendency to perceive a thing as a whole. This tendency towards the whole is also known as the tendency towards the perception of good figures. Accordingly, we eliminate the irregularities in a given figure and fill up the gap to give it a complete meaning. Thus the tendency to the perception of good figures or wholes leads sometimes to the perception of material actually absent in the picture.
4. *Perspective Theory:* This theory states that the distant object emerges smaller in size than the nearer objects. Hence an individual balances for such learning even though they may be equal. As a result he perceives the objects at a distance to be bigger in size than the nearer ones.
5. *Emotion:* In an emotional state, perception often becomes false and leads to an illusion. An individual in a frightened state takes a rope to be a snake.
6. *Contrast of Stimuli Theory*: It has been a common observation that a fair face looks fairer if looked at in contrast to a dark face. This is illusion is called contrast of stimuli theory.

7. *Preconception*: Preconception is another cause of illusion. Let us assume that Hari is a first B.H.M.S. student, who regularly attends class without any break. If he remains absent on a given day, the teacher will not notice it. The teacher may feel that Hari has attended his class on the day when the student has not actually put in an appearance.
8. *Habits:* Habits also cause illusion as is exemplified by the mistakes of the inexperienced proof-readers.
9. *Defects of Sense Organs*: Defective sense organs cause incorrect perception and is followed by an illusion. A person suffering from high temperature finds that most of the food tastes bitter.

II. Hallucination

Hallucination is dissimilar to illusion. Hallucination implies false sense of perception without any external object or stimulus. Some people see a ghost in a dark place. This is an example of hallucination. Some people relate strange incidents of hallucination e.g., an individual may narrate that a beautiful woman dressed in a white saree came at midnight and sat down on his bed and she patted his head with love and affection. Some factors like drug abuse, injury to the head, high temperature may generate hallucinations. In hallucinations, there is no apparent external stimulus, as is found in an illusion. The prey perceives it as some object or figure and put across experiencing hallucination.

Classification

Hallucination has been classified below as per the sense organs. Out of these classifications, first two are very common hallucinations.

1. Visual Hallucination

In this condition of delusion, the victim visualizes sights, which do not exist. He watches those things, which are not at all present in front of him. He may cry and say that he can see Lord Krishna or Christ who is calling him to visit heaven.

2. Auditory Hallucination

The victim in this condition claims that he hears voices or sounds without their presence. Clairvoyance of *Medorrhinum* comes under auditory hallucination.

3. Olfactory Hallucination

The sufferer smells something without the presence of anything. Here, exists a false sense of smelling.

4. Gustatory Hallucination

Here the victim experiences taste of food and drink having no discoverable sources.

5. Tactile Hallucination

In this condition the victim complains of a crawling sensation, like that of an insect over his body without it actually happening.

6. Psychomotor Hallucination

The classical example of *Baptisia* (also *Thuja*) can be illustrated for this condition. Here the sufferer feels movement of a part of the body; say legs or hands, although in reality there exists nothing as such.

According to psychologists, hallucinations represent our inner conflicts, fears, anxieties, etc. In schizophrenia, hallucination is a common symptom. The schizophrenic patient may try to sweep you with hallucinations, illustrating visual scenes and auditory receptions. He will claim that he has seen such and such God, who has ordered him to do this and do that and others must follow him. Caution must be taken in understanding hallucinations in rural set ups; where public take such things as normal. Very often they worship a schizophrenic patient without having knowledge of the disease. We must know that these are the outcomes of our repression of intense desire and aspiration.

Salient Differentiating Points Between Illusion and Hallucination

Hallucination differs in many ways from illusion. Let us discuss the salient differences.

1. Illusion usually occurs to ordinary people whereas hallucination occurs to people who are intoxicated and people who are mentally upset, distressed and tired.
2. Generally illusions are related to physiology while hallucinations are related to pathological conditions.
3. In illusions there generally exist distinct external stimuli, which are not found in hallucinations.
4. In illusions there exist external stimuli while the stimulations in hallucinations are in the individual himself, which makes the latter a kind of subjective perception.
5. An illusion may become common perception to all, like the illusion of merger of railway tracks at a distance, geometrical illusions, seeing water

in a sunny desert (or even on a pitch road in summers), Muller Lyer illusion, etc. The perception of a given situation is identical to every individual in case of illusion; whereas in hallucinations, the perception differs. For example, in a state of intoxication, Ram may see a ghost, Shyam may see a giant with a sword, while Hari may see a woman dressed in black saree, etc.

We can sum up the above as follows:

	Point	Illusion	Hallucination
1.	Nature of stimulus	Explicit	Not clear
2.	Source of stimulus	External	Internal
3.	Condition	May occur in in normal conditions	Usually occurs in abnormal conditions
4.	Experience	Experience is identical for everyone in a given situation	Experience varies in different people in a given situation

III. Delusion

Delusion is a false belief in something without having a basis. It can occur to both sane and insane individuals. Delusions can be removed from the mind of a sane person by providing him rational explanation and demonstration of falsity of belief, whereas no amount of explanation or demonstration can remove delusion in case of an insane individual.

Types of Delusions

Delusions are classified as per the nature of belief.

1. Delusion of Grandeur

This is also known as delusion of exaltation. The sufferer remains in a state of exalted feelings of greatness, power and riches. There occurs extravagance of thinking and action. By this he may squander money and property and may even commit a crime.

2. Delusion of Persecution

In such type of delusions, the patient believes that something bad is going to happen (*Calc.*) He may also think that he is going to be killed. He suffers from imaginary troubles (*Naja*). Such patients may commit the crime of killing with a feeling of utter helplessness.

3. Delusion of Influence

The sufferer from this delusion believes that he is under some external power or supernatural power (*Med.*). The sufferer may become a self-styled Baba or incarnation and may adhere to unlawful acts.

4. Hypochondriacal Delusion

In this delusion, the sufferer believes that there exists some abnormality or pathological condition inside the body, which cannot be detected in reality. This delusion may give rise to delusion of persecution.

5. Nihilistic Delusion

Nihilism means denial of existence of self and the universe. The sufferer does not believe in the existence of worldly matter or occurrences. He even condemns his own existence. These individuals are prone to accidents and may commit suicide.

6. Delusion of Infidelity

Usually a male patient strongly believes that his wife or lover has betrayed him by having some illicit relation with others, having no background or evidence. He also thinks that his wife does not love him. Such patients resort to torturing or killing their wife. Sometimes, the patient may commit suicide also.

7. Delusion of Self-reproach or Self-criticism

In this delusion, the sufferer censures himself for some imaginary offence or misdeed. In extreme cases, he is likely to commit suicide.

8. Delusion of Reference

In this delusion the patient believes that he is being referred by various media people and other agencies. By this belief he enters into a state of conflict with others. This affair may lead the sufferer to do some undesirable and unacceptable acts.

IMAGES

Let us assume that the principal of your college directed you to carry out the arrangements for the celebration of Hahnemann's birthday in your college. What will you do now? How you will plan the arrangements like making the dias, decorating the auditorium, fixing the sound system, inviting the dignitaries, entrusting the responsibilities, etc. for the celebration? For this you need a mental imagery to plan the celebration. Because, mental images are important tools for solving such problems.

An image is a kind of symbol which includes faint recollection of perceptions. Past experiences of an individual move around in his mind in the form of images. Image means mental pictures; a picture in an individual's mind or an idea of how someone or something is.

Mental images resemble but are not identical with a percept-visual, auditory, olfactory, etc. These mental images may be memories of previous events, scenes, etc. Imagery is the ability which differs from individual to individual.

Images play a crucial role in our life. Our life cannot move forward without its manipulation. Activities like dreams, daydreams, imagination, thinking, etc., come under purview of images.

An image is a symbol. But its stability, vividness and intensity are less in comparison to perception. Frequently, one may confuse images with concepts. Hence we should know its chief differences, which are delineated below:

1. Concept is general despite the fact that image is specific.
2. Concept is formless while image has a form.
3. Concepts are generally associated with thinking whereas images do not form an indispensable part of thinking.
4. Images are generally related to imaginations but concepts are used comparatively infrequently.

Types of Images

Followings are the major types of images:

1. **Imagined Image:** Imagined images are the outcome of distorted perceptions. It is a reorganization and re-interpretation of previous experiences. The image of a mermaid, an imaginary creature described in stories, with the upper body of a woman and the tail of a fish will be an imaginary image because we do not find it in the objective world, which is formed by the distortion of the perceptions of an woman and fish. In day dreams such imagined images are created in abundance in human life.

2. **After Image:** Our sense organs have a capacity to feel sensations from objects for some time after the sensation has been received. This is

called after sensation or after image. This remains only for a few seconds after the disappearance of the stimulus. Suppose you passed by a garden and smell the fragrance of roses. The after image of fragrance of roses remains for some moments and then it disappears.

3. **Eidetic Image:** These images are as steady, dramatic and powerful. These types of images are found among children and are equally powerful to perception.

4. **Memory Image:** It is a weaker image in comparison to Eidetic image. We posses the largest amount of memory images in comparison to other images. These images are residues of our past experiences of various places, persons and things.

5. **Dream Image:** Dream images are the images that occur in dreams and are related to the unconscious state of mind. These images are often symbolic. According to Freud, images of mountains, trees, etc. that occur in dreams represent the male sex organs whereas images of valleys, wells, etc. are the symbols of female sex organs.

6. **Hypnogogic Images:** As the name suggests, these images are aroused when the person enters into the subconscious state. This state may develop from a waking state or may be induced by a professional hypnotist. The subject feels these images as if it were real, distinct and intense in a state of trance

7. **Sensory Images:** These images are concerned with sensory images. These sensory images differ from person to person. Sensory images are of the following types:

   i. *Visual Imagery*: images related to the eyes. An individual with intense visual imagery can remember various experiences for a long time.

   ii. *Auditory Imagery* : These images are related to sensations received by the ears.

   iii. *Gustatory Imagery*: These images are related to sensations in relation to taste, which can be internal experiences even in the absence of external stimuli.

   iv. *Tactile Imagery*: These are the images related to the skin. The feeling or experience of heat or cold or weight are felt even in the absence of external stimuli.

   v. *Mobile Imagery*: This imagery induces an individual with the feeling of doing something or as if in motion even when either or both are not taking place.

Chapter 6

LEARNING

(Scientific Study of Behaviour: Pavlov, Skinner & Watson)

It was a festive occasion in the month of May (Savitri Amavasya) in 1971, when I was a student of standard VII and ate a lot of ripened Jackfruit with greed without bothering about its outcome. I ate a lot with greed. A few hours after consuming jackfruit, I suffered from vomiting and diarrhea (most probably it was cholera with fishy smelling rice watery stools). I had to suffer a lot and ultimately a doctor was summoned. I was given some injections along with some medicines. Since then I have never dared to take a piece of ripened jackfruit till date.

Once, one of my friends, Mr. B. became exceedingly afraid and nervous of seeing a taxi of a specific brand, say "A". After careful investigation and interrogation I came to know that the syndrome started since the day he found out that his beloved girl friend had eloped with another guy in the said brand taxi.

Let us take another example from the book "An Introduction to Psychology" by Norman L.Munn, L.Dodge Fernald Jr. and Peter S. Fernald mentioned below for better comprehension.

"*In late May of my junior year in high school, just after my last semester exam, I went for a drive in the country to celebrate the beginning of summer. While enjoying the fresh air and heavy fragrance of yellow jasmine, blooming at the time, an oncoming car careened from his side of the highway directly into my lane. There was no head-on collision, but the impact sent my car to the right into a field of yellow jasmine, the other car, whose driver had fallen asleep, ended up with me in the same field. No one was seriously hurt, except* the cars, but now whenever I smell yellow jasmine, I feel my stomach tightening up as when something frightens me and I have chills..."

From above, it is crystal clear that learning is not restricted to formal education or educational institutions only. Even an illiterate man from the country side is capable of counting coins or a given sum or rupees without undergoing any formal learning. Learning is constantly influenced by almost all phases of life.

Learning: Defined

Learning is a way of life. All living creatures learn everyday in every way. We all learn from the day of our very birth to the very day of death. Anyhow, the main aim of learning is to instill the desired and required changes in the pattern of behavior.

We learn new skills with fresh information, which is followed by beliefs and attitudes. We have formal education in schools and colleges. We also learn a lot from non-formal sources like cinema, TV, internet, software, etc. We also learn through other ways like, social interaction with a neighbor or at a shop, inter-relationship with parents or teachers.

When you (or I or anybody else) takes birth, your mind is like a clean slate. Then you are told that you are Rama or Rahim or Romeo. Then you are baptized and told that you belong to such and such religion, etc. Subsequently, when you grow up, you greet your teacher with "Good Morning" or by "Namaskar" or "Salam" as per your instilled learning. Similarly, you (or we) learn and the learning goes on continuously. You have to pass through several metamorphosis from birth to death. This happens due to learning. Melvin H. Martix justifiably says, Learning is a relatively enduring change in behavior which is a function prior to behavior, usually called practice."

Moreover, learning modifies our personality

Gardener Murphy (1968) defines "The term learning covers every modification in behavior to meet environmental requirements."

Woodworth (1945) defines, the same in a better way : " Any activity can be called learning as far as it develops the individual (in any respect, good or bad) and makes him alter behavior and experience different from what they would otherwise have been."

Another impressive definition is given by Henry P.Smith (1962): "Learning is the acquisition of new behavior or the strengthening or weakening of old behavior as the result experience."

Explanation

1. Learning is a process and not a product. You may learn driving and a you may also learn a lesson from an accident. But cramping due to an accident cannot be attributed to learning.

2. It involves all those experiences and training of an individual (right from birth) which help him to produce changes in his behavior. It may have ups and downs, but still it is learning. Suppose, few years back I had adopted a type of teaching which fetched good results but due to some reason or the other I changed the pattern and felt that the present pattern is not effective and again I adopted the former. All this can be attributed to learning.

3. Obviously from the former point it is clear that learning leads to changes in behavior but this does not necessarily mean that these changes always bring about improvement or positive development. One has an equal chance to drift to the negative side or acquire new behavior.

4. Instead of a change in the existing behavior or acquisition of a new behavior, learning may also result in discontinuance or abandonment of existing behavior. Though it is referred to as unlearning, actually unlearning in itself is also a learning process.

5. Learning prepares an individual for adaptation, adjustment and fitness that may be necessary to a given situation.

6. Learning is purposeful and goal-oriented. In case there is no purpose, there would hardly be any learning. The "knee jerk" reflex response to a knee hammer cannot be attributed to learning.

7. The scope of learning is too wide to be explained in words. It is a very comprehensive process which covers nearly all fields of behavior: Conative, cognitive and affective.

8. Learning is universal and continuous. It extends from womb to tomb. Every creature that lives, learns. In human beings it is not restricted to any particular age, sex, race, religion or culture.

9. Learning involves new ways of doing things but there is no limit to adopting these ways and means. All learning does not take place in the same manner. Therefore, learning as a process is of different types and involves different methods.

10. As maintained by Hilgard, the concept of learning excludes changes in behavior on the basis of native response tendencies like instincts reflexes, etc. Instinctive or specific programmes cannot be termed as learnt

behavior. Similarly, reflexes are the innate involuntary responses to stimulation e.g., blinking as bright light and the infant's suckling behavior cannot be attributed to learning.

11. Learning does not include changes in behavior on account of maturation, fatigue, illness or drugs.

Theories of Learning (Scientific Basis of Behavior)

We can broadly divide learning under two headings:

1. Connectionist or Behaviorism or Stimulus – Response theories.
    a. Pavlov's Classical Conditioning or Associative theories.
    b. Watson's theory of Behavior.
    c. Operant conditioning theories:
        i. Thorndike's trial and error learning.
        ii. Skinner's operant condition.
    d. Miller's theory of learning.
    e. Hull's theory of learning.
    f. Gutheri's sign learning.
2. Cognitive or Gestalt or Organismic or Purposive theories.
    a. Gestalt or Insight theory by:
        i. Koffka.
        ii. Kohler.
        iii. Wertheimer.
    b. Field theory of Kurt-Lewin.
3. Synthesis of above two.

In the first chapter, we read the definition of psychology, its evolution and a detailed description of its various branches. We also read how it freed itself from the clutches of philosophy and moved to the arena of science. Since then, many scientific studies have been carried out for the basis of behavior. Among prominent exponents in this field are Pavlov, Watson, Thorndike, Skinner, Miller, Hull, Gutheri, Koffka, Kohler, Wertheimer, Kurt-Lewin, etc. We will focus our study only on the following three:

I. Ivan Pavlov
II. John Watson
III. B.F. Skinner

I. IVAN PETROVICH PAVLOV

Ivan Petrovich Pavlov was born on September 14th, 1849 at Ryazan, Russia. He was the Russian physiologist who discovered and propounded the concept of the conditioned reflex. He developed a method, which emphasizes the importance of conditioning in animal behavior. In an experiment, he trained a hungry dog to salivate at the sound of a bell, which was earlier associated with the sight of food. He was awarded the Nobel Prize in 1904 for his work on physiology of digestion, exclusively for secretion of salivary (reflexive), gastric and intestinal secretions. He died on February 27th, 1936 at St. Petersburg.

Pavlov's Classical Conditioning*

Classical conditioning is a simple way of learning. It consists of the development of association between the response and the stimuli which are present when those responses are made.

Pavlov was initially interested in studying the physiology of digestion in animals. He chose a dog for experimentation. While studying the relative automatic reflexes associated with digestion, Pavlov noticed to his surprise that the dog salivated not just when food was put in its mouth but also at the mere sight of food. He interpreted the flow of saliva to food placed in mouth

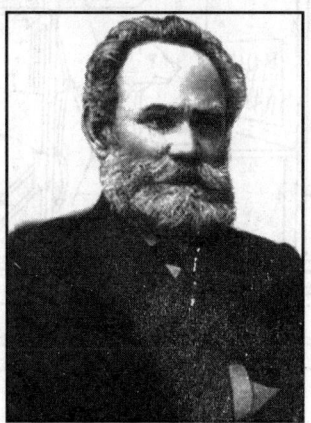

Fig. Ivan Pavlov

---

* **Note:** In translation, the Russian word **"ouslovnye"** has been used, which means conditioned rather than conditional behaviour.

as an unlearned response (unconditional response). He also interpreted that the response to the sight of food has to be learned (conditioned response). Gradually Pavlov carried out various experiments and taught the dog to salivate in response to various signals like onset of light, tone foot steps, ringing of a buzzer, etc. Later he established a new stimuli response association in the laboratory.

Pavlov's Experiment

As already mentioned, Pavlov took a dog for experimentation. A minor operation was carried at the cheek of the dog so that a part of the salivary gland was exposed to the surface. Then the cheek was attached to a measuring capsule. Next, the dog was taken into a sound proof laboratory and positioned in a harness on a table in such a way that the dog could be supervised through the glass windows. Then the dog was given meat powder in a bowl. After that, the salivation was recorded automatically in the measuring capsule. Care was taken so that the dog is not disturbed from extraneous sources like noise, light, smell, etc.

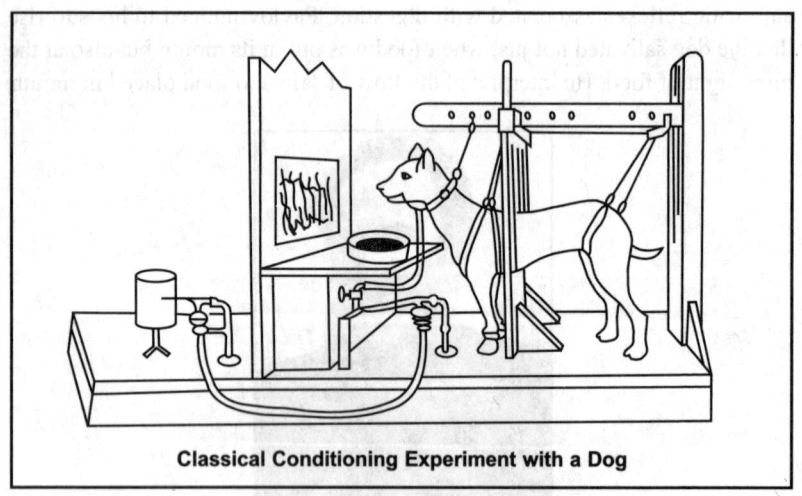

Classical Conditioning Experiment with a Dog

First a particular type of music (called conditioned stimuli) was turned on. By this the dog might become disturbed a bit and might move. But the dog would not salivate. After a few seconds, meat powder as food was administrated to the dog. Now the food would be consumed by the hungry dog. The secretion of copious saliva is collected in the capsule. Some more trials were conducted in which the sound was always followed by food and the food in turn, by salivation. This following of the conditioned stimuli (CS) by unconditioned stimuli (US) was called reinforcement. After several reinforcements the dog started salivation when the sound was produced even with absence of food i.e., plus or minus supplement of food. When this occurs, a conditioned response is established.

The above experiment could be represented under the following diagrams:

1. UCS ———————— UCR
   (Food)   (Salivary response)
2. CS ———————— No salivary response
   (Bell)
3. CS ———————— UCS ———————— UCR
   (Bell)   (Food)   (Salivary response)

This step must be repeated several times before arriving on the following step:

4. CS ———————— No Food ———————— CR
   (Bell)   (Salivary response)

The above pattern of condition response has three basic features:

a. A conditioned stimuli that does not initially evoke the unconditioned response.
b. An unconditional stimuli can evoke an unconditioned response.

c. Paired presentation of the conditioned and unconditioned stimuli is an internal CS-UCS pattern, i.e., the CS must precede the UCS always.

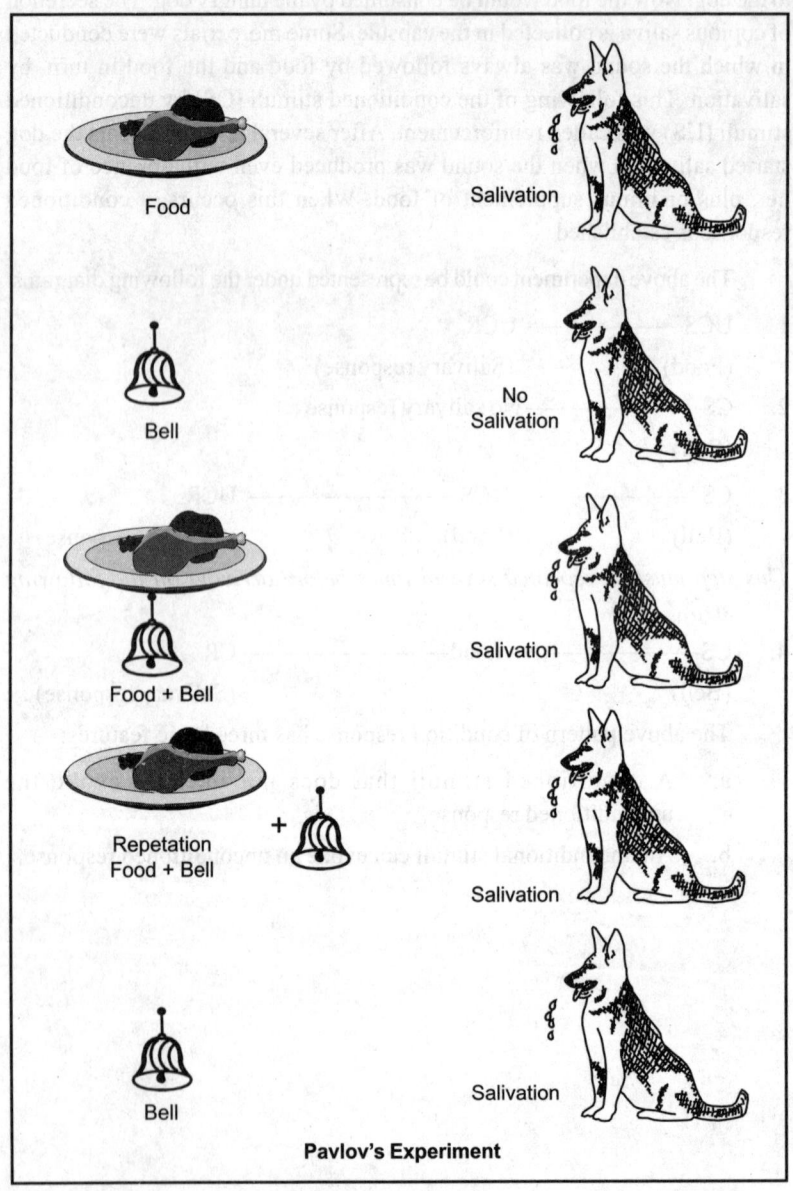

Pavlov's Experiment

Important Points to be Noted
1. Conditional stimuli must precede the unconditional stimuli.
2. Unconditional stimuli has got to be of greater intensity.
3. Maintain appropriate uniformity between the presentation of conditioned stimuli and unconditioned stimuli.
4. Reinforce the unconditioned stimuli after the conditioning has been set up.

Laws of Classical Conditioning

We have observed that classical condition is a process in which a neutral stimuli by pairing with a natural stimuli acquires all the characteristics of the natural stimuli. Pavlov and his followers carried out intense research with great variation in this field and evolved several phenomena, which can be termed as *Laws of Classical Conditioning*.

1. Law of Latency

Pavlov observed that there is a positive correlation between the intensity of stimuli and magnitude of response. The greater the intensity of conditional stimuli, the more rapidly conditioning will occur.

The above law can be represented as:

CS............High Intensity....................CR (Strong)

Pavlov also observed that the opposite of the above case can occur case if there exists negative correlation between intensity of the stimuli and latency of the response. The less intense conditioned stimuli results in sluggish conditioning. The following expresses the above phenomena:

CS............Low Intensity....................CR (Weak)

It is also observed that if the conditional stimuli is too weak, it may not evoke any response at all, which can be represented as follows:

CS............Weak Intensity.................... No CR

2. Law of Temporal Relationship Between CS and UCS

It has been also observed that an interval of 0.5 seconds between CS and UCS results in the greatest amount of conditioning. If the interval is shorter than 0.5 seconds then dramatic failure typically ensues.

3. Law of Extinction

If CS (say, ringing of the bell) is not followed by UCS (food) it means reinforcement is lacking. This leads to failure of secretion of saliva and this law is called the law of extinction. This can be represented in the following diagram:

- UCS———————UCR
  (Food)   (Salivary response)
- CS——————No salivation
  (Bell)
- CS—————UCS—————UCR
  (Bell)   (Food)   (Salivary response)

  (This step must be repeated several times to obtain the following step)
- CS—————No Food—————CR
  (Bell)   (Salivary response)

  (This step must be repeated several times to obtain the following step)
- CS—————No Food ————CR
  (Bell)   (Drops of saliva reduced)

  (This step must be repeated several times to obtain the following step)
- CS————For Food——————————No CR
                              (Extinction)

4. Law of Spontaneous Recovery

It has also been noticed that when the dog is brought out of the experimental arrangements, and again exposed to the same experimental arrangement even after a lapse of time, the dog responds to conditioned stimuli again. This is called spontaneous recovery. It has been observed that complete extinction does not occur due to interval of time.

- CS—————No Food———————————CR
                              (Spontaneous recovery)

(**Note:** To obtain this stage Step no. 6 as mentioned above must be repeated several times followed by a period of rest and then CS.)

5. Law of Inhibition

Inhibition is defined as a process by which a stimuli inhibits a response that would have occurred in a given condition. Pavlov recognizes two types of inhibitions:

a. External.
b. Internal.

In external inhibition, the conditioned reflex (CR) is inhibited by external factors like noise, high intensity of light, etc. In the said experiment, the dog may not evoke the response of salivation in case it is upset or alarmed by the external disturbing factors.

In internal inhibition, the condition reflex (CR) is inhibited by not giving food to the dog.

(**Note:** But spontaneous recovery is possible if the experiment is tested after 24 hours of rest.)

6. Law of Generalization

Generalization is a process where a condition reflex (CR) to a stimuli is generalized to a similar category of stimuli. In the experiment, CR results at the sight of food along with its associated stimuli, like appearance of light, ringing of the bell, foot steps of the feeder, etc.

Factors Controlling Conditioned Methods

1. Factor of Effect of Motive

Motive has an important effect in the conditioned response. The stimuli must have the potentiality to evoke the response. In Pavlov's experiment, the dog was hungry and it made an association between the sound of the bell and the food.

2. Factor of Effect of Time

The time relation of the two stimuli is also an important factor for conditioning, since conditioning of response depends upon association with each other. It is of paramount importance that the new stimuli must be perceived along with its natural sequence before the response subsides. We have observed this phenomenon under three steps:

Step I- Making the sound of bell before giving food.
Step II- Food must be given after the ringing of bell.
Step III- Food must be given after ringing of bell but before response subsides.

If there is too much interval or lapse of time between the two stimuli, it will be difficult for the animal to find the relation between the two.

3. Factor of Repetition of Stimuli

The third factor controlling conditioned response is the repetition of the stimuli. In Pavlov's experiment, the dog was given food only after the ringing of the bell. The saliva started to flow from the mouth as soon as the bell rang. Such repetition is necessary to establish the condition.

4. Factor of Absence of Disturbing Stimuli

It has already been mentioned that during the experiment, disturbing stimuli like noise, light, etc. should be avoided. These disturbing factors interfere in the experimental procedure and impede the evoking of the conditional response or desire.

II. JOHN B. WATSON

The full name of Watson is John Broadus Watson. He took birth on January 9th, 1878, at Travellers Rest, near Greenville, South Carolina, U.S.

He was the professor of psychology at John Hopkins University, Baltimore, Maryland. He propounded that psychology is the science of human behavior, which, like animal behavior, should be studied under exacting laboratory conditions. He also promoted conditioned responses as taught by Pavlov. In 1918, Watson ventured into the relatively unexplored field of infant study. In one of his classic experiments, he conditioned fear of white rats and other furry objects in an 11 month old infant named Albert, which will be described soon. In his magnum opus *"Standpoint of a Behaviorist"* (1919), he sought to expand the principles and methods of comparative psychology to the study of human beings and with certainty promoted the use of conditioning in research. His association with academic psychology ended suddenly. In 1920, in a dramatic scandal surrounding his divorce from his first wife, he had to resign from John Hopkins. Later he signed up in the business of advertising in 1921. Watson devoted himself wholly to the business until his retirement (1946). He died on September 25th, 1958, in New York.

His name will always remain in the annals of history of psychology for his great contribution of freeing psychology from the mechanist and mentalist warfare. He put forward psychology as the study of overt and observable behavior which can be measured objectively. He categorically discarded the introspective or subjective way of studying the behavioral process. Hence he was able to promote psychology as close as possible to science. He stressed the objective study of behavior. He attributes that all behavior is guided by the interaction of mind and nervous system with the influence of external environmental stimuli. He is criticized for over-emphasizing the importance of environment in relation to the development of various behaviors in an individual.

Watson's Theory of Behavior

Watson developed a simple theory of learning. Watson's theory was primarily a protest against Thorndike's theory. He postulated that when a stimuli and response occur simultaneously in close contiguity, the bond between them is strengthened. The strength of connection between stimuli – response (S-R) is guided by the frequency of S-R connections, which has been propounded by Thorndike, but Watson rejected the role of reinforcement and laws of effects. Rather, he attributed his views to law of frequency. He emphasized the importance of frequency or exercises in learning.

The second law which he proposed is of recency. The most recent response is strengthened more by its frequent occurrence than the earlier response. He made conditioning the basis of learning. Learning for him is the shifting of old responses to new stimuli.

Watson's Experiment

Watson took Albert, an 11 months old infant for experimentation purpose. The baby was exposed to tamed white rats (they were not harmful) to play with. Albert loved them and played with them. He liked to touch the fur of the rats. Watson carefully observed the pleasant responses of the infant.

In the course of the experiment, a loud noise was made as soon as Albert touched the rat. The loud noise was produced repeatedly as a part of the experiment whenever the infant touched the rat. This induced a fear response in Albert. After some time, the baby began to fear the rats, even in the absence of the loud noise. This way the infant learned to fear the rabbit also through conditioning. The original neutral rat became a "conditional stimuli" to fear. Moreover, Albert further expressed his fear to other similar white objects like his mother's fur neckpiece. Albert's fear was generalized to objects that were similar to objects in some respect to the rat.

In another experiment, Watson experimented with a child called Peter as a subject. Peter was afraid of rabbits. At first the rabbit was placed at a distance from the boy so that it would not cause any intimidation to Peter. Progressively, on the successive day, the distance between Peter and the rabbit was reduced. Eventually the rabbit was allowed to sit on the dinner table. Then the rabbit was put on Peter's lap. This way Peter enjoyed the pleasure of eating with rabbits and got rid of his fear. Next, he began to touch its fur and played with it. Thus, through a simple treatment of conditioning, the child learned to get rid of his fear of rabbits.

III. B.F. SKINNER

Burrhus Frederic Skinner was an American psychologist and an influential exponent of behaviorism. He was born on 20th March, 1904 at Susquehanna and died on August 18th, 1990 at Cambridge. He was a promoter of scientific study of behavior. He views human behavior in terms of physiological responses to the environment. He also asserts that scientific study of response is the most direct means of explaining man's nature.

Skinner was fascinated by psychology through the work of the Russian physiologist Ivan Pavlov on conditioned reflexes, articles on behaviorism by Bertrand Russell, and the ideas of John B. Watson, the founder of behaviorism.

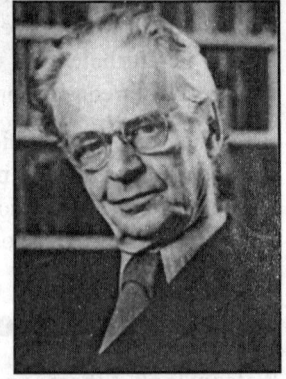

B.F. Skinner
(1904-1990)

As a professor of psychology at Harvard University (1948 and emeritus 1974), Skinner contributed a lot to psychology. Using various kinds of experimental equipment that he devised he conducted experiments with animals in laboratory to perform complex and sometimes quite exceptional actions. The example of his genius can be judged from his pigeons that learned to play table tennis. He is also credited with one of his best-known inventions called the "Skinner Box" which has been adopted in pharmaceutical research for observing how drugs may modify animal behavior.

Skinner's Operant Conditioning

Skinner used the term operant conditioning because this learning occurs while the learner is operating in the environment.

He emphasized the role of instrumental conditioning or operant conditioning as the process in which learning takes place and undesirable behaviors are also modified. In agreement with Pavlov, Skinner holds that by controlling the environment one discovers order in behavior that becomes predictable and controllable. But operant conditioning differs considerably from the classical conditioning sponsored by Pavlov in many ways. We observed that in Pavlov's experiment, the conditioned response resembles the response elicited by the unconditioned (reinforcing) stimuli. i.e., salivation is a dog's normal response to food. In Skinner's operant training, the reinforced behavior has no resemblance to the behavior normally elicited by the reinforcing stimuli. Operant condition involves two types of behavior:

A. Respondent behavior.
B. Operant behavior.

A. Respondent Behavior

Respondent behavior is directly under the control of stimuli, like classical conditioning of Pavlov.

Examples:

i. The flow of saliva to food in the mouth.
ii. The contraction of the pupil to a flash of light on the eye.
iii. The knee jerk to a tap on the patellar tendon.

Roughly speaking, it is a sort of automatic response to a stimuli, where an individual has no direct control. The behavior often appears simply to happen.

B. Operant Behavior

The word operant derives from the fact that the operant behavior "operates" on the environment to produce some effects. The relationship between operant behavior and stimuli considerably differs from above. The ringing of a calling bell invites one to open the door. It tells that the calling bell is answerable, but it does not force you to respond. Here the behavior does not occur automatically. For example, you may or may not respond to the telephone ringing. The ringing of the bell or telephone is categorized under discriminative stimuli. The stimuli that may influence operant behavior is called a discriminative stimuli.

In classical conditioning, reinforcement (reward) is paired with a stimuli while in Skinner's operant conditioning, reward is dependent upon a response emitted by the organism.

In Pavlov's classical conditioning, anticipating events is done in its environment. Contrary to this, in instrumental conditioning, the organism changes its environment. Responses are emitted rather than elicited. This technique was developed by Skinner.

The study of the response elicited by classical conditioning is less important to understand complex behavior that the study of responses which are not reflexively or mechanically evoked.

Before proceeding further it would be relevant to understand two types of responses used by Skinner in this respect:

i. *'Elicited' response means by the known stimuli which he called 'respondent behavior'.*
ii. *'Emitted' response means by the unknown stimuli which he called 'operant behavior'.*

Skinner's Instrumental Conditioning

Instrumental conditioning can be divided into two parts:

a. Instrumental reward conditioning.
b. Instrumental aversive (escape and avoidance) conditioning.

a. Instrumental Reward Conditioning

Skinner designed a number of boxes for conducting various experiments. The apparatus is known as Skinner box. A Skinner box consists of a cubic box with a bar. Below or to the side of the bar is an opening from which pellets of food can be ejected.

A hungry rat is placed in a Skinner box. Now the rat moves around the box often seeking escape from it. By this movement the rat ultimately stumbles on the lever. By this, the lever is depressed and a small pellet of food is delivered through the opening of the box. The rat moves about some more times and happens to press the bar again; another pellet of food is delivered. After few such trials, the rat learns that pressing the lever brings food.

Psychologists prefer to represent the instrumental reward by the following way:

$S_1 \ldots R_1 \ldots S_2$

S1 stands for Skinner box that evokes a bar pressing response R1, which in turn produces food (reinforcement) S2.

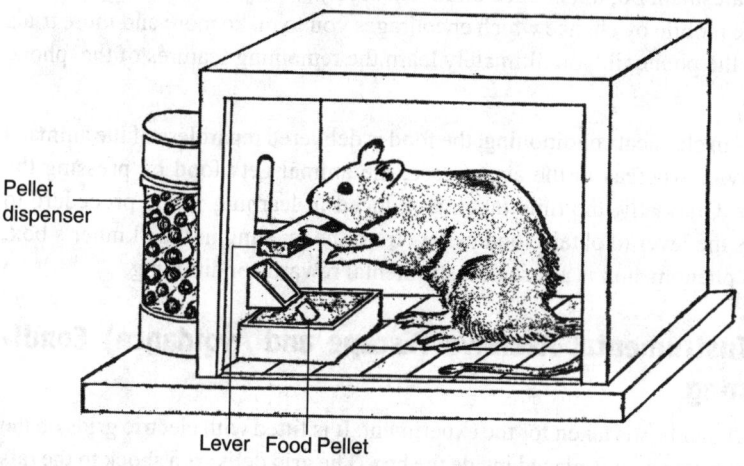

Skinner Box 1

In recent days, psychologists have developed a practical and simple device called a cumulative recorder (like an ECG) to measure animal behavior as counting the lever process (or even Pavlov's salivary response of the dog) is tedious. Now a days, sophisticated computers have been developed for cumulative recordings.

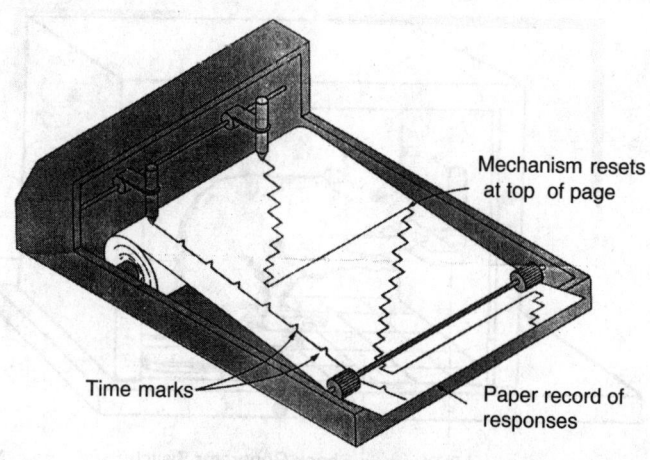

Cumulative Recorder
(Source: Lefton, 3rd ed.)

In our day to day life this happens with us also. When you purchase a brand new mobile, you may shy from asking about its various features from the salesman. So, under such circumstances you may discover some feature of the mobile by chance which encourages you to make more and more trials with the phone till you ultimately learn the remaining features of the phone also.

In classical conditioning, the food is delivered regardless of the animal's behavior whereas in the above case, the animal gets food by pressing the lever. Gradually, the time taken is reduced in learning in the procedure to press the lever to obtain food pellets from the opening in the Skinner's box. This phenomenon is a case of instrumental reward conditioning.

b. Instrumental Aversive (Escape and Avoidance) Conditioning

A Skinner box is taken for the experiment. It is fitted with electric grids on the floor. Again a rat is placed inside the box. The grid delivers a shock to the rats paws when it is placed inside the box. The shock can be terminated only when the rat depress the lever. It was observed that when the rat was shocked for the first time, it showed varied behavior like bending down or diving. By this movement the rat inadvertently pressed the lever and the shock was terminated. In this way the rat learned to press the bar whenever it was given a shock, in the course of this behavior. This kind of instrumental conditioning is known as escape conditioning.

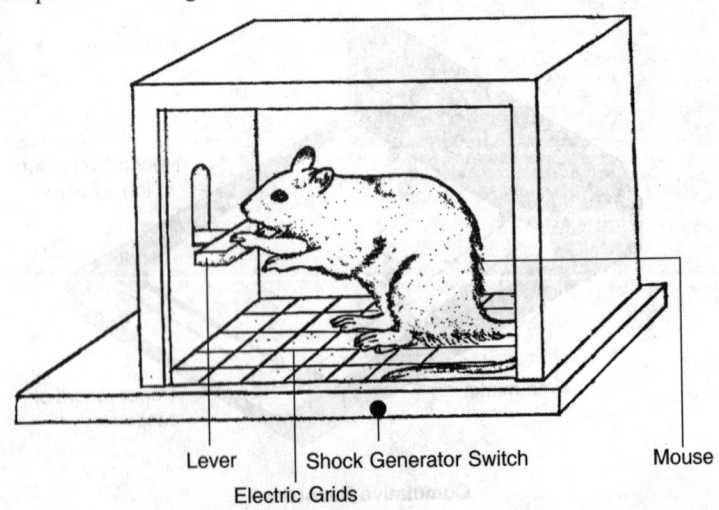

Lever | Shock Generator Switch | Mouse
Electric Grids

Skinner Box 2

Avoidance conditioning is very akin to escape conditioning. In avoidance conditioning, a warning signal is initiated prior to the onset of the shock. The warning signal may be a sound. By this, gradually, the rat will learn how to avoid shock by pressing the lever, even before the generation of shock, by just hearing the warning signal say, a sound.

From this it is clear that in escape conditioning the rat presses the bar to escape from the shock whereas in case of avoidance conditioning the rat avoids the shock stimuli by pressing the bar by just listening to the sound.

Mechanism of Operant Conditioning

In operant conditioning, the process may start with a natural response. In case natural responses are occurring, then trials are taken to make them happen. To make this occurrence, a process called shaping is adopted. Shaping is building a chain of responses that is made step by step.

Skinner was able to train a pigeon to walk in a figure of eight by giving a small amount of grain reward (reinforcement) whenever it followed the path of direction of figure eight (8).

Let us discuss the steps of mechanism under:

A. Shaping.
B. Other aspects like:
   1. Extinction.
   2. Spontaneous Recovery.
   3. Concept of reinforcement.

A. Shaping

Shaping involves sensible employment of selective reinforcement to bring definite and desirable changes in the behavior of the organism. Hence it adheres to successive approximation to the desired behavior. By this, Skinner was able to train a pigeon to play table tennis, making eight, pecking a particular disk, etc. Let us take one of them as an example i.e., how the pigeon was able to make an eight.

First the pigeon was given the reward of food pellets for a single turn— its head moving towards the right direction. Then it was trained for the movement of right direction. Gradually step by step with reinforcement i.e., the reward of food pellets, the pigeon was taught to walk the complete figure of eight. Thus, shaping is a successful technique that can be imparted to an individual to learn the complex and difficult behavior by adopting simple procedures, step by step.

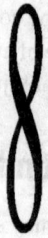

This process of successful shaping involves two psychological principles:
   a.   Generalization.
   b.   Chaining.

1. Generalization

It means to use a particular set of facts or ideas in order to form an opinion that is considered valid for a different situation. It also means to apply a theory, idea, etc. to a wider group or situation than the original one. According to Skinner, "Generalization' has been divided into the following two types:
i.   Response generalization
ii. Stimuli generalization

i. Response Generalization

It means when the responses are repeated, they are likely to vary over a range of more or less similar acts. Hence, response generalization forms an important part of shaping. This principle has been induced in the pigeon to make the figure '8' which is clear from above. Here the pigeon repeats the previously reinforced response in exactly the same way so that it ultimately forms the figure '8'.

ii. Stimuli Generalization

Stimuli generalization occurs when a particular response elicited by a particular stimuli also becomes elicited by other similar stimuli. It is obvious from Watson's experiment of Albert and Peter.

2. Chaining

In this process, the task is broken down into small steps for effective learning. In this sort of chain reaction, one action gives rise to the next action and the recent action to the next, and so on. In other words, chaining is initiated when one response leads the organism to get in touch with stimuli that do two things simultaneously: First, it rewards the last response and secondly, it initials the next response. The response in turn triggers the organism to experience the stimuli also does two things simultaneously: First, reward the response and secondly, cause the next response, and so on.

B. Other Aspects of Mechanism

1. Extinction

Let us assume that in the Skinner box, the rat presses the bar but does not get food pellets. The rat may try again and again. After repeated efforts, the rat will stop pressing the bar as it is not getting any food pellets by doing so. This process induces extinction. Extinction means disappearance of the previously established relationship that had resulted from withholding the reinforcer, subject to the condition that it (i.e., reinforcer) had generated the accurate response.

In an operant conditioning, an operant is strengthened by its reinforcement or weakened by its extinction. Extinction is opposite, rather reverse of reinforcement. When a reinforcement stimuli fails to occur following a response, the frequency of response diminishes. It becomes less and less frequent; this is called operant extinction.

2. Spontaneous Recovery

This is almost similar to Pavlov's condition of spontaneous recovery that we have read. When an organism is displaced from the situation for a while after occurrence of extinction and then again restored to the former situation, his performance will be improved in comparison to the performance that had occurred prior to the onset of extinction. However, we have to remember that an operant habit is directly related to the length of period since the termination of extinction. Moreover, the strength of reinforcement occurrence (or training test) that preceded extinction also effects the magnitude of spontaneous recovery.

3. Concept of Reinforcement

Concept of reinforcement forms one of the important edifices of Skinner's operant conditioning. This has been divided under the following three categories:

i. Positive reinforcer.
ii. Negative reinforcer.
iii. Punisher.

A positive reinforcer includes stimuli like food, water, sexual contact, etc., the awarding of which enhances the probability of a particular behavior.

A negative reinforcer is any stimuli, the removal (or withdrawal) of which enhances the probability of a particular behavior. An electrical shock, a loud noise, etc. are considered negative reinforcers.

A punisher is an aversive stimuli which follows a response and suppresses it. Punishment weakens the behavior. This must not be confused with negative reinforcer, because the negative (as well as the positive) reinforcer strengthens the behavior. Moreover, a negative reinforcer precedes the response.

CLASSICAL CONDITIONING AND OPERANT CONDITIONING : A COMPARISON

Sl. No.	Point	Classical Conditioning	Operant Conditioning
1.	Orientation	Stimulus oriented	Response oriented
2.	Organism's behavior	UCS is given regardless of the organism's behavior	Organism's behavior is decided whether or not the UCS will be offered
3.	Factor of time interval	Time interval between CS & UCS is strictly behavior	Time interval depends on the organism's own set
4.	Relationship of CR & UCR	CR & UCR are similar but not identical	Similarity is the exception and not a rule
5.	Response mode with nervous system	Responses involuntarily medicated by autonomic nervous system	Responses is under voluntary control medicated by central nervous system
6.	Emphasization	Emphasization is put on time control	Emphasization is put on Role of motivation and reward.
7.	Response	CR is reflexively forced by UCS	Response is more voluntary and spontaneous

Sl. No.	Point	Classical Conditioning	Operant Conditioning
8.	Organism's learning	Stimulus substitution is the core of learning	Response modification is the core of learning
9.	Reinforcement	Precedes to food presentation	Succeeds foods presentation
10.	Association	Between stimulus response (S-R) is on the basis of law of	Between stimulus response (S-R) is on the basis of law of effect.
11.	Factor of Reward	The UCS occurs independent of reward	The reward is dependent upon the occurence of response

CLINICAL APPLICATIONS

We, the homeopaths can take the best advantage of learning theories or behavior mentioned above. We can use it for case taking. Our case taking has its own specialty and it differs to a greater extent to other modes of case taking for treatment. For us, case taking in detail to determine the totality of symptoms is of paramount importance. It is said that a well taken case is half the job of the physician is done. But the fact is that if you are not able to take the case in a proper way, then every effort and toil of yours goes to oblivion. Hence, leaning can make you an expert in case taking.

Learning may also help you in developing an amicable interpersonal relationship with your patients and their attendants, hospital staff, seniors, colleagues, etc. Bedside, examination of patients along with dealing with people or patients can also be developed thorough learning. Clinical skills can be learnt through imitation, modeling and role-playing. Cognitive learning methods can also be learnt, developed and applied in clinical settings.

In our day to day, life most of us live in emotions. Emotion has its plus points as well as minus points. Sometimes an emotional reaction may cause havoc not only for the individual but also for a mass or society. Most of these feelings are found to be conditioned responses. These emotions cannot be traced to their origin, which have become so generalized. Hence, these emotions can be unlearned through principle of learning.

Programmed learning is one of the important aspects of learning. This can be introduced in our homeopathic curriculum. In this method, a lesson is divided into various parts. The parts are arranged in a step by step manner.

The main aim of arranging it in a step by step manner is to gradual unfold the study material in a manner that the learner is guided from known (or easy subject) to unknown (or difficult subject) in a flexible way. We have seen the pigeon training. If you direct the pigeon to make the figure eight without exposing it to a programmed learning (as mentioned above), then you would fail utterly. Moreover, in programmed learning, the learner is allowed to master the lessons at his own pace.

Maladaptive behaviors are those behaviors that have detrimental effects on the individual like gambling, smoking, over-eating, various addictions, etc. These behaviors are the result of conditioned responses which can be de-conditioned through learning. Additional instances of maladaptive behaviors are non-compliance of treatment of a patient, abnormal illness behavior, which too can be modified by learning techniques.

praiseworthy. She was to bear six children, one whom was Anna Freud, who later became a psycho-analyst in her own right. Moreover, Anna was an empathetic companion to Freud. She took care of Freud right from 1923 when Freud was undergoing treatment for oral cancer till his departure for the heavenly abode.

During the Second World War, Freud was attacked in Austria by Nazi regime as a non-Aryan. He was rescued by the Princess of Greece by paying a ransom of 250,000 shillings to the Nazi regime.

Freud was a hero, who virtually changed the very course of humanity and paved a new path for psychology, but he died a pauper in London on 23rd September, 1939 at the age of 83 with great anxiety, agony as he was devoid of home, property and paper.

Let us bow down our head for a few seconds before this great man, paying a tribute. Remember my dear friend, if you understand Freud even a little, you can read many behavioral patterns of humanity accurately and exactly.

Some Important Works of Sigmund Freud

1. The Interpretation of Dreams, 1913.
2. Psychopathology of Everyday Life, 1914.
3. Three Contributions to the Sexual Theory, 1910.
4. The History of the Psychoanalytic Movement, 1917.
5. Resemblances Between the Psychic Lives of Savage Neurotics, 1918.
6. A General Introduction to Psycho-analysis, 1920.
7. Beyond the Pleasure Principle, 1922.
8. The Ego and the Id, 1927.
9. Inhibition, Symptoms and Anxiety, 1927.
10. The Problem of Lay-analyses, 1927.
11. The Future of an Illusion, 1928).
12. Civilization, Its Discontents, 1930.
13. New Introductory Lectures on Psycho-analysis, 1933.
14. Studies in Hysteria, 1936.
15. Moses, Monotheism, 1939.
16. The Origin and Development of Psycho-analysis, 1949.

17. The Complete Psychological Works of Sigmund Freud, 6 vol., 2nd ed. (1984).
18. Sigmund Freud's Writings: A Comprehensive Bibliography, (1977).

(**Note:** *These are the translated works of Freud. The original contributions (in Germany ?) date much earlier.*)

From above it is clear that the contribution of Freud to humanity are immense. Therefore, it is neither desirable nor feasible for us to study everything of Freud. We will study his psychoanalysis under the following heads within reasonable dimensions.

I. Structure of mind.
II. Daily psycho-pathology and defence mechanism.
III. Psycho-dynamics – Behavioral process.
IV. Psycho-analysis as a therapy.
V. Criticism to Freud's works.
VI. Dreams (see Chapter IX).

(**Note :** Psycho-analysis was initiated by Freud and hardly anybody shared responsibilities with him at the earliest stage of its development. Therefore, Freud and psycho-analysis has become almost synonymous with each other and he is regarded as the Father of Psycho-analysis. All of above topics mentioned except the last one comes under psychoanalysis.

PSYCHO-ANALYSIS

I. Structure of Mind

Freud divides mind (also personality) into two different parts:

1. Topographical aspect, by arranging it into three layers, viz:
    a. Conscious mind.
    b. Sub-conscious mind.
    c. Unconscious mind.

2. Dynamic aspect of mind, postulating three other components:
    a. Id.
    b. Ego.
    c. Super ego.

1. Topographic Aspect of Mind

Now let us start with the topographic aspect of mind.

a. Conscious Mind

Conscious mind is the superficial or surface layer or upper most layer of mind. It is the sum total of the individual's experiences at a given time and his ability to know the external objects that influence them. It is the conscious mind through which we listen, talk, see, etc. Various ideas, thoughts and images that we are conscious of at any moment belong to the conscious mind. This portion of mind is concerned with immediate awareness only. Now you are reading this book. You are aware that you are reading this book. You are not aware of the sound of the ceiling fan under which you are carrying out the study of this book. Similarly, when you watch cricket on TV, you are only aware of cricket at that given time. This is the function of the conscious mind.

b. Sub-conscious or Pre-conscious Mind

This is the second layer of mind. This is the store house of all types of information. All the experiences and knowledge which have been gained or learned are stored in this second layer. From this portion of mind one can recall past experiences. You are reading this book. You are not aware of the sound of the ceiling fan, under which you are carrying out your study. Let us assume that due to some reason or the other, the fan stops, you immediately become aware of it. This happens so because the sound of the fan was in the margin of your conscious mind. You may read or experience a thing in your conscious mind, but in the margin, there may exist so many things to which you may not have an immediate awareness.

c. Unconscious Mind

This is the 3rd or last layer of the mind. It is the most important part of mind. This third layer is related to a vast part of mental life, which is hidden and usually not accessible to the conscious state of mind. It hides all the repressed wishes, desires, feelings, drives and motives of an individual. This unconscious mind is very significant for our study. As a homeopath we can do wonders in understanding the patient's unconscious mind. Unconscious mind contains all repressed and forbidden desires and ideas. But the unconscious mind cannot contain all these feelings and ideas till eternity. These forbidden and repressed desires strive to come up to the upper layer of mind. These desires very often come up in disguised forms, in dreams and reveries. The importance of prescribing on dreams to homeopaths is well known since a century, back to the advent of Freud. Now we can approach this concept in a more systematic and precise manner. Moreover, this mind is also responsible for all our behaviors. Freud asserts "What we do, how we do, we behave is always determined by the forces residing in our unconscious mind and not by the choice of conscious mind." All the normal or abnormal behavior and mental illnesses are the outcome of the unconscious mind. As a homeopath we can bring this relevant information from the unconscious to conscious mind with specific techniques like catharsis and psycho-analysis along with giving anti-miasmatic treatment for a permanent solution to a given behavioral disorder.

Anyhow, the concept of unconscious mental process was recognized long before Freud. German philosophers like Gottfried Wilhelm Leibnitz (1646-1716), who was also a mathematician, Herbart Johann Friedrich (1776-1841), who was also an educator, Gustav Theodor Fechner (1801- 1887), who was also a physicist, Arthur Schopenhauer (1788- 1860), etc. were aware of the unconscious mind, which can be discovered referring their respective literary contributions. Still, it remained for Freud to give a new dimension to the concept of unconscious mental process. Freud was the first to relate its tremendous impact in the development of human personality. He was also credited for bringing forth its significant role in various mental abnormalities. In fact, Freud gave it a new tint and a new recognition to the term unconscious mind.

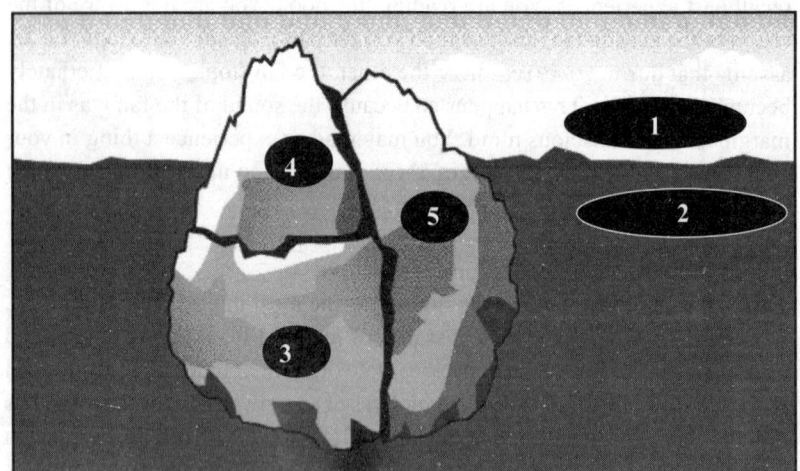

Structure of Human Mind Compared to an Iceberg
1. Conscious Mind 2. Unconscious Mind 3. Id 4. Ego 5. Super Ego

(Freud compares the human mind to an iceberg phenomenon. The tip above the water surface corresponds to consciousness, and the huge region below the surface represents the unconscious mind. Note that the Id is totally unconscious of the three basic personality structures)

2. Dynamic Aspect of Mind

Freud ushered a new era in psychology exploring the dynamic aspect of psyche or mind. He attributed Id, Ego, Super Ego to the dynamic aspect of mind. According to him, all the conflicts are generated and resolved through these three aspects of mind. Moreover personality of an adult is related to the result of interaction of these aspects of mind. The study of dynamic aspects of mind is highly essential for us as a homeopath. We can understand a patient in a better way through this concept.

a. Id

It is situated in the unconscious mind. It comes with birth. It operates on the animal level. It is the source of mental energy, which when pent up produces frustration. It only knows the subjective reality of mind. It,

- is biological in nature and seeks pleasure and gratification
- pursues pleasure only
- follows no rules or regulations
- is selfish
- is concerned with own means and end
- avoids pain
- does not accept reality
- cannot differentiate between good and bad
- stands for all anti-social and moral wishes, desires, motives, etc.
- is the storehouse of jam-packed excitement and wild passion
- is the reagent of unconscious and the stockpile of instincts

b. Ego

Ego is psychological and examines the reality. It develops gradually out of Id. A child comes to this earth as just a mass of protoplasm at the time of birth. Gradually he undergoes various forces and develops the sense of 'I', 'me", 'mine', which is the expression of Ego. It acts as an intermediary role between Id and Super Ego.

- Ego can distinguish between subjective reality and the things that exist in the external environment
- It is called the executive of personality
- It maintains balance between the two fighting forces of 'Id' and 'Super Ego'. Id seeks direct instinctual gratification whereas Super Ego acts as

an internalized checking agent or policeman to guard Id not to do immoral acts
- Very often Id and Ego are compared to a horse and its rider respectively. Ego is the rider, who decides the direction of the horse
- Ego integrates the conflicting demands of Id, Super Ego and the external world
- If Ego fails in keeping the balance between Id and Super Ego, there occurs the disintegration of personality
- If the Ego is strong it can control the ruthless Id. Freud's whole attempt is to strengthen the Ego, so that a positive personality can be evolved
- If Ego joins hands with Id and defeat the Super Ego, then the individual may become anti-social, delinquent and may commit a crime
- It also satisfies the nutritional need of the body and protects against injury
- It reinforces repression

c. Super Ego

It does not come by birth. It appears at about the age of 4 to 5. It is also situated in the unconscious mind. Very often it is referred to as conscience. It is the direct antithesis of Id. It is developed progressively by the reward and punishment meted out by the parents. It is the Super Ego in an individual that desists the individual to commit an evil. Super Ego—

- is social-self and strives for perfection
- is ethical and moral aspects of psyche
- follows the moral standard authorized by the society
- gives judgment within
- is not guided by any instinct or primitive drive
- stands for ideal rather than the real and strives for perfection
- prevents destruction
- opposes the action of Id

Interrelationship of Id, Ego and Super Ego

In a nutshell, we can describe Id as biological which seeks pleasure, the Ego as psychological, examines the reality and Super Ego is social-self who strives for perfection.

Moreover, these concepts explain the genesis of neurosis (and anxiety) see the Chapter XVIII.

II. Daily Psycho-pathology and Defence Mechanism

In day to day life, activities like slip of a pen or tongue or other actions are taken by us as normal. We very often consider these actions as a chance happening. But according to Freud, such incidents do not occur by chance; rather they bear special significance in expressing the language of unconscious. Such languages are the deliberate and planned expressions of the unconscious mind. It carries unique significance in psycho-analysis.

Whenever, an individual encounters a situation that threatens to cause mental imbalance or leads to a state of conflict or an injury and he fails to make any direct adjustment with that situation, then in order to attain such an adjustment he adopts a group of mental processes that enables the mind to reach a compromising solution to the problem is called defence mechanism. The process is usually unconscious, the compromise generally involves concealing from oneself internal drives or feelings that threaten to lower self-esteem or provoke anxiety. The defence mechanisms are those adjustment mechanisms which are adopted by ego autocorrectively and unconsciously to save itself from defeat.

Some of the major defence mechanisms described under psycho-analysis are:

1. Repression

Repression is the withdrawal from consciousness of an unwanted idea, affect, or desire by pushing it down into the unconscious part of the mind and are prevented from re-entering into the conscious mind by constructing a blockade. The concept of repression was evolved by Freud during his treatment of hysterical patients. He found that many patients exhibit signs of paralysis and approaching blindness without having any physical basis. These patients were not able to remember the painful experiences which could not be brought out by psychotherapy. Repressions have the effect of either attaining a complete forgetfulness with regard to these memories or of at least reducing their intensity for the time being. In hysterical amnesia, the victim completely forgets the act itself and the circumstances surrounding it. However, a psycho-analyst can bring back those repressions, so that the mental conflict can be removed. It helps to clear the conscious part of mental conflict.

2. Reaction Formation

Sometimes an individual conceals a motive from himself by giving expression to its opposite. Such a tendency is called reaction formation. It is the fixation of an idea, affect, or desire in consciousness that is opposite to a feared unconscious impulse. Let us assume that a girl became pregnant through an illicit relationship. Now she is carring an unwanted child. She may react to her feelings of guilt by not opting for an abortion and by becoming extremely solicitous and over-protectiveabout the child, in order to convince both the child and herself that she is a good mother.

3. Projection

Projection is a form of defence in which unwanted feelings are displaced onto another person, where they then appear as a threat from the external world. In projection we protect ourselves from recognising our own undesirable qualities by assigning them in inflated sum to other people. A common form of projection occurs when an individual, threatened by his own angry feelings, accuses another of harboring hostile thoughts. A bad workman quarrels with his tools. A dishonest person sees dishonesty everywhere, by which he convinces that he is not the only dishonest person on this earth. But these types of projections cut the self-insight and prevent the individual from progressing.

You will soon observe this projection with your classmates. If one of your classmates fails in the examination; he will blame the teacher concerned for his failure. At the root of projection there lies the desire to protect one's self-esteem. Hence, whenever you find a person constantly criticising others, be sure that at least some of the traits that he criticises are within him also.

4. Denial

Denial is the conscious refusal to perceive the existence of painful facts. It is specially found amongst children and psychotic regression. In denial, the individual denies the latent feelings of acts like homosexuality or hostility, and by this the individual escapes from intolerable thoughts, feelings or events. It operates in the conscious and subconscious mind. It is considered as a common source of back-up against anxiety, helplessness, inadequacy, etc.

5. Identifications

When an ego is weak to stand alone, he picks up some hero from the environment. The individual tries to renovate his ego or self to the hero he likes. In other words the individual identifies himself with the hero picked up by him. By this, his ego satisfies the desire to be somebody he likes most. You can observe many street Romeos, who style themselves with a particular film star or cricketers (in recent days). By this they identify themselves with their corresponding hero.

6. Regression

Factually, regression means going back. Regression, as a defence mechanism implies a return to earlier stages of development. Through this mechanism, the person wants to avoid the realistic and controlled thinking. Generally, regression is the outcome of a severe frustration of an individual and it generates anxiety and stress in him. As a result the person resorts to less mature, less realistic and more childish behaviour. For example, a young wife might retreat to the protection of her parents' home after her first quarrel with her husband. Similarly, you might have observed one of your friends, who had wept loudly like a child due to a failure in B.H.M.S. examination.

7. Sublimation

Sublimation is the diversion or deflection of instinctual drives, usually sexual ones, into non-instinctual channels. The process of sublimation is a positive one and not negative. It is the healthy solution to problems that crop up in an individual's adjustment. Psycho-analytic theory holds that the energy invested in sexual impulses can be shifted to the pursuit of more acceptable even socially valuable achievements, such as artistic or scientific endeavors.

8. Rationalization

In your childhood you might have read the story of "The Fox and the Grapes". When the fox cannot jump high enough to get the grapes and it realised that the grapes are beyond his reach, he satisfied himself by thinking the grapes are sour and hence not worth the effort. This is called rationalisation.

Rationalisation is the substitute of a safe, reasonable explanation for the true (but threatening) cause of behavior. This rationalisation does not mean "to act rationally"; it means assigning logical or socially desirable motives to what we do so that we seem to have acted rationally or properly. Rationalisation serves two purposes:

a. It eases our disappointment when we fail to reach a goal.
b. It provides us with acceptable motives for our behavior.

Rationalisation is to put forth the "good" reasons rather than the "true" reasons. A person practices rationalization mainly for the following three purposes:

i. *Liking or Disliking as an Excuse* : The college student who was not allowed to take a part in a play for annual function says he would not have participated even if asked because he did not like some of the students involved.
ii. *Blaming Other People or Circumstance as an Excuse*: "Mother failed to wake me up." "I had too many other things to do." Both reasons may be true, but they are not the real reasons for failure to perform the behavior in question. If the individual had been really concerned, he could have set his alarm or found the time.
iii. *Necessity as an Excuse*: "I brought this new model because the old car needed a lot of expensive repairs."

9. Compensation

Demosthenses (384 B.C.-322 B.C.), a contemporary of Plato and Aristole, is considered as one of the greatest orators of Greece. He was a stammerer. He overcame his defect by hard toil and determination. This a typical example of 'compensation'.

When an individual assembles an attempt to make up for a deficiency by coverging his energies to another aspect of his personality in which there exists no deficit, then he is applying the mechanism of compensation. The individual attempts to overcome a failure or deficiency in one sphere by achieving recognition in another venue, and is thus able to boost his self-esteem which has been under a threat. You might have observed one of your friends who has not done well in studies, might have shown his extraordinary abilities in singing or dramatics.

The compensatory reaction may operate in another way too. A person having weak muscles and short stature, may try hard to become a prominent athlete or sportsman.

A compensation mechanism has an also adverse affect too. A perosn who is physically too weak may turn into a great wrestler or boxer and later may torture and extort the people who are weaker to him.

10. Substitution

It is another mechanism of adjustment, where a superior goal (or desire) of an individual is substituted wiht another inferior goal (or desire) due to presence of some deficiency with the individual. First an individual desires and accordingly sets a higher goal for achievement, but due to having some shortcomings, he fails to achieve the goal. Now he understands his limitations and substitutes it with another goal, which is generally of same line. For example a lady who desires to be a doctor after failing in her effort, opts for a nursing career. Similarly, a person who wants to be an officer goes for a clerical job after his failure in the interviews.

11. Fantasy or day dreaming (*see the chapter Dream*)

12. Sympathism

In this mechanism, the individual avoids necessary efforts to solve a given problem and in reverse he desires sympathy from others. He tries to draw the attention of others and secures sympathy of concern over his difficulties. For example some of your class mate may deliberately avoid to attend the classes throughout the academic session (but may roam here and there, pass time watching movies and TVs unduly etc.) and when he fails in examinations, then he tries to draw the attention of friends and teachers by explaining that the study material were too tough, that his family burdens him a lot, that he is unlucky etc.

13. Intellectualization

In day to day life, this mechanism may prove a great boon to you. You may come across a dying cancer patient. He may seek your help and compel you to cure him. You know that the patient has no chance of recovery. you are in a turmoil situation of emotion. You cannot say the attendant or patient that you are sorry or that the patient is destined to die etc. Here you may state that the vital force of the patient is not giving any cooperation. Here you try to use some complicated professional terminology to shut up the mouth of the patient (or client) and at the same time you want to get rid of the professional jam. This mechanism is called intellectualization which means to detach oneself from an emotional or threatening situation by giving an explanation through intellectual terms. In other words your explanation remains obscure under the term of intellectualization for the cilent (or patient). In other words you separate yourself from professional crisis. But frequent adoption of this style may make others take you as a very cold detached individual devoid of healthy experience.

III. Psycho-dynamics – Behavioral Process

We will discuss this portion under four heads:

A. Life and death instinct.
B. Infantile sexuality and psycho-sexual development.

C. The flow of libido.
D. Anxiety, conflict and disintegration of personality (see Chapter XVIII).

A. Life And Death Instinct

Freud was a biologist, who subsequently become a clinician. His contribution comes from clinical study. The great contribution of Freud is that he tried to explain human behavior through conflicting and clashing forces. He firmly believed in the role of instincts or urges in human behavior. He postulated two basic urges which are

i. *The Instinct of Eros* – Life Instinct. It is also known as love instinct or sex. It is also called pleasure principle. This is the source which makes one to develop the need for self preservation.

ii. *The Instinct of Thantos* – It is also known as death instinct. This is related to impulse for destruction. It is expressed through acts of aggression, cruelty and even self destruction by suicide.

[**Note:** You must remember that the above two instincts are not mutually opposed to each other. Freud maintains that when we analyse the desire for love, we find also some desire for aggression. That is the reason very often our best friend become the bitterest enemy. Behaviour originated by life instinct is not necessarily free from death instinct. Similarly, behaviour motivated by death instinct may incorporate the components of life instinct. These principles of love and hatred can be compared to the oscillation of pendulum. Hence, when you love less somebody, you also hate less to him. Similarly, when you love somebody extremely, you also hate him extremely (in a hidden form, which may be expressed later). This phenomenon is also called ambivalent attitude. According to Freud, all our attitudes towards a person are ambivalent in nature.]

B. Infantile Sexuality and Psycho-sexual Development

If you ask a layman some information regarding sex, his answer will probably be:

i. Sexuality is connected to only sexual organs.
ii. One can perform sexual act only after onset of puberty.
iii. Children have no sexual instinct or erotic pleasure.

Contrary to the above mentioned beliefs, Freud was the first psychologist who postulated that sex begins from the birth of an individual.

He subscribed the following three principal erotic zones which give pleasure to an individual:

i. Mouth
ii. Anus and
iii. Genital organs.

He also asserts that any part of the body surface of an individual may become an excitatory centre that demands relief and provides pleasure. He further maintains that these three zones are of paramount importance for the development of personality because these zones are the first important sources of pleasure.

Freud opined that the ultimate end of the instinct of love (or life) can be attributed to sex. But this pleasure is not limited to genital organs only, rather before puberty our instinct of love may be satisfied by other zones of the body too.

The personality of an adult depends upon the experiences of infancy and childhood in relation to the various stages of psycho-sexual development.

In future course of action, the infant has to face the world, and undergo various frustrating experiences corresponding to the satisfaction of sexual and aggressive urges.

His personality is determined by his inner urge and the interaction with various environmental conditions.

From birth to puberty, the process of personality development is divided into the following five stages, out of which the first is again divided into two stages. Anyhow, there does not exist any water tight compartment for distinction between the stages. Very often these stages may overlap one another.

1. Oral stage
   a. Oral sucking.
   b. Oral biting.
2. Anal stage
   a. Anal expulsive.
   b. Anal retentive.
3. Phallic stage.
4. Latency period.
5. Genitalia period.

Now let us discuss the above mentioned stages.

1. The Oral Stage

The oral stage starts at birth and continues up to the 2nd year of life.

After birth, the child has to undergo a strong frustrating experience. The newborn baby has to breathe, has to acclimatize the body to the surrounding temperature, to search for food; etc. The infant at birth is basically a physiological organism. He is mostly Id, has no sense of time and place. Id is devoid of organization, logic or reasoning. It functions entirely according to the pleasure-pain principle. So, for the satisfaction of his physical needs, he has to depend upon others. Others may or may not satisfy his needs. When his physical needs are not satisfied, he experiences a feeling of psychological dissatisfaction.

Mouth is the primary organ that gives pleasure to an infant during this oral stage.

The oral stage is divided into oral sucking and oral biting stage.

a. Oral Sucking Period

It is initiated with birth and continues up to 8 months of age. Sucking has two purposes:

  i. Self preservation.
  ii. Initial expression of sexual impulses.

The later point may look absurd and ludicrous but this can be judged from the fact that many a times a child likes to suck the breast before sleep although he is free from pangs of hunger. Freud maintains that at this stage the libido or the pleasure principle is to be found in the mouth (or oral zone). The child at this stage desires oral satisfaction because his erotic steer is confined to mouth, lips and tongue. He derives erotic pleasure through sucking. Moreover, all the frustrating experiences of the child are relieved through sucking. Ego emerges at about the end of this period. The stage of sucking continues up to eruption of teeth.

b. Oral Biting Period

This period starts from the age of six months and extends up to the 18th month. The main region of pleasure at this stage is teeth and jaws.

During this stage, the infant is discouraged or not allowed to suck mother's breast. Sucking is substituted with other foods. Hence, the infant experiences an overwhelming frustration by feeling that he is being taken away from his loved object physically.

Until this time, he was utterly reliant on the mother. Now, he develops some ideas about his outside reality. At this time, the teeth erupt and he obtains pleasure by aggression, i.e., by biting. By this he expresses his frustration of weaning. Though the oral biting period usually starts at the age of 8 months, one should note that oral sucking does not disappear at the 8th month. Instead, oral sucking and oral biting stages overlap each other; some of the behaviors of oral sucking period may also continue at this stage.

In the oral biting stage, the libido is fixated on the physical self and erotic pleasure is primarily derived from the sucking, swallowing, biting and devouring activities. During this stage the child becomes autoerotic and narcissist. His behavior towards his mother becomes that of oral sadistic attachment.

In the oral biting stage, the child shows ambivalent tendencies (i.e., symptoms of love and aggression) towards the mother. He loves his mother because she caters to all his needs. At the same time, he hates her because she has neglected him by physical separation.

At this stage he builds up narcissism or self love. According to Freud, this narcissism is also an expression of his libido. Naturally, the Ego becomes stronger and can be discriminated from Id. The child becomes more and more aware of the reality of his outer world. If another child is born at this time, the child becomes more frustrated and develops a sense of jealousy to the care and attention paid to the younger child.

PERSONALITY TRAITS DEVELOPED AS A RESULT OF DEPRIVATION OF ORAL STAGE

It is commonly observed that the behaviors present in the oral sucking and oral biting period have a tremendous impact on the adult in the development of their personality.

a. Early oral eroticism is represented by eating habits and interest in food in adulthood or later part of life.
b. Extreme fixation at this stage is framed in adult life by:
   i. Kissing.
   ii. Smoking.
   iii. Gum chewing.
c. Fixation in the oral stage may lead to:
   i. Acquisitiveness.
   ii. Tenacity.
   iii. Determination.
d. Oral aggressiveness, represented by biting becomes the sample for direct, displaced and disguised aggressions. The child who bites with his teeth may as an adult bite with verbal sarcasm, scorn and cynicism. He may also have the aptitude to become a lawyer, politician or journalist.

2. Anal Stage

The anal stage is divided into two parts:
a. Anal expulsive.
b. Anal retentive.

a. Anal Expulsive Period

This phase starts from the age of 8 months and continues up to 3 years. Hence it is obvious that it overlaps with the oral biting period.

In this phase, location of pleasure or libido is transformed from the mouth to the anus and adjacent areas. The child gets pleasure in passing stools and urine here and there. Expulsion of feces and urine gives him pleasure by reducing tension. Moreover, the child likes to go over this mode of action so that he can become free from the tension that has accumulated in other parts of the body. According to Freud, expulsive elimination is the representation of emotional outbursts, anger, irritability, peevishness, rages and other primitive discharge reactions.

The child belonging to this age group gets physiological pleasure and psychological satisfaction from toilet habits because till now narcissism or self love has not faded and autoeroticism of the oral period exists and tends to shift to the anus. Gradually his toilet training is guided by some dos and don'ts. This interferes with his freedom. By this he has to undergo the first crucial experience with external authority and discipline. Toilet training initiates and represents a conflict between the wish to defecate and an external barrier imposed by parents or society. Anyhow, the child learns about the reality principle. Now he has to compromise the pleasure principle to reality principle. Consequently, the child becomes conscious of himself as a self-regulating individual and continues to direct his libido upon himself as a psychological entity. He feels that he is an individual of his own right, but has certain responsibilities to perform. This also creates conflict, stress, tension and finally anxiety in him, Hence he derives pleasure physically by stimulation of mucous membrane in the excretory function and psychologically, satisfaction from parental incentive and attention during toilet training at a directed place. During this stage, Super Ego develops. The child is also able to differentiate between the two sexes.

Factors like toilet training, parent's attitude towards defecation, cleanliness, etc. leave indelible impressions on the development of the child's personality. Hence during this stage, judicious employment of toilet training is very crucial for the child.

If toilet training is very rigid and rigorous disciplinary measures are adopted, then there is maximum chance that the child will become rebellious and will oppose by deliberately soiling himself. Hence this conflict must be settled in an amicable manner, otherwise it leaves its adverse effect upon the personality structure. In future the child (especially during his adulthood) may become untidy, awkward, irresponsible, disorderly, wasteful and extravagant. Other frustrations during this stage lead to their corresponding traumatic experiences which have their repercussion upon the later personality.

b. Anal Retentive Period

This stage starts from the 12th month, and may last up to the fourth year of life in an individual. During this stage, the child gets pleasure by retaining and controlling feces and urine. Here the chief area of obtaining pleasure is the anus but the act of expulsion is replaced by retention. Now, the child does not pass stool and urine here and there, it is passed at a fixed place. Through this he learns and realizes the social value of retaining, possessing and controlling them. Again, parents and other alike agencies of society give importance to personal hygiene and cleanliness, the child develops the habit of cleanliness, as it is rewarded by praise and other incentives.

Around the 4th year, the child is exhorted to give up his anal pleasure by parents. By this, he undergoes severe conflict and frustration and thus ends the anal retention period.

EFFECT OF FIXATION IN THE ANAL STAGE ON ADULT PERSONALITY

Fixation in the anal period leads to awkwardness in later life. This may lead to:

i. Excessive cleanliness.
ii. Pendentry.
iii. Obstinacy.
iv. Petulance and miserliness.

(All these behaviors are indications of some kinds of reaction formation due to excessive fixation in the anal stage.)

Strict toilet training in the anal stage may bring about a reaction formation against uncontrolled expulsiveness in the form of:

    a. Meticulousness.
    b. Neatness.
    c. Fastidiousness.
    d. Compulsive orderliness.

e. Disgust.
f. Fear of dirt.
g. Strict budgeting of time and money.
h. Other over-controlled behavior.
i. Constipation is a common defence reaction against elimination. But if the child is praised or given some incentive the child learns the value of bowel movement and elimination, and practices it to get praise and incentive. In later life, he may be motivated to produce things:
   i. To please others.
   ii. Charity.
   iii. Generosity.
   iv. Philanthropy.
   v. Giving presents may be an outcome of basic experience.

But if much stress is put on the value of elimination, the child may feel that he misses something valuable when he eliminates. Thus, as a result of this missing, he will feel depressed and anxious. In later life, he will become thrifty, economical and would like to retain everything.

Excessive fixation in the anal stage also leads people to develop the tendency to be:

i. Teachers.
ii. Opera singers.
iii. Actors who usually demonstrate exhibitionistic and narcissistic tendencies.

Gradually, the anal period ends and phallic period sets in.

3. The Phallic Stage

Freud fixes the age between 3 to 7 for the phallic stage. Accordingly, at this age, the sex energy or libido shifts to the genital organs. Children become interested in their own genital organs. They obtain pleasure by caressing and fondling their genital organs. During this period, the child's sexual cravings also intensifiy due to which a number of crucial changes occur in them.

Now we will discuss this caption under two heads because the sex organs of male and female are significantly different from the anatomical and physiological point of view. Moreover, they have also specific and peculiar impacts in the development of their personality.

a. Male Phallic State

After birth, the infant first comes in contact with his mother. The first object of love for the child is not the mother as such, but only her breasts which give him nourishment. Gradually it shifts to the mother as a whole and the desire for possessing the mother grows. She also becomes the first loved object because the mother gratifies his need for preservation. She also gives him close physical contact that satisfies his psychological necessity for pleasure.

Secondly, during this phase he also identifies his father and becomes frustrated by the relationship between his parents. The child has to tolerate the idea that his loved object is to be shared by somebody else. This leads to severe jealousy towards his father hence, considers him as his rival.

Now he has to undergo two simultaneous experiences of object love (i.e. mother) and identification (i.e. father) which brings about modifications in his personality structure. But the child has to imbibe the values of his parents and integrate them with his own individual views to develop a pre-oedipal ego organization, which later develops into the Oedipus complex (see below). Thus, before the arrival of Oedipus complex, there are long dynamic interactions between the child and the parents. These interactions, along with the child's infantile sexual maturation leads to the development of Oedipus complex.

OEDIPUS COMPLEX

[Background: This reference is derived from Greek mythology. Laius, was the king of Thebes territory. He was forewarned by an oracle that his son would kill him. When his wife Jocasta (also called as Locasta) gave birth to a son, Laius ordered to have the baby killed. The agent pinned his ankles (that caused swelling of feet, hence the name Oedipus) and left him on Mount Cithaeron. A shepherd saw the baby and brought him to his house. In due course of events, the baby was adopted by King Polybus of Corinth territory. The Queen and King brought him up as their son, Oedipus.

Once, at his early age, Oedipus visited the famous Delphi temple, where another oracle warned him that he is destined to kill his father and marry his mother. This forewarning deeply disturbed Oedipus. He decided to leave the territory and never to come back again to Corinth. The fact is that he was not aware of his real parents.

In course of time, Oedipus drifted towards Thebes, encountered and killed Laius and married the widowed queen (i.e., his own mother) Jocasta. Later Jocasta committed suicide with a sense of guilt and remorse after discovering the truth. Oedipus was also bewildered with the whole sequence of events. He left his borther-in-law Creon on the throne. Then he had his eyes removed. Thus he became blind, went into exile with his two sons Antigon and Ismene. Oedipus died at Colonus near Athens, where he was gulped into the earth and treated as a guardian hero of the land.]

Oedipus complex is defined as a sexual attachment towards one of the parents (of the opposite sex) with a concomitant jealousy towards the other parent. It is also described as love for the parent of the opposite sex and death wishes for the parent of the same sex.

As mentioned above, the child figures out that parents love each other and he is being neglected. So during this phase when the sexual urge increases, the child's love for his mother which is merely oriented towards physical pleasure, makes him jealous of his father. Hence, he considers his father his rival. Thus, the craving of the boy for the exclusive sexual possession of the mother leads to the development of the Oedipus complex. Anyhow, this Oedipus complex gets a set back and is ultimately resolved for the following reasons (the fourth point is very important as it plays a crucial role in the development of the personality of the individual):

i. The practical impossibility of fulfilling the sexual wish for the mother.
ii. Disillusionment from the mother.
iii. Development of maturation.
iv. Castration anxiety.

CASTRATION ANXIETY : WHAT IS IT?

Oedipus complex is not an isolated phenomenon. It generates castration anxiety in the child. The child feels that if he becomes sexually attached to his mother, his sexual organs will be castrated or removed. He also observes that his female counterpart lacks something that he possess. He thinks that the sexual organs of the female child have already been castrated. At the same time he deems that sex organs are the most precious organs and they should preserved at any cost. He also takes it for granted that castration of sex organs may be carried out in case he persists on Oedipus complex. Moreover, he remains in a stare of quandary about what to do: First, if he chooses love of mother, then he has to loose his sex organs or give up mother's love to save his organs from castration. Finally, after a terrible conflict, he decides to abandon mother's love. As a result, the boy represses the developed incestuous wish and resentment towards his mother and father respectively. Thus, the Oedipus complex is resolved or repressed chiefly due to three threats:

more than his expectations. Anyhow, he ultimately became a doctor in medicine after graduating from the University of Vienna in 1881. Initially he too was not interested in medical practice and still hoped to become a scientist. However, he had to abandon this aspiration chiefly due to two reasons, first, during those days Jews had limited opportunities due to the discriminatory attitude of the social structure and secondly, the burden of the family led Freud to start a practice. Freud was blessed with a very sensitive and creative mind and he quickly became very successful in the medical profession. Despite his busy practice, he found time for research and documentation, which fetched him a solid reputation.

Freud took special interest in the treatment of neurological disorders. During that period, Jean Martin Charcoat was a celebrity in France for treating various nervous and psychic disorders including paralysis with the help of hypnotism. Charcoat had gained a solid reputation for the treatment of hysteria. He was treating such diseases exclusively with the help of hypnosis. This drew the attention of Freud. In 1885, Freud left Vienna and proceeded to Paris where he worked under the guidance of Charcoat. He stayed there for about six months, and during this stay he was not very impressed with the efficacy of hypnosis. Frequent relapses occured after the treatment of hypnotism. Ultimately he left Paris in February 1886 with great disappointment. However, during this period he had conceived the seeds of his future revolutionary psychological methods. After returning from Paris, he came in contact with physician Joseph Breuer (of Austria), who was a physiologist and physician. Joseph Breuer was a celebrity for his famous discovery of "catharsis". In this method, the patient was allowed to talk to himself in a closed room, so that the pent-up feelings would come out and the patient would get rid of his neurological problems. This catharsis of pent-up feelings is the blockage at the root of pathological behavior. Breuer's theory was that neurotic symptoms result from unconscious processes and disappear when these processes become conscious. Subsequently, Breuer and Freud collaborated in writing some of their cases histories; those that had been treated by the said process of catharsis. Soon Freud's point of view started differing from Breuer's in bringing the sexual conflict as the basic cause of hysteria to which Breur did not concede. Ultimately, destiny made the two great men separate on the ground of sexual factor in hysteria. Freud become all alone but he still developed his ideas further which later became – *psycho-analysis*.

In the year 1886, he married Martha Bernays, the daughter of a prominent Jewish family, whose ancestors included a chief rabbi of Hamburg. Martha's life long devotion to her husband, especially during his tumultuous career, is

Chapter 7
FREUD & PSYCHOANALYSIS

The Jews are wonderful people. Today they take away lion's share in Noble prize. You may be surprised to note that today's world is controlled by three Jews – Christ, Freud and Marx. Christ was a Jew not a Christian. Today, majority of people belong to Christianity. Marx was the Father of Communism (i.e., with vision of socialism) and a reasonable majority of people of this world are under the rule of communism. In the world of psychology, the impression led by Freud is unique, original and dominating. His theories concern one and all.

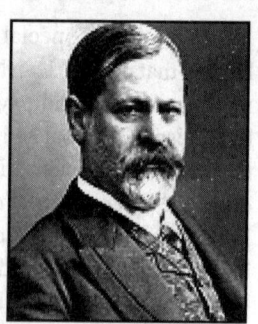

Sigmund Freud
(1856-1939)

AN INTRODUCTION TO FREUD

Sigmund Freud was born at Freiberg, a small town in Moravia, Austrian Empire (now, Pribor, Czech Republic) on May 6th, 1856. He belonged to a middle class Jewish family. Freud's Father, a Jewish wool merchant, was forty at the time of birth of Freud. His mother was Amalie Nathansohn, who was the second wife of his father. Freud was like the cream in a sandwich, as he had to adjust between his father, an authoritarian figure and mother, a symbol of emotion and affection.

In 1859, his family had to shift to Leipzig (can you recall Hahnemann and the first psychological laboratory by Wundt?) due to financial reasons. Then they had to move to Vienna in 1860. Freud remained there for about 78 years till the annexure of the state by Nazi regime.

Freud graduated from the Spiral Gymnasium in the year 1873. As a young guy, he aspired to be a scientist. But he was destined to be something

i. First, development of guilt that sexual attachment towards his own mother cannot be recognized legally by the society.
ii. Secondly, genitals would be cut off if he plays with them or attempts sexual attachment with his mother.
iii. Third, he observes that women do not have visible genitalia like male genital organs.

Anyhow, he experiences the greatest trauma of his life and this introduces a period of latency with all its punishment.

Freud further holds that every person is constitutionally bisexual in nature, where every individual is neither hundred percent masculine nor hundred percent feminine. An individual is an amalgamation of feminine and masculine qualities. After the fading of the Oedipus complex, the boy may identify with any one of the parents depending upon the relative strength of their masculine or feminine nature and qualities. He will identify with the mother if his feminine tendencies are relatively stronger. Otherwise he will identify with the father having a masculine disposition. But here also we should not count hundred percent of either behavior. Generally we find some identification with both the parents, though the degree of identification depends upon the dominance of masculine and feminine qualities. The relative strength and success of identifications plays a decisive role in his attachments, antagonisms and degree of masculine and feminine tendencies in later life. The identifications give rise to the configuration of the Super Ego, another important concept of Freud that appears after the end of the Oedipus complex. Subsequently, Super Ego becomes closely connected with Id. The development of Super Ego assists in the repression of the childish and abnormal attachment of the boy towards the parents. Super Ego also helps to subdue abnormal cravings of Id and directs him to follow the social norms, traditions and values of the ages that have been handed down from generation to generation.

b. Female Phallic Stage

In this stage, for the girl, like the boy, mother becomes her first love. She soon comes to know that she does not have sexual organs like her male counter part. So she takes for granted that she has already been castrated. She makes her mother responsible this state. She also feels that she is being neglected by her mother. She thinks that her mother does not give her love and attention as compared to her brothers. Thus, she starts loving her father. But this love is tinted with envy as the father possesses something that she does not possess. This is popularly known as *Penis envy*. This is called *Castration complex* because she feels that she has already been castrated. This castration complex is also called Electra complex (see its background, mentioned below).

In case of the male counterpart, this castration creates anxiety and is hence called castration anxiety.

(Backgorund : Electra – the literary meaning in Greek is 'bright red'. According to the Greek legend, Electra is the daughter of Agamemnon and Clytemnestra. Agamemnon was the commander of the Greek forces during the Trojan war. Clytemnestra took Aegisthus as her paramour and upon the return of Agamemnon, Clytemnestra along with Aegisthus murdered Agamemnon. Electra saved the life of her brother, Orestes by sending him away. Later, upon the return of Orestes, Electra helped him slay their mother and their mother's paramour. Afterwards Electra married her brother's friend Pyledes).

(**Note:** *Initially Freud used the term 'Oedipus complex' for the love of the son towards his mother and hatred for his father and 'Electra complex' for the love of daughter towards her father and hatred towards her. Later he dropped 'Electra complex' and applied 'Oedipus complex' for both.*)

This castration complex and penis envy is responsible for the formation of Oedipus complex in the female child. Because of the castration complex, she loves her father and becomes jealous of her mother. We have to note another point that in case of the boy, the castration anxiety is the primary cause of the disappearance of Oedipus complex, whereas in case of the girl, the castration complex and the penis envy are responsible for the appearance of Oedipus complex (or Electra complex). But as she grows up, she becomes aware that a father-daughter relationship is not sanctioned legally in society. She also finds that it is impossible to fulfil her sexual desire with her father. Thus the Electra complex disappears gradually.

Similar to the boy, the girl's identification with the father or the mother is related to the relative strength of her masculine and feminine characteristics. However, generally there is some degree of identification with both of the parents. Again the strength and success of these identifications influence the nature of her attachments, hostilities and the degree of masculinity and femininity in later life.

The phallic stage continues up to the age of six or seven. They become conscious of their sexual differences and develop a segregating attitude.

EFFECT OF OEDIPUS COMPLEX ON PERSONALITY PATTERN

Excessive fixation during the Oedipus stage affects a man to choose a wife who resembles his mother. He wants to find his mother's various qualities, virtues, merits, etc. in the woman that he marries or proposes to marry. If the Oedipus complex is not resolved successfully during childhood and if the fixation is carried to adulthood, the man will expect motherly affection from his wife, and hence can only be happy by marrying an elderly woman who resembles his mother in physique and behavior. Similarly, excessive fixation in this stage affect the woman to choose a husband who resembles her father and she tries to find and appreciate the qualities of her father in her husband. Females expect fatherly affection from their husbands. If they fail to obtain their corresponding expectations, married life becomes endangered. Therefore, people having tremendous or great parent fixation usually lead a poor and unhappy married life.

It is clear that the Oedipus complex generates all sorts of neuroses. The presence of Oedipus complex seems to be normal after a certain age. But its latency is also pathological. Homosexuality develops in case the Oedipus complex is not properly resolved. Homosexuality also leads to unhappy marital life.

Castration anxiety and complexity may lead to impotence in males, frigidity in females and practice of homosexuality in both the sexes.

EFFECT OF FIXATION IN PHALLIC STAGE ON PERSONALITY

Generally, the healthy and educated parents line up a male child with appropriate behaviour pattern, which distinguishes between the masculine behaviour and aspirations of the preoedipal boy. Similarly, They also train a female child to distinguish between the feminine behaviour and aspiration of the preopedipal girl. They restrain themselves from expression of love to each other in front of their children. They sublimate their love and openly expressed love to their children so that a boy may learn to set up his masculine identity and the girl to set up her feminine identity before the oedipal phase starts. Sometimes on the contrary, a child may not receive love from his parent, which may lead to an imbalanced sexual life in future. Lack of parental love is observed amongst parents who are—not educated, emotionally immature, posses a pathological and abnormal personality, follow their respecture are Super Ego, incapable of expressing or showing normal and sublimated parental affection to the child, etc.

If the interaction between the child and the parents during the pre-oedipal phase is amicable and healthy, then the oedipal situation can be successfully met.

4. Latency Period

This period develops at the age of 6–7 years and lasts up to 12–13 years. This state is the sequel of child's repression of infantile sexuality and castration anxiety. During this period, the urges are sublimated in the process of education. The child goes to school and most of his time is utilized for academic purposes. In this stage, eroticism and narcissism decrease. Also, at this stage, the boys and girls prefer to be in their own gender and they hate the company of the opposite sex. Girls become more lovable for the reason that they accept the castration anxiety whereas boys are still afraid of being castrated.

5. Genitalia Period

This stage starts at the onset of puberty. The adolescent stage begins with the onset of puberty. It is the longest period that lasts from the age 12–20. During this period, sexual instincts develop with the aim of reproduction. The adolescents begin to get attracted by the opposite sex. There is gradual revival of oral, anal and phallic interaction, but with more maturity. During this stage, society allows a sexual outlet. Adolescents adhere to dirty and sexual jokes. Falling in love during this stage is attributed to the phallic stage instead of the genital stage. This stage is characterized by various aspects of a human being like socialization, group interaction, marriage, establishing a home, raising a family, etc.

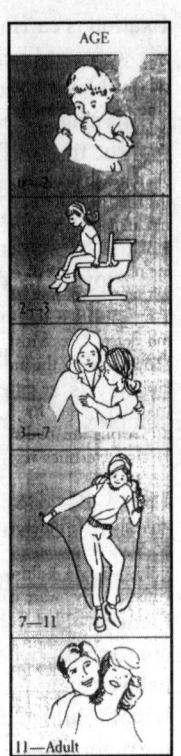

C. The Flow of Libido

According to Freud, all the instincts are related to love which can be grouped under two classes:

a.   Self-preservation or Ego.

b.   Race preservation or Libido.

Later Freud fused both under libido. The flow of libido is one of the cornerstone concepts of Freud. According to him, libido is the life maintaining energy which seeks pleasure through sexual gratification. Freud maintains that libido is always present in all the organisms. He further asserts that the intensity of libido differs from person to person, age to age and under various physiological conditions. Libido can be stimulated through various zones like oral, anal, genital, etc.

The fundamental need of libido is expression. There is a possibility of six types of expression:

1. First when the libido flows outward to love or for sexual gratification, life becomes normal due to gratification.
2. Second, if the flow moves inside then the individual may develop narcissist or self love type of personality.
3. Third, if the flow of libido is arrested or blocked at some particular stage of development (like oral, phallic, etc.) there may be fixations giving rise to various personal traits which already have been discussed.
4. Fourth, if the flow is blocked, repressed or made to travel backward, then the individual may develop a regressed personality. They tend to behave in the manner and ways related to that developmental stage at which they encounter frustration over the pleasure seeking desire.
5. Fifth, when the flow is condemned or repressed by the dominance of ego with respect to the Super Ego, it may give rise to anxiety and conflict leading to neurotic and psychotic behavior.
6. Sixth, if the flow is deflected, it may lead an individual to seek sexual gratification through channels of social value i.e., sublimation.

IV. Psycho-analysis as a Therapy

It is obvious from above that psycho-analysis is a method of study of behavioral processes. Hence we can adopt psycho-analysis as a drugless therapeutic measure in our day to day practice. This therapy involves the following steps:

A. Establishing the Rapport

Rapport means a friendly relationship: An emotional bond or friendly relationship between people based on mutual liking, trust, and a sense that they understand and share each other's concerns. Hence, there should be a reciprocal bond of emotion and trust between the physician and the patient. In the language of psycho-analysis, the former is called psycho-analyst and analysand. But for easy comprehension we will use the word patient for analysand.

The patient should accept the psycho-analyst whole heartedly with trust. The qualification of the analyst presupposes to have a humane, empathetic and understanding human nature.

B. Analysis

Analysis means close examination: The examination of something in detail in order to understand it better or draw conclusions from it.

It also means separation into components; the separation of something into its constituents in order to find out what it contains, to examine individual parts, or to study the structure of the whole.

Moreover, it also means assessment, an assessment, description or explanation of something, usually based on careful consideration or investigation

The aim of analysis is to explore the etiologies of problems plaguing the patient. According to psycho-analytical theory, mental illness is the outcome of repressed wishes and desires leftover in the subconscious mind. Hence the examination of unconscious mind is done by psycho-analysis.

The patient is directed to recline in a relaxed posture on a couch in a semi-dark room. The analyst should be seated towards the back of the patient. Techniques are employed to determine the reasons for the present precipitations of trouble.

Generally, three types of psycho-analysis (techniques) are carried out:

i.   Free association.
ii. Dream analysis.
iii. Daily psycho-pathology.

In *free association*, the patient is instructed to speak whatever he likes to speak what comes to his mind without any inhibition. While the patient is talking, the analyst does not interfere at all. The analyst should not make any correction to any statement made by the patient, however ludicrous or illogical the statements may be. The analysts role is only to watch the whole expression as a silent observer. By this, all the pent up feelings will come out gradually and the patient will be relieved.

In *dream analysis,* the unconscious mind is revealed which often leads to the root of the abnormalities as dreams are considered to be desires that have been repressed during conscious time.

Analysis of the *daily psycho-pathology* reveals the repressed desire or experience hidden in the unconscious mind.

Thus by these three practical steps the analyst fairly and squarely meets the unconscious mind. By this the root cause of disorder is exposed and the mental illness of the patient is alleviated.

C. Synthesis

Synthesis means result of combination: A new unified whole resulting from the combination of different ideas, influences or objects. It also means combining of various components into a whole—the process of combining different ideas, influences or objects into a new whole.

After the analysis is over, the steps of restructuring and restoration of psyche or mind is taken into account, which involves the following steps:

i. *Abreaction of the whole play with special focus on the precipitating factors.* Abreaction means release of tension by recalling trauma; to release unconscious psychological tension by talking about or reliving the events that caused it. By this the patient is informed about the factors that precipitated the present problem.

ii. *Discussion of the genesis of the trouble* as per the tenets of psychoanalysis as mentioned above.

iii. *Acceptance of the reality principle.* The patient is informed that pleasure and pain are part and parcel of life and cannot be separated. Moreover, he should be told that acceptance of the reality principle is also essential for human growth.

D. Breaking the Rapport

Finally the rapport of the temporary emotional bond formed between the analyst and the patient (or analysand) during the course of the treatment is broken amicably, so as to enable the patient to stand on his own feet. The analyst takes back the emotional crutches which he had supplied to the patient for a temporary period. In this way the rapport is broken and the patient is allowed to face the realities of life.

V. Criticism to Freud's Works

Freud has given his best for the mankind. Some grains of truth that have been discovered by Freud has been absorbed by medical as well as other branches of humanity. His work has been shown new vistas for humanity. However, his works are still subject to criticism.

i. First, it has over-emphasised the role of sex in human life.

ii. Secondly, it misses other aspects of life.

iii. Third, role of the unconscious mind has been exaggerated.

iv. Fourthly, it treats mankind to be a self-centred, gratification seeker and animal – like rather than being social and humane.

Despite the above criticism it can still be asserted that Freud was in pathology and talks of pathology, which is true. It seems that he had not understand a Rama or Buddha or Mahavira or Christ. They belong to the physiological expression of existence. The pathological state has imbued almost all the humans so Freud's contribution have emerged relevant today, especially after the advent of movies, TV channels and internet. Another thing we must know is that Freud has pointed his fingers to moon and we should not hold his fingers. Let us try to understand his sense not words. Anyhow, we have to go a long way to evolve a synthetic approach of Hahnemann, Kent plus Freud and neo Freudians.

Although almost a century has passed, yet it has not received a potential response in India. Indians never believe in theoretical aspect. They believe in "being" not in "doing". Whatever may be the teachings of psychology, the moment somebody accepts something in toto, the role of the therapeutic aspect of psychology seems to finish. Indians are practical people who are basically interested in meditation instead of medication. In every house you will find simple home remedies. These remedies are auxiliary to them. Indians believe that they are puppets in the hands of destiny. Hence, diseases as well as death are easily accepted by them. They are free from anxiety, conflict and repression. It is the advent of western culture that has shattered the Indian values and tradition. Moreover, Krishan, Rama, Buddha, Mahavira, Kabir, Meera, Nanak, etc. along with the teachings of Patanjali Yoga Darshan had been a solid block to Freudian practice. In recent days, with the advent of computer, TV channels, multimedia, etc., Indian culture has been devastated. It is being replaced with pornography and crime which are subtly injected to the soft and innocent minds. Hence the role of Freud and Neo-Freudian has become relevant.

Chapter 8

NEO-FREUDIAN PSYCHODYNAMICS

Freud was ahead of his time. He did wonderful work on human psychology, which brought laurels to him along with a natural concomitant variation: Criticism. The chief criticism came from his disciples. Some of his close disciples deviated from him but explained their theories from as psychoanalytic approach. These people are called Neo-Freudians. Among various differences, the characteristic difference is that all the Neo-Freudians categorically reject the theory of 'libido' and pan sexuality as propounded by Freud. The Neo-Freudians have their own individual explanation for the development of personality: Some put stress on the culture factor, some on social experience, etc. Let us explore the following prominent Neo-Freudians:

I. Alfred Adler
II. Carl Gustav Jung
III. Erich Fromm
IV. Karen Horney
V. Sullivan
VI. Erikson

I. ALFRED ADLER

Alfred Adler was born on February 7, 1870, at Penzing, Austria and died on May 28, 1937, at Aberdeen, Scotland. Throughout his life, Adler concerned with a strong awareness of social problems, and this acted as a prime motivation in his work. He was a physician (M.D., University of Vienna Medical School, 1895). He considered a patient with reference to the total environment with a humanistic and holistic approach.

Adler, being a physician became interested in the psycho-pathology in the genesis of various illnesses. Ultimately he was drawn to Freud and became closely associated with him in the year 1902. Nevertheless, divergence between the two became irreconcilable, when Adler rejected the pan sexuality and suggested that people try to compensate psychologically for a physical disability and its attendant feeling of inferiority. Unsatisfactory compensation results in neurosis. Adler strongly condemned Freud's basic argument that sexual conflicts in early childhood cause mental illness, and he further limited the role of sexuality to a symbolic part in human strivings to overcome feelings of inadequacy.

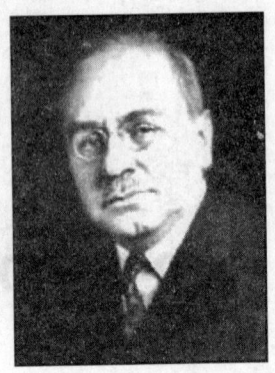

Adler (1870-1937)

Adler's Individual Psychology

Alfred Adler was a prize disciple of Freud. As mentioned earlier, Adler had to break off with Freud for denying over-generalisation of sex motive as an explanation for behavior determination. He was the first psychologist to de-emphasise the concept of inborn instincts and gave full stress to social factors in the development of personality. He built up his own school and developed an individual psychology.

Concepts of Individual Psychology

The major concept of Adler's individual psychology revolves around two aspects viz,:

A. Power motive and striving for superiority and excellence.
B. Style of life.

A. Power Motive and Striving for Superiority and Excellence

According to Adler, every child is born an unaided individual in himself and has to depend on others for his various needs and wants along with growth and development. This helplessness develops a feeling of insecurity, inferiority and inadequacy within him. Obviously, he wants to become powerful enough to supersede others so that he can quash his feelings of insecurity, inferiority and inadequacy. Secondly, his rearing environment might have generated him to run after power to rule others. Thirdly, his upbringing may also be in negligence, which might have induced a sense of inferiority in him. He seeks power as a compensation to this feeling of inferiority.

By superiority, Adler means striving for perfection or self-actualization. In his early writings he stressed on 'will to power' as a motive but in later writings he changed 'will to power' to 'striving for superiority'.

B. Style of Life

This is one of the important catchphrases of Adler's personality theory. According to him, style of life is the principle by which the individual personality functions. It is the whole that commands the parts (can we recall Hahnemann and Kent, who are much before Adler). Everyone has a style of life but no two individuals develop the same style (again recall Hahnemann and Kent). *Everyone develops his own individual style of life.*

Adler maintains that every person has a goal that is to prove himself superior to others. But the mode and means of adoption to reach that goal differs from person to person. One person may be superior by writing poems while another tries to prove his superiority by weight lifting. The poet has a specific life style. He remains aloof and leads a sedentary life. He visits places of scenic beauty for inspiration. The weight lifter leads an active life. He shuns a sedentary life. He visits various places where weight lifting competitions take place. He consults his seniors and experts, who can give him tips and tricks for future participation. Both of them learn and retain that course of action, which fits their life style and ignore, everything else. You might have observed such things in your class room. One of you may not be interested in politics. So, you avoid those things which are related to politics like campaigning, political propaganda, building political relationships with others, visiting party offices, etc. On the other hand, another person, who is interested in politics avoids classes but does the jobs mentioned in relation to politics. Both of them have joined the B.H.M.S. course but adopt their life styles individually in different manners.

Adler asserts that the life style is formed by the age of four or five. This style adoption ultimately leads to final blooming of the personality and style of life. His attitudes, feelings and judgment become fixed and built at an early age. In future the person may get hold of some new ways for the style of life but the early style fixed, runs all through life. The latter becomes only a decorum on the former life style which acts like a solid foundation.

Adler made some empirical studies and observed that it is the innate urge in all individuals to seek power. So an individual adopts a particular type of life style, so that he can excel and become superior to others. This concept is the key concept of Adler's system of *Individual Psychology*. Accordingly, an individual tries to become a political leader or a doctor or an engineer or a writer or alike. The individual adopts a specific type of life style in relation to one's time schedule, habits of work, personal and social contacts, attending institutions, etc. to achieve this goal.

Adler divides life styles for the development of personality under four heads, viz.,:

1. The ruling type.
2. The go- getting type.
3. The escaping type.
4. The struggling type.

Anyhow, the mentioned life styles are guided by some factors, which can be comprehended below:

a. Order of Birth

According to Adler, the order of birth plays a vital role in moulding the type of personality and life style. He observed that most of:

i. The eldest children became neurotics, timid, shy or drunkard, or criminal.

ii. The second, middle child became ambitious and also envious. But by and large, the second child got better adjusted than the elder one despite his rivalry and envy towards the older child.

iii. The youngest child was found to be a spoiled one.

Adler assigns very important reasoning for the above. The first born child is given great care and detailed attention for all his activities with great affection and love. This affair is maintained till the birth of the second child. After the birth of the second child, the attention of parents (others) is shifted towards the second one. Now the first child is dethroned from his favored position and compelled to undergo with limited shares as prescribed by parents. Now the elder child feels that his importance has become less and hence protects himself against sudden setbacks and insecurity by developing a negative attitude towards life as mentioned earlier. The youngest child is paid more attention and pampering, which makes him a spoilt child.

Hence Adler advises parents to handle such situations wisely and judiciously.

b. The Type of Children

It is obvious that the unwanted or neglected child may become timid, shy or criminal as mentioned above. Similarly the pampered child may adopt a life style of dominance (ruling type). He wants be obeyed like a king. Hence, he commands others to get his wish fulfilled.

c. Fiction Finalism

Adler brought this concept from Hans Vaihinger's work *The Psychology 'As If'*. In this book, Vaihinger maintained that men live in many fictions, which have no counter parts. His proposition of fiction highly influenced Adler. Adler modified it in his unique style and stated that fiction finalism can also amend a life style. Fiction finalism means that man's actions are caught in fictional ideas which necessarily do not confirm to reality. Adler also made fiction finalism responsible for shaping one's life style. Adler maintains that fiction finalism seems to help to cope more successfully with life. These fictional propositions cannot be tested as these are mere assumptions. Had these statements been categorised as hypothesises, then these could have been verified for concrete utility for future. These notions are only of limited use and become invalid after dispension. Some examples of fiction finalism are given below:

    i. All men are created equal.
    ii. Honesty is the best policy.
    iii. Stars decide the fortune of a man.
    iv. The end satisfies means.
    v. Female child is a curse to the family.
    vi. Women are created to serve men.

The role of such fiction finalism can be observed in our day to day life. We live in such a prejudiced state that our life style is modulated by these fictions. Such statements play a terrific role in an individuals life. Very often these fictions serve as a prism through which an individual's life style has to pass leading to a mirage. These fictions may be of limited use, but adoption of these statements in life has a profound impact in developing a personality and life style.

d. The Creative Self

Adler also accepts the creative power of an individual. He consigns that the power of the creative self accounts much in shaping the life style of an individual. The doctrine of creative self postulates that man is the maker of his personality. The genesis and growth of this creative self is determined by heredity and environment. Heredity gives the ability and environment for impression for this creative self. The abilities and impressions are the edifices of life style. 'The creative self gives meaning to life. It determines the mission of life. It creates the goal as well as the means to goal. The creative self should not be confused with the old concept of soul. Soul is the active principle of human life. An individual tends to solve problems and act according to the commands of his creative self. His life style is therefore said to be shaped in accordance with the development of his creative self.

This concept has a positive outcome. By this, man does not remain in a passive state by becoming a victim of luck or destiny. Man tries to make his own destiny adopting a possible life style.

e. Compensation for Inferiority

An individual may suffer from a feeling of inferiority, inadequacy or incompleteness as a result of frustration arising from:

   i.   Physical defects.
   ii. Low social status.
   iii. Pampering or neglect during childhood.
   iv. Other causes encountered in the course of life.

An individual meets the above aspects of personality through the mechanism of compensation:

   i.   In the form of striving for superiority by developing their skills and abilities.
   ii. Less healthily, they may develop an inferiority complex that dominates their behavior.
   iii. Over-compensation for inferiority feelings can take the form of an egocentric striving for power and superior behavior at others' expense.

f. Social Interest

During his early writings, Adler preached about the compensatory theory of an inferior complexity. He also extended this theory further and propounded that aggression and the power hungry nature of man is the masculine overcompensation for feminine weaknesses. This theory was widely criticised from every quarter for its parochial trend, selfish drive and ignorance of social interest.

Adler, being a champion of social justice and adherent of social democracy broadened the early concept and stressed on social interest in relation to life style.

He asserted that to strive for superiority, an individual had to take social interest. It is the society that gives recognition to an individual for superiority. Hence striving for superiority in this connection becomes socialisation instead of a selfish need and the life style gets shaped through one's innate social interests. During this progression, the individual has to make three adjustments in life: Adjustment with society, adjustment with vocation and adjustment with love. Thus, Adler was able to meet the criticisms made by opponents fairly and squarely.

The strive for superiority co-exists with another innate urge: to co-operate and work with other people for the common good, a drive that Adler termed social interest.

Adler maintains that an infant enters into social relation from his very birth. His interaction with his mother results in social transaction. Gradually this transaction develops into an inter-personal relationship, which ultimately spreads to a social network. Thus he enters into social interest, which contributes in his efforts for superiority. Now the parochial and limited ambition of striving for superiority of the individual is changed to building up an ideal society. Social interest comprises of the individual's service to society, to arrive at the goal of an ideal society. Social interest is the final compensation for all the natural weakness in an individual. Adler further held that social interest is innate and not attained by habit. But this innate quality does not appear abruptly or spontaneously. This quality of an individual has to be motivated for enjoyment by guidance and training. In this sense, Adler proved himself an exemplary icon by starting a child guidance clinic for educating the common man about appropriate methods of rearing children.

II. CARL GUSTAV JUNG

Analytical Psychology

Carl Gustav Jung, physician by profession was born on July 26th, 1875, in Kesswil, and died on June 6th, 1961 at Kusnacht, both the locations situated in Switzerland. He was a very ardent disciple of Freud. He was declared his 'beloved son' and 'crown prince' by Frued with a view to keep up the legacy of psycho-analysis. However, Jung was destined to do something else. He founded analytic psychology, which was erected as a reactionary measure to Sigmund Freud's psycho-analysis Jung developed the concepts of the extroverted and introverted personality archetypes, and the collective unconscious. His work has been significant in psychiatry and in the study of religion, literature and related fields.

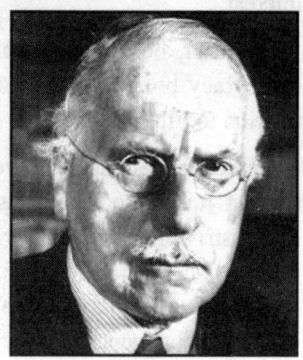

Carl Gustav Jung
(1875-1961)

A. STRUCTURE OF PSYCHE OR MIND

According to Jung, there exists conscious mind. He differs from Freud in many respects, which are obvious from the following lines.

Jung accepted the concept of unconscious and conscious in the structure of one's psyche or mind or self. But he differs to a greater extent in his concept of unconscious to that of Freud. Jung states that one's mind has the following layers:

1. Conscious Mind

This is the uppermost or superficial layer of mind. Memory, thoughts, feelings, etc. are related to this layer. It is the seat of Ego and conscious behavior.

2. Unconscious Mind

Layer next to conscious lies the unconscious mind. It also has two layers:

a. Personal unconsciousness.
b. Collective unconsciousness (also called Primary or Racial unconsciousness).

a. Personal Unconsciousness

This is the immediate layer to consciousness. It is highly individualistic and personal in nature. It preserves all the repressed desires, feelings, ideas, guilts, fears, anxieties, dreams, fantacies, etc. along with other experiences.

b. Collective Unconsciousness

This is the layer next to personal unconsciousness. This layer is neither private nor personal. This layer is universal to all individuals. Jung maintains that the mode of thinking, feeling and doing are transferred from generation to subsequent generation as a legacy. This becomes part and parcel of one's unconsciousness. The individual takes over enormous stores of ancestral characters or racial memory, so they are conditioned to perceive the world in the similar fashion as the previous generations did. Jung stresses that one's collective unconsciousness stores experiences of the whole race gathered over millions of years.

Jung further asserts logically that the entire human race has the same origin and common ancestral history. Hence the images are held and contained in our unconscious mind. These images are called *archetypes.*

Archetype is derived from the Greek word 'archetypos', "original pattern". Archetype means a primordial image, character or pattern of circumstances that recurs throughout.

In a better way, we say archetypes are the roots and bases. They represent eternal inherited ideas and forms which are common to every generation and culture since time immemorial. *His concept somehow resembles genetic coding and transference to successive generations.*

These archetypes are handed down with the evolving brain in the form of inherited nervous processes or may be gained through direct or indirect experiences. Let us explore various archetypes.

According to Jung, there exists three types of archetypes:

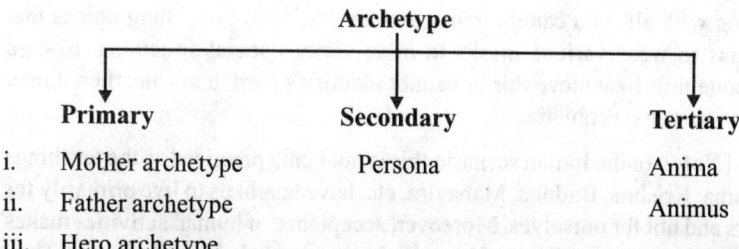

	Primary	Secondary	Tertiary
i.	Mother archetype	Persona	Anima
ii.	Father archetype		Animus
iii.	Hero archetype		

1. Primary

i. The Mother Archetype

The image or archetype of a mother has always have been a symbol of kindness, love, protection, nourishment and warmth. This is common to and universal to all cultures and religions. It is an eternal image or archetype handed down from generation to generation. In almost every culture, the earth, plants and rivers are associated with the symbol of mother.

ii. The Father Archetype

The image archetype of a father is unlike that of mothers. It symbolizes strength, authority and power. The sky, the sun, the ocean, lightening, thunder are equated with the image of a father.

iii. The Hero Archetype

Very often we pay respect to a person who is an ideal, unselfish, heroic figure. Similarly, in almost every culture or race we find many other universal and identical likenesses to the image of God, birth and death, demons and devils, saints and wise men. Also there exists some energy that moves this world, which is also taken as hero archetype.

2. Secondary

Persona

The term, coined by Carl Jung, is derived from the Latin persona, referring to an actor's mask, and is thus etymologically related to the term dramatis personae, designating the characters in a drama.

According to Jung, the persona enables an individual to interrelate with the world around him by reflecting the role in life that the individual is playing. This way one can arrive at a compromise between one's innate psychological constitution and society. Thus, the persona enables the individual to adapt to society's demands. One has to wear different masks to cope with different situations. Society also demands the same. It does not accept a stereotype dealing with all. You cannot treat a servant like your boss. Jung opines that one has to wear various masks to meet various social situations. In case someone fails to achieve this or cannot identify a particular role, then it may lead to personal problems.

[**Note:** In the Indian scenario this is not being practiced as the teachings of Rama, Krishna, Buddha, Mahavira, etc. have taught us to live primarily for others and not for ourselves. Moreover, acceptance of human activities makes you free from personality problems. In India, people believe in *destiny*. They believe, whether right or wrong, that destiny is the sole authority in shaping everything including breathing. Hence, this acceptance has made them free from conflict. However, after the advent of various gadgets like TV, computer, etc. which display objectionable ideas, the youth of this country has been misguided. Hence the need of Freud and Neo-Freudian, like Jung Adler, etc. has become very relevant.]

3. Tertiary

Anima and Animus

Anima is the female archetype and animus is the male archetype. Jung asserts that every male has a female in him, and every female has a male in her. He clearly states that the characteristics of both anima and animus lie within every individual. *Strictly speaking, this concept is not a new one. Hakim Sanai, the Sufi prophet has already exposed this concept in his "The Hadiqa", which means garden. Osho has also dealt with it exhaustively in his book "Unio Mystica".*

The Concept of Libido and Personality Development

Ordinarily we understand libido as sexual gratification. Jung in contrast assigns a very comprehensive meaning to this term. According to him, libido means 'life urge' or 'life energy' which may flow both ways – inward or outward. When the life energy flows inwards of a person, he is called an introverted person. The scientist, philosophers, writer, poets etc. may belong to this category. In contrast persons in whom the life energy flows outwards, are termed as extroverts. Politicians, advocates, speakers, salesmen etc. come under this group. But we cannot draw a Chinese wall between these two. We can find some combinations of above in many persons. Anyhow, Jung links following four behavioural functions to these two orientations – extroversion and introversion.

1. Thinking
2. Feeling
3. Sensational
4. Intuition

Thus he describes personality under following heads:

1. Thinking Type:
    a. Introverted.
    b. Extroverted.

2. Feeling Type:
   a. Introverted.
   b. Extroverted.
3. Sensational Type:
   a. Introverted.
   b. Extroverted.
4. Intitutive Type:
   a. Introverted.
   b. Extroverted.

Characteristic Features of Jung's Personality Types

1. The Introverted Thinking Type:
   a. Theoretical.
   b. Remains aloof.
   c. Afraid of external realities.
   d. Tactless.
   e. Cold.
   f. Absorbed in his own intellectual pursuit.
2. The Extroverted Thinking Type:
   a. Realistic.
   b. Practical.
   c. Propogates his views with insistence and vehemence.
3. The Introverted Feeling Type:
   a. Day dreamer.
   b. Feelings : Strong.
   c. Desire and aversions : Strong.
   d. Inexpressive of his sufferings.
4. The Extroverted Feeling Type:
   a. Social.
   b. Objective oriented.
   c. Admires others.
   d. Helping nature.
   e. Empathetic.
   f. Expressive.
5. The Introverted Sensational Type:

a. Choosy.
   b. Fussy.
   c. Physical constitution : Lean and thin.
   d. Does not eat well.
   e. Dissatisfied.
   f. Brooding in solitude.
   g. Sad.
6. The Extroverted Sensational Type:
   a. Voracious eater.
   b. Easily satisfied.
   c. Demands constant emotional sensation.
   d. Carefree.
   e. Friendly.
   f. Talkative.
   g. Does not have patience for abstract and theoretical ideas.
7. The Introverted Intuitive Type:
   a. Subjective.
   b. Concerned with probabilities rather than actuality.
   c. Moody.
   d. Unstable.
   e. Temperamental.
   f. Behaves like a theoretical scientist and prophet.
8. The Extroverted Intuitive Type:
   a. Outwardly.
   b. Optimistic.
   c. Takes risks.
   d. Quite set in intuitive judgement.

III. ERICH FROMM

Erich Fromm, was a German-born U.S. psycho-analyst and social philosopher who was born on March 23rd, 1900, in Frankfurt and died on March 18th, 1980, in Muralto, Switzerland.

He explored the interaction between psychology and society. By applying psycho-analytic principles to the remedy of cultural ills, Fromm believed, mankind could develop a psychologically balanced "sane society."

In the year 1922, he received his Ph.D. from the University of Heidelberg. Then he underwent training in psycho-analysis at the University of Munich and at the Psycho-analytic Institute of Berlin. He began practicing psycho-analysis under the tutelage of Sigmund Freud. As time passed he differed from Freud. He opposed Freud's fixation of unconscious drives and ignoring of the role of society in human psychology. Fromm propounded that an individual's personality was the product of his culture as well as biology. Fromm viewed that an understanding of basic human needs is indispensable to the understanding of society and mankind itself. He also gives reasoning regarding social conflict which may play a key role in the development of a personality. A man has many desires which cannot be fulfilled due to existence of our social systems, by which social conflicts are generated.

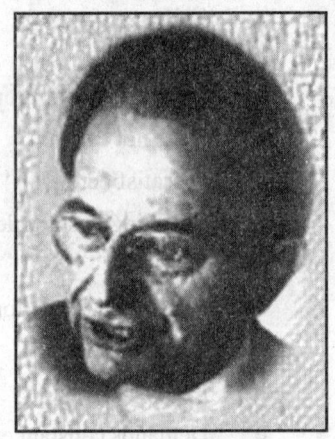
Erich Fromm (1900-1980)

Two concepts of Erich Fromm are very important and they deserve our attention:

A. Basic nature of human beings.
B. Development of personality.

A. Basic Nature of Human Beings

Fromm maintains that man has dissociated himself from Nature by violating its laws with the illusion of gaining freedom and happiness. This dissociation has brought all misery and troubles unto him. Hence, Fromm strongly exhorts to be back with Nature and urges human beings for a renewal of affiliation with Nature. He also believes that although man possesses an animal nature, he has to rise above it. He also highlights the role and relation of an individual with the society. He states that man has a deep desire to be a part of society with a sustainable relationship with others while maintaining identity as a distinct individual.

B. Development of Personality

Fromm is silent about any specific developmental stages. The learning of distinction between 'I' and 'not –I' through social interaction induces the child with the idea of individualisation and separation. This separation from parents gives birth to the feeling of isolation and doubts in the mind of the child. Fromm also accepts importance of early childhood experiences in the development of personality but states that the personality can also be modified during adulthood, provided the external stimuli are pretty powerful to effect changes in adults.

IV. KAREN HORNEY

Karen Honey, born on September 16th, 1885, in Blankenese, near Hamburg, Germany died on December 4th, 1952, in New York, U.S.A.

Karen studied medicine at the Universities of Freiburg, Göttingen and Berlin, taking her M.D. degree from the last in 1911.She joined the teaching staff of the newly founded Berlin Psycho-analytic Institute in the year 1920.

Karen Horney was also a Neo-Freudian, who accepted the outlines of Freudian theory but departed from some of the basic issues like:

1. Female psychology, which is built as an offshoot of male psychology.
2. Concepts of:
    - Libido
    - Death instinct
    - Oedipus complex
    - Penis envy
3. Freud's disregard of environmental, cultural and social basis for the development of personality and its disorders.

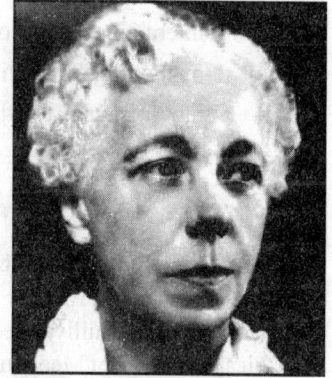

Karen Horney (1885-1952)

She was a dynamic and straight forward lady. She had to pay a heavy price for her rejection to hold fast to strict Freudian theory in the form of expulsion from the New York Psycho-analytic Institute in 1941.

She revealed that several female psychiatric disturbances are due to the male-dominated culture. She introduced the concept of womb envy, suggesting that males envy pregnancy, nursing, motherhood, etc. She maintained that this envy leads men to claim their superiority in other fields.

She categorically rejected the instinctual or biological drive in the development of personality as propounded by Freud. She stressed that it is environmental and social conditions, that determine much of the individuals personality and are the chief causes of neuroses and personality disorders. She advocated that an infant's experience of basic anxiety, isolation and helplessness in this aggressive world is responsible for the later development of neurosis. The child adopts various irrational strategies to cope with this anxiety, which eventually becomes the cause of personality disorder.

Her ideas on female psychosexual development were given particular attention after the posthumous publication of '*Feminine Psychology*' in the year 1967.

The main postulations of Horney are stated below:

a. Man has many positive qualities.
b. Biology (genetic endowment), environment and socio-cultural influences have a great impact on the development of personality.
c. She stresses that it is the self-concept of an individual which acts as the directing force in life.
d. She accepts the role of conflict in human life and suggests remedial measures for it by:
    - interacting with people or,
    - by moving away with the conflict or,
    - moving against with conflict.

V. SULLIVAN

Dr. Harry Stack Sullivan was born on February 21st, 1892, in Norwich, N.Y., U.S. and died on January 14th, 1949, in Paris. Sullivan received his M.D. from the Chicago College of Medicine and Surgery in 1917 and subsequently adopted Sigmund Freud's psycho-analysis and extended it to the treatment of severely ill, hospitalized psychotic patients rather than restricting them to the more functional neurotics treated by traditional Freudian analysts of the time.

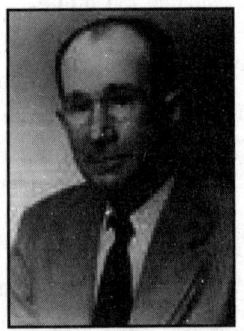
Sullivan (1892-1949)

Sullivan is another Neo-Freudian who emphasised the importance of social factors in the development of personality.

Sullivan puts stress on the early childhood relationship with his mother, the first social interaction in the development of the personality of an individual. He states that mother is the first and most important person to an infant. When this relationship is disturbed, anxiety is generated. The child then develops a mode of behavior with a view to reduce this anxiety. This mode of adoption establishes the characteristics of personality that would continue during adulthood. Hence the early social interaction with the mother forms the basic pattern of the personality.

Again, when the child is exposed to the external environment, he begins to form social relationships with other children and starts a social interaction. It is the social interaction that builds the personality of an individual. Sullivan maintains that personality is the outcome of interaction of the individual with the society. Personality is a matter of how we look at ourselves and how others look at us. Future development to a greater extent depends on early experiences of a child and how he relates with others. If a person accepts himself to be a 'bad-me' relationship with others it will generate a lot of anxiety because people are likely to reject him.

He also postulated that rules and norms of society are extremely restrictive and do not allow even reasonable freedom to an individual. These enforced rules and norms frequently lead to personality problems. If an adolescent does not find sufficient self-growth during this period and lacks reasonable freedom, then he is likely to become a homo-sexual, because to him that seems to be a safer relationship than one with the opposite sex.

He considered that anxiety and other psychiatric symptoms crop up in fundamental conflicts between the individual and his relationship with the human environment. He stresses that personality development takes place by a series of interactions with other people. He even extends this to the genesis of schizophrenia claiming that both normal and abnormal personalities stand for lasting patterns of interpersonal relationships with social environment.

VI. ERIKSON

The full name is Erik Homburger Erikson. He was a German-born American psycho-analyst. In 1927, he was requested by Anna Freud, the daughter of Sigmund Freud to teach art, history and geography at a small private school in Vienna. There he developed interest in psycho-analysis with Anna and underwent training to become a psycho-analyst himself. In 1933, he emigrated to the United States. He became a professor of psychology at the University of California, Berkeley in 1942 and remained Professor Emeritus from 1970 until his death. Erikson combined his interest in history and psycho-analytic theory, and called it Psycho History. Even he was able to interpret Gandhiji non-violence through this psycho-history.

Erikson also laid emphasis on the value of social factors in personality development. He developed the concept of 'developmental milestones'.

Erikson attempted in his theory to bridge the gap between Freudian theory of psycho-sexual development and present day knowledge of children's physical and social development.

Erikson conceived eight stages of development, where each stage deals, with the individual and its psycho-social requirement that continues into old age. Personality development, according to Erikson, takes place through a series of crises that must be overcome and internalized by the individual for the future developmental stage.

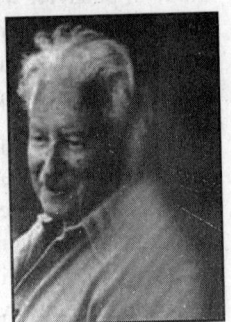

Erikson (1902-1949)

He introduced eight stages of development in which he emphasised the importance of interaction between biological and social factors in the development of a personality.

He distinguishes three aspects representing the personality:

a. Somatic or body.
b. Ego or self.
c. Social or the influence.

His theory is systematic and comprehensive in its approach and integrates social, anthropological and biological factors into personality.

Erikson proposed a psycho-social theory of development. This means that the stages of a person's life from birth to death are formed by social influences interacting with a physically and psychologically developed organism. In Erikson's words, there is a mutual fit of individual and environment – that is, of the individual's capacity to relate to an over-expanding life space of people and institutions, on one hand, and on the other, the readiness of these people and institutions to make him part of an enjoying cultural concern.

Erikson's Eight Developmental Stages

Out of eight stages, as advocated by Erikson, the first four stages occur during infancy and childhood, the fifth stage during adolescence, the sixth and seventh during adult years and the eighth stage in old age. Erikson puts special emphasis to the period of adolescence as it is the crucial period of transition between childhood and adulthood.

These successive stages are not arranged according to a firm sequential schedule. Erikson only provides a functional period or stage, and therefore it would be misleading to specify an exact duration for each stage. Each stage does not pass through one after the other. Instead, each stage plays a role in the formation of the total personality, with an overlap between stages. Each of these stages possesses its own type of crisis, or conflict which must be studied to understand the development of personality.

1. Trust vs Mistrust (Birth to 18 Months)

Erikson designates the first developmental stage as the 'sensory stage'. This stage starts with birth and continues up to one and half a years. This stage corresponds to Freud's oral stage. In this stage, there generates the crisis of learning of basic trust or mistrust of other people. During this period of life the infant has to totally depend on his mother or caretaker to meet his various needs. The mode by which he is nourished, handled and protected at this stage may provide the infant with a sense of security or insecurity. By this a feeling of trust or mistrust with regard to the environment is developed. If, for any reason, the mother is incoherent in satisfying the infant's needs, the infant may carry suspicion and doubt through the rest of its years.

2. Autonomy vs Shame and Doubt (18 Months to 3 Years)

This stage starts from the eighteenth month and lasts up to three years. This second stage subscribed by Erikson's corresponds to the anal stage as described by Freud. After gaining the sense of trust and security in the environment, the baby acquires physical skills and language ability. Now he wants to make experiments with strength and limitation for achieving a sense of autonomy. So he makes experiments during toilet training. During this training, the child learns to control its own muscles and begins to assert its individuality. The crisis here is that of autonomy, or the ability to control one's own bodily functions. Success leads to autonomy and in case of failure, there develops shame and doubt about his own abilities.

3. Initiative vs Guilt (3-6 Years)

This is the third stage of Erikson's psycho-social development. This stage is related to locomotor control and is similar to Freud's phallic stage. Now the child attempts to develop its own way of claiming its needs and gaining its rewards. Now generates the sexual instinct. He wants to possess the parent of opposite sex at least in imagination and accept the parent of his sex as a rival. Now the child has to undergo the crisis of inner urges versus society's norms of morality. Erikson suggested that if the child could channelise its sexual needs into socially acceptable behaviors, then the child acquires initiatives, otherwise the child develops a strong sense of guilt which may last throughout his life.

4. Industry vs Inferiority (6 to 12 Years)

Both Freud and Erikson called the fourth developmental stage that of latency. During this period, the child has to undergo educational curriculum. The school environment generates pressure on him to excel. Now he has to compete with peers in terms of achievement. The crisis the child faces is that of competency or failure. If the child does well in school, he will be motivated to become successful and thus becomes industrious. If his performance becomes poor then he develops a sense of inferiority complex.

5. Identity vs Role of Confusion (12 to 19 Years)

This stage begins with the advent of puberty. Erikson asserts this puberty crisis as that of either finding one's identity, or of developing what he called role confusion. Now the adolescent makes attempts in search of his identity by redefining his own socio-psychological identity. The development of identity depends largely upon the degree of success he gains in resolving the early crises. Failure in resolving the old crisises may lead to a state of confusion. He may become bewildered and confused. Even he may fail in choosing a career or profession.

6. Intimacy vs Isolation (19 to 45 Years)

This is the sixth stage of psycho-sexual development. During this stage, the individual tends to develop a sense of intimacy or a desire for company. He wants to have intimate personal relationships with others.

The intimacy may develop under two aspects. First, the successful relationship with the opposite sex attaining orgasm that may leads to intimacy. The second intimacy is seen in dedications made for one's close friends or any individuals like brother, sister, father or mother or even a teacher.

But when the relationship cannot be built or it deteriorates for any reason or the other, there develops a sense of isolation.

7. Generativity vs Stagnation (45 to 65 Years)

Erikson believed that adults often experience the "growth" crisis during their middle years. An individual's life is spent in trying to establish himself in a professional career. Hence he satisfies his need for generativity and becoming a guide to the next generation. He must be creative, resourceful and helpful to his fellow beings. He should contribute to the society. This gives a sense of satisfaction to him. Contrast to the sense of generativity, an individual may develop a sense of selfishness and ego. This leads to stagnation.

8. Ego Integrity vs Despair (65 Onwards)

This is Erikson's eighth and final stage of psycho-social development. During this stage, an individual is confronted with ego integrity versus despair. According to Erikson, ego integrity refers to the integration of the successful resolution of all the above seven stages in the course of life. Successful resolution of the last seven phases of life gives the individual a sense of fulfilment and perfection. He becomes free from various hangovers and remains in a state of serenity. On the other hand, individuals who have not been able to resolve successfully the crisises of the developmental stages become despaired. If the individual fails to resolve the early crisises, he feels that life has become useless, incomplete and wasted. They feel miserable and succumb to the feeling of despair and dejection.

Summary of Erikson's Eight Developmental Stages

No.	Stage	Stage & Age	Psycho-social Crisis	Major Concern
1.	Oral	Infancy (0-18 months)	Trust vs Mistrust	The infant develops a sense of trust / mistrust in relation to basic needs.
2.	Anal	Early childhood (18 months -3 years)	Autonomy vs. Shame & doubt	Learns self-control as a means of being self-sufficient, e.g., toilet training. Shame and doubt may crop up if it fails.
3.	Genitalia	Play age (3-6 years)	Initiative vs Guilt	Investigates adult activities, may develop the feelings of guilt about trying to be independent and daring.
4.	Latency	School age (6-12 years)	Industry vs Inferiority	Develops learning skills and becomes industrious. The feelings of inferiority complex develop if he fails in a given assignment.
5.	Adolescence	Adolescence (12-19 years)	Identity vs Identity confusion	Try to identify who he is, how he is unique, how he can establish his career amd identity. Confusion can arise in these decisions.
6.	Young	Young adulthood (20-45 years)	Intimacy vs Isolation	Seek companionship and intimacy or being a failure in relationship, develops the tendency to become isolated.
7.	Adulthood	Adulthood (46-65 years)	Generativity vs Stagnation	Need to be productive or become stagnated.
8.	Maturity	Mature (age 65+)	Integrity vs Despair	Efforts are directed to make sense of one's life. Despair may be induced when last seven phases are not resolved successfully.

Chapter 9

PSYCHO-SOMATIC MANIFESTATION OF DREAMS

Do you not dream?

Do I not dream?

Yes, we all see dreams. A dream is a sequence of mental images that occurs during sleep: a sequence of images that appear involuntarily in our mind while we are in sleep, often an assortment of real and imaginary characters, places, and events. Every one of us (except a snorer) sees dreams. Simply because we do not remember dream does not mean that we do not see it. Dreams are indispensable for our life. A lack of dream activity generally indicates towards a personality disorder or protein deficiency.

Very often we enjoy our dreams. The crude meaning of dream is 'joy' and 'music'. The word "dream" is traditionally traced back to 13th century word 'dreme' (Anglo-Saxon), which means joy, gladness, or mirth. However, the word 'dream' more likely came from the Sanskrit, meaning deception. Thus, when we dream, is it a joy or a deception. We remember some of them and we forget the rest. We spend at least 5-6 years in dreaming throughout our life. One-thirds to four-fifth of our sleep is spent on dreaming.

We dream 4-7 dreams for one or two hours every night. If we wake up just after REM sleep, then we can recall our dreams more vividly in comparison to dreams that occur in our sleep from the night until morning. Again, we forget 50% and 90% of dreams within 5 minutes and 10 minutes respectively after the end of the dream.

Physiological research has revealed that males experience erections and females experience increased vaginal flow during dreaming REM sleep. Anyhow, "wet dreams" may not necessarily happen together with overtly sexual dream content. Nightmares or frightening dreams are common between early childhood and beginning of late childhood of life i.e. during 3-8 years of age.

Interestingly animals like cats and dogs see dream. Even a blinds dreams, whether visual images will occur in his dream is related to the period when he became blind: blind by birth or became blind later in life. We should know that vision is not the only sense that represents a dream. Other sensations like sounds, smell and tactility become hypersensitive for the blind and their dreams are based on these.

It seems that the dream might be known since the very birth of human beings. We can trace back its history to 5000 years. The importance of dream has been referred by Maharshi Patanjali in his magnum opus '*Patanjali Yoga Pradeep*'. References regarding dreams is also found in '*The Atharva Veda*'.

In ancient days, the Greeks and Romans strongly believed in dream interpreters. Even their military campaign was guided by interpretation of dreams. It is said that the wife of Julius Caesar, the Roman emperor (100-44 B.C.), had dreamt the assassination of Julius Caesar prior to the night of the assassination. Julius Caesar was forewarned by his wife regarding this much before the time of assassination. The forewarning was disregarded by Julius Caesar and subsequently the dream proved to be true. He was assassinated by a group of nobles in the Senate House on the Ides of March.

Man has always been probing about the sense of dreams since its appearance. Before Aristotle, people attributed dreams to be supernatural power. It was Aristotle, who for the first time stated that dreams are related to psychological problems. Nevertheless, it was Freud who gave the first systematic interpretation of dreams. Freud's interpretation of dreams is a classic treatise and must be read by every one of us. He vividly explores the unconscious mind and explores the reasons behind the pathological states of mind in relation to dreams. Although Freud has been credited for the exploration, Hahnemann had given glimpses regarding the importance of dreams in the treatment of various diseases much before Freud. Even today, a single dream of intensity or frequency can build a totality in the treatment of various illness from a homeopathic point of view.

NATURE OF DREAMS

Exploring the nature of dreams is highly essential for us. This knowledge helps us in the evaluation of symptoms and decisiveness of dreams for a successful prescription in our clinical practice.

1. Dreams Manifest Desires

The role of dreams for our mental life cannot be denied. The repressed or restrained and frustrated desires that generate in the conscious mind shift to the unconscious mind and stay there in a latent form. Later they are manifested in the form of dreams. Dreams may be expressed in various forms. Thus, by the expression of repressed and frustrated desires, the person achieves mental tranquility.

2. Dreams are the Expression of Repressed and Forbidden Desires

We are not yogis or saints who can renounce the desires or the world completely. We also cannot digest the advice of Buddha that all the sorrows are the cause of desire. We are worldly people and full of desires. We also want all the desires to be fulfilled. Some of those desires are weak and some are strong. Some of them do not affect at all whereas some deeply affect us. Some of them are within our reach and some are out of control. Let us take your example. You want to have a talk with your classmate of the opposite sex. You also want to have an affair with him or her. But due to some reason or the other you cannot propose it. Now this desire will not vanish in the air. This will move from the conscious mind into the sub-conscious mind. Now this desire is repressed. Repression is a psychological protective mechanism by which it protects us from threatening thoughts by blocking them out of the conscious mind. Later, these repressed desires manifest themselves in the form of dreams.

Just as in a cinema or film is examined by the Censor Board before its public exhibition, the dream has to pass the censorship of Super Ego before its manifestation during sleep.

During our conscious state, we are successful in avoiding the desires. By this we push those desires in the process of repression, which moves to the unconscious mind. During a state of sleep, we loose hold over the unconscious mind and the repressed desires express themselves in the form of dreams only in a changed form. According to Freud, most of the desires expressed in the form of dreams are sexual by nature.

3. Most Dreams are Wish Fulfillment

Psycho-analysis has done much work in the direction of the analysis of dreams and has postulated many hypotheses explaining dreams. According to Freud, dreams are wish fulfillment. Most of our desires can not be fulfilled in the waking state. For example, a diabetic patient wants to eat sweets but he is not in a position to do so. His desire is strong but he cannot take sweets out of fear of raising the blood sugar. In such a state, his desires are not satisfied but repressed. These repressed desires do not disappear but manifest themselves in the form of dreams. At night, he sees the dream of eating sweets. But we must remember that all dreams are not wish fulfillment because:

a. Some dreams are meaningless.
b. In some dreams, several objects are distorted and bewildered.
c. Some dreams might be entirely self-contradictory.
d. Some dreams are the reflections of physical illness.
e. Dreams may be the expression of our reactions to particular things in life and not necessarily wish fulfillment.
f. Human psychology and dreams are complex phenomenon and cannot be attributed to such simple explanation.

Hence we have to remember that wish fulfillment is one of the various aspects of dreams.

4. We Sleep because of Dreams

In our clinical practice patients come and complain that dreams disturb their sleep. We also listen to such statements in day to day casual discussions. These statements are erroneous. The fact is that dreams are helpful in sleep.

Let us take an example of a dream of drinking water. This is the reaction to thirst that occurs while we are sleeping. But what happens is that we dream of drinking water and go on sleeping keeping the thirst at abeyance for some time. Here dreaming of drinking water plays a crucial role. In such a condition; had there been no dream we could not have slept. It may also happen that the dream may not quench the thirst. Then, we wake up and drink water. Thus dreams help us in meeting physical needs.

Mental desires and tendencies are also satisfied through dreams and sleep continues.

For example, a businessman immersed in the fear and worries of financial loss, dreams about it and continues to sleep. If these dreams were not there, the businessman could not sleep. Thus in the dreams our painful and pleasant desires get expression and we achieve mental serenity. If these dreams of expression were not there, the same desires would express themselves in some abnormal behavior and there may be difficulties in the individual's adjustment with the situation. Dream is the safest outlet for the appearance of desires.

From homeopathic point of view, we should look to another side. In case of enuresis, the patient may dream of urinating (*Kreosotum*) and may also urinate in reality without conscious awareness. Here homeopathy has a tremendous role to play and the selected simillimum may restore the sick individual to health.

5. Dreams Disclose our Unconscious Mind towards Life's Problems

In our day to day life we have to encounter many problems of life like:

a. Our many desires are not fulfilled.
b. Our self-assertion with power motive may get a set back.
c. Current problems may not be solved and take the shape of a monster.

All these events are related to our unconscious mind. These events are expressed in dreams. Thus, dreams reveal the unconscious mind towards problems of life.

6. Pathological Conditions are Detected through Dreams

(See below under 'Freud on Dreams'.)

CLASSIFICATION OF DREAMS

Klein's Classification

Klein Melanienée Reizes was an Austrian-born British psycho-analyst. She was born on March 30th, 1882, at Vienna and died on September 22nd, 1960, in London.

Klein expressed an early interest in medicine but abandoned her plans when she had an unhappy marriage with three children and she had to undergo psycho-analysis under Sándor Ferenczi, a close associate of Freud. Ferenczi urged Klein to study psycho-analysis of young children, and in 1919 she produced her first paper in the field. Two years later she was invited by Karl Abraham to join the Berlin Psycho-analytic Institute, remaining there until 1926, when she moved to London.

Her classification on dreams is widely accepted, which is produced as below:

a. *Premonitory Dreams*: Those dreams which leave the impression of some future significance.
b. *Prophetic Dreams*: It is direct indication or a clue regarding future events.
c. *Pradromic Dream:* When a prophetic dream conveys distorted meaning, it is called pradromic dream. You may see a dream of extraction of teeth. You wake up and find your teeth hale and healthy.
d. *Recurrent Dream*: Recurrent dreams are those dreams that recur from time to time. Recurrent dreams occurs in neurotic people who have suffered a lot during a given period of time, say a soldier who has terrifying war experiences. The author was a patient of asthma since the age of seven. He had to suffer from asthma till the age of 23. He was cured from asthma after undergoing homeopathic treatment. Although he has been free from asthma for 25 years, he dreams of the asthmatic attack occassionally, which terrifies him. Such type of dreams are called recurrent dreams.

There also exists another classification that deserves our attention, which is highlighted below:

i. *Collective Dreams*: The dreams which are seen by more than one people at a given time.
ii. *Kinesthetic Dreams*: Dreams related to floating, soaring, falling, etc.
iii. *Paralytic Dreams*: Where an individual becomes almost paralyzed after experiencing a horrifying dream.

THEORIES OF DREAMS

There exist many theories of dreams out of which following are important:
1. The Supernatural Theory of Dreams.
2. The Physiological Theory of Dreams.
3. Psycho-neurological Interpretation of Dreams.
4. Psycho-analytical Interpretation of Dreams
   A. Freud's Theory of Dreams.
   B. Adler's Theory of Dreams.
   C. Jung's Theory of Dreams.

5. Perls's Theory of Dreams.
6. Activation-synthesis Theory of Dreams.
7. Mark Solm's Theory of Dreams.
8. Jie Zhang's Continual-activation Theory of Dreams.

1. The Supernatural Theory of Dreams

Dreams having supernatural significance come under this category. In olden days and even now, on many occasions the future events are sent as a premonition. With the advent of the modern era, frequency of such dreams has dropped significantly. Although it may look unscientific, on many occasions the prediction comes true. In villages, females have premonitions in dreams which often come true. It is claimed that early morning dreams come true. Anyhow, many psychologists do not agree with it.

2. The Physiological Theory of Dreams

According to this theory, dreams are simply a reaction to the physical stimuli that occurs in sleep. They put forward those internal and external stimuli as the cause of dreams. It is also known that an individual is never free from these stimuli and hence he dreams. An Individual cannot dream in the absence of these stimuli. Dreams are caused by the sensory impressions collected in the brain due to the restraint during day time. In other words, we can say that suppressed sensory impressions of an individual manifest themselves as dreams. Dreams put away the brain from the weight of sensory impressions.

No one can deny the influence of physiological sensations in the process of dream, but physiological interpretation alone is not sufficient. Dreams have a mental as well as psychological aspect. Hence we dream happenings that had occurred twenty or thirty years back. It is true that physical sensations bear some influence on dreams but due to psychological differences, the same physical sensations can create different expressions in the dreams of different people. For example, if a knife or some hard thing is placed on the neck of some sleeping person, a farmer may dream of the stroke of his sickle while a student of French history may dream of a gullitive. The physiological theory cannot explain this difference. Dreams, however, not only remove the load of sensory impressions, but also individualize mental frustrations to which physiological explanation has no answer.

3. Psycho-neurological Interpretation of Dreams

The chief exponent of this theory is Harton. He interpreted the theory of dreams on the basis of psycho-neurology. Accordingly, if some water is poured on the feet of a sleeping individual, the person may dream of walking on ice. Similarly, an individual sleeping in a running train may dream of a storm or typhoon. This is the result of physical sensations caused by the noise of the train. Thus according to Harton's theory, the individual dreams in accordance with external stimuli working on his body.

The theory of psycho-neurological interpretation of dreams is a narrow one. This fails to interpret individual dreams and dreams of long past memories. It also fails to explain meaningless dreams.

4. Psycho-analytical Interpretation of Dreams

Despite a long history of dreams, since time immemorial, the most substantial contribution came from Freud and the school of psycho-analysis. Till date this is considered the best.

A. Freud's Theory of Dreams

Freud's psycho-analytical theory of dreams stands as the most valid and fundamental among all the theories of dreams. It would not be an exaggeration to consider Freud's mammoth work as Goliath whereas others to Liliputs. Freud was the first person to state that we sleep because of dreams which is contrary to the general belief that people cannot sleep because of their dreams. Freud asserted that dreams are not a barrier for sleep, in fact they aid it. Now let us discuss the views subscribed by Freud on dreams:

i. Dreams are Wish Fulfillment

We have already discussed about it. Let us explore it further.

Freud emphasized that when an individual's desires, which are not satisfied in the external world or are repressed due to some cause, they do not get extinguished, but go to the unconscious plane and from there try to manifest themselves at an appropriate time. This individual manifestation of dreams is one of the most surface means of expression of the unconscious desires.

It may be questioned here that if dreams are wish fulfillment, why does one see painful and traumatic dreams? Freud has explained this by pointing out that these dreams are the distorted forms of the latent content of the dreamer. For example, if a young individual dreams that a lady has got severely hurt and the lady resembles his mother, Freud will interpret the dream by pointing out that the young individual actually desires that his mother should get hurt. Every young individual would revolt against this interpretation. But according to Freud, in the individual's mind there are mutually conflicting desires; where there is love there is hate, where there is a wish for life there is a desire for death as well. However, occasionally in a state of traumatic neurosis, the dreams often stop in the state of worry and appear to be unsuccessful in the fulfillment of desire. Hence, Freud later modified his theory and called the dreams "attempted wish fulfillment" and not wish fulfillment itself. Thus later on, Freud divided dreams into three classes:

a. Wish dreams.
b. Anxiety dreams.
c. Punishment dreams.

ii. The Significance of Sexual Wishes in Dreams

According to Freud, the most frustrated desires of an individual are sexual desires. Gratification of sexual desire is universal. First an individual has to satisfy the norms and other standards of code of conduct in the society and at the same time satisfy his sexual wishes. Thus, there generates tendency for conflicts in the individual's mind. In other words, there occurs a clash between Id and Super Ego. Id is ruthless and always in a state of seeking pleasure. It seeks the satisfaction of sexual desires by hook or by crook. Super Ego in turn, is the representative of social morality and it tries to persuade Id to refrain from such an attempt. Super Ego attempts to control sexual impulses. Later, Super Ego edits the dreams for its manifestation in varied forms.

iii. Pathological Conditions are Detected Through Dreams

Freud's psycho-analysis opened new vistas in the realm of dreams. Freud was able to detect many mental abnormalities through analysis of dreams. Dream analysis along with free association is a real asset for a physician to discover the mental pathological conditions. This association shows the unconscious causes by which mental abnormalities are identified.

iv. Dream Work

It has already been described above that frustrated desires become latent contents of the dreams. Due to censorship this desire cannot manifest itself in the dream in its original form. Thus the dream wishes turn into distorted forms. This process of dreaming is called dream work through which the latent contents become manifested in the form of dreams. Freud postulated that dreams may adopt any of the following five mechanisms:

a. Condensation

In condensation, a major part of the latent dream fades away before its manifestation.

b. Displacement

In this mechanism, the primary things in the latent dream become secondary and vice versa. Here the censorship fails to recognize the real desires.

c. Dramatization

Here the abstract desires express through concrete form in the dream. This dramatization is expressed in the altered form. Hence, due to this phenomena of dramatization, the dreams, feelings, emotions, etc. are manifested in a concrete form.

d. Symbolization

In this mechanism, the symbol represents another matter. Freud has done extensive work on this aspect. He has given a detailed description of different symbols of various sexual organs and tendencies. For example, a light pole in a dream may symbolize a male organ whereas a well may represent female organs. In this process the censorship remains static and does not interfere. Hence, most frustrated desires manifest themselves in the form of symbols.

e. Secondary Elaboration

Here, the real form of dream is concealed. In fact it is added with some imaginary statements by an individual. We know that a human being wants to express a continuity and meaningfulness in everything. So when he awakens after the dream, he cannot correlate those dreams in a logical manner because it is not mandatory for a dream to express itself in a logical manner. Moreover, the individual may forget the total content of the dream. Hence he elaborates the dream with logical continuity so that the dream becomes meaningful. This mechanism is known as secondary elaboration.

v. We Sleep Because of Dreams

Freud was the first to assert that we sleep because of dreams. Thus dreams help in the continuation of sleep. This has already been discussed earlier.

vi. Dream Interpretation

The interpretation of dreams is attributed to the assumption that every phenomenon has a cause. Freud maintains that dreams are an expression of unconscious information. He has tried to analyze the meaning of dreams with the help of:

a.   Free association.
b.   Dream symbols.

a. Free Association

In free association the dreamer freely associates his ideas with the places, persons and things witnessed in dreams. The procedure of free association is conducted by making the patient lie on a couch. The analyst is seated out of his sight but close enough so that he can hear everything clearly. The patient is also allowed to talk whatever he likes. The psycho-analyst does not interfere with the patient. The analyst should not point out anything as being wrong or over-exaggerated by the patient. By this, the subconscious state of mind of the patient is revealed from which the dream is analyzed. Thus, the dreamer comprehends the real sense of the dream by freely associating without any restrain of the intellect.

b. Analysis of Dream Symbols

Freud interprets most of the dreams in the form of symbols. These symbols have been embraced from mythologies, folklores, scriptures, etc. Some of the examples of these symbols are as follows:

- Water symbolizes birth
- Queen is a symbol for mother
- Cloth is a symbol for nudity
- A voyage or expedition represents death
- Snake is related to sex
- Climbing a hill or a ladder is a symbol for sexual intercourse

Criticism of Freud's Theory

Humanity cannot disregard Freud for his various contributions. It does not matters so much as to what he said. What matters is that he opened the eyes of mankind in the field of psychology. Despite all this, he too was not immunized against criticism. He is criticized under the following grounds:

1. *Putting Much Stress on the Unconscious Mind*: It has been pointed out

by Woodworth that Freud has laid too much emphasis on the role of the unconscious mind in dreams. Most of the desires which are ignored and rejected still remain in the conscious mind. It is not true that all the frustrated desires reside in the unconscious mind.

2. *Putting Too Much Emphasis on Sex*: It has been pointed out that Freud has laid too much emphasis on the role of sexual impulse in relation to dreams. Again, some dreams are meaningless while some are mere responses to physical stimuli. Hence it is clear that only a small percent of dreams can be subscribed as sexual.

3. *McDougall's Criticism*: McDougall objects that Freud tried to interpret abnormal by the normal and normal by abnormal. He further criticizes that Freud's attempt regarding the interpretation of dreams may be helpful in understanding of some cases of neurosis, but that cannot be generalized.

Anyhow, we have to understand the limitation of Freud's interpretation of dreams as they mostly:

   a. Belong to subjective experience.
   b. Synthesized from empirical observations.
   c. Come from study of abnormal cases.
   d. Data is furnished by sick individuals.

Inspite of so many protests in opposition to Freudian hypothesis, it should be remembered that Freud's interpretation establishes to be the most successful and useful in the interpretation of individual dreams. His thesis on repressed desires in dreams, wish fulfillment in dreams, symbols in dreams, the dream mechanism, adoption of free association are wonderful and its benefits will be utilized for humanity till another alternative rises in the horizon of psychology.

B. Adler's Theory of Dreams

Adler maintains that the most important elements in dreams are the mental conflicts and repressions. Adler emphasizes the impulse of self-assertion as the genesis of dreams instead of sexual impulse as emphasized by Freud. Adler also differs from Freud in the interpretation of dreams. Adler attributes dreams to the future whereas Freud connects them with the individual's past. He cites the example of a worried young man who wants to get married. The worries may induce a dream of arrest and threatened imprisonment between the precincts of two countries.

C. Jung's Theory of Dreams

Jung, like Freud, accepts the importance of dreams. He also agrees with certain aspects of Freud and in other instances he gives his own verdict.

Jung asserts that dreams are the natural outcome of the whole psyche. According to him, psyche means a self-regulating system that maintains an equilibrium as the body does. Some psychologists interpret this as general life energy. Jung states that dreams are the natural product of the whole psyche.

He agrees with Freud that dreams have a genesis from the unconscious mind. But he rejects them as being representations of repressed desires. Moreover, he also rejects Freud's unconscious mind as the primary factor in the genesis of dreams. He ascribes collective or racial unconscious instead of unconscious mind as the genesis of dreams. Of course, he further asserts that dreams are due to motivation of the unconscious mind. He justifies by giving the example of a father and son who can have a similar dream since both come from the same stock and their racial conscious is of the same nature. For Jung, dreams are a common mental process in which the archetypes of racial characteristics, present in the collective unconscious are manifested.

Another important difference between the views of Freud and Jung is that Freud maintains that repression is must for dreams whereas Jung maintains that dreams can happen even without repression.

According to Freud and Adler, dreams are connected with the past and future respectively, while according to Jung they are connected with the present. Thus according to Jung's theory, dreams are the expression of an individual's unconscious approach towards his present problems.

Let us illustrate a dream to highlight the Jungian theory. Jung cites an example – a bachelor of a certain university who developed psycho-neurosis due to unemployment. He dreamt that he was climbing a ladder with his mother and sister and the moment they reached the highest rung of the ladder, he was informed that his sister is about to give birth to a child. Jung interpreted this dream by stating that mother symbolizes the sense of duty, sister represents true love and the child symbolizes rebirth. Hence accordingly, the whole phenomenon of dreams stands for the young individual's mode of adjustment to the present life situation.

Jung further directs the subjective and objective interpretation of dreams. Accordingly, dreams that occur from personal unconscious should be interpreted objectively, while dreams from the racial unconscious should be interpreted subjectively.

5. Perls's Theory of Dreams

Friedrich (Frederick) Salomon Perls (July 8, 1893 – March 14, 1970, Chicago), better known as **Fritz Perls**, was a renowned German-born psychiatrist and psychotherapist. He alongwith his wife Laura started 'Gestalt Therapy' in the 1940s. This *gestalt therapy* must not be confused with *Gestalt Psychology* although the former is somehow related but not identical to the later. The underlying endorsement of *Gestalt Therapy is awareness, the awareness of the unity of all present feelings and behaviours, and the connection between the self and its environment.*

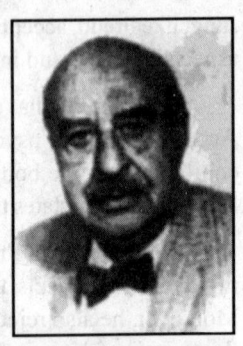

Fritz Perls (1893-1970)

Perls categorically rejected the idea that dream imagery was a part of universal symbolic language. He postulated that dreams embrace the unwanted, discarded, disowned part of the self. Each and every character or object that appears in dream is related to the individual who dreams it. Again each dream is unique to the individual who dreams it. Hence according to Perls it is important to initiate a dialogue with one's dream object despite living or non-living aspect and express in the present tense so that he can discover what aspect of his self is being disowned or rejected. By this one may be able to recognize and realize his unnoticed or masked feelings.

6. Activation-synthesis Theory of Dreams

In the year 76-77, Allan Hobson and Robert McCarley disregarded the Fruedian view of dream as subconscious wishes. They proposed a neurobiological theory of dream which is known as "Activation-synthesis theory of dream". According to them rapid eye movement, is produced druing REM (rapid eye movement) sleep, caused by stimulation of mid brain and forebrain cortical structures by ascending cholinergic PGO (ponto-geniculo-occipital) waves. Dream is produced by the activated forebrain out of this internally generated information. The activation-synthesis theory answers all the questions about the meaning of dreams by the simple means of announcing them meaningless. They also denied that dreams have meaning or are related to our real world environments.

Anyhow, this theory was very much citicized by various dream experts. Hence Hobson submitted a modified version of this theory acknowledging that dreams do reflect past memories, fears, hopes, and desires.

7. Mark Solm's Theory of Dreams

Initially Marks Solms accepted the theory given by Hobson by examining the dreams of patients who have come for the treatment of brain injuries in the neurosurgey departments of hospitals in Johanesburg and London. He conformed that the patients having damage to the parietal lobe stopped to dreaming. But Solms did not come across with cases of loss of dreaming with patients having brain stem damage. Then he reached to the conclusion that dreams are generated in the forebrain, but dreaming is not directly related to REM sleep.

8. Jie Zhang's Continual-activation Theory of Dreams

Jie Zhang suggested a theory of dream which combined Hobson's activation synthesis hypothesis with Solm's findings, the continual-activation theory of dreaming. He asserted that dreaming occurs as a result simultaneous brain activation and synthesis. To understand him let us go through the following points. According to Jhang

a. The function of sleep is to process, encode, and transfer the data from the temporary memory to the long-term memory.

b. Non-REM sleep processes the conscious-related memory (declarative memory).

c. REM sleep processes the unconscious related memory (procedural memory).

d. REM sleep is controlled by different brain mechanisms.

e. During REM sleep, the unconscious part of the brain keeps itself engaged in processing the procedural memory; in the meantime, the level of activation in the conscious part of the brain will fall down to a very low level. This will trigger the "continual-activation" mechanism to generate a data stream from the memory stores to flow through the conscious part of the brain.

DAY DREAMS

Day dreams can be compared to a type of imagination. We dream in sleep whereas in day dreams an individual dreams in an awake state. A day dream typically looks towards the future as if planning for possible action, only it is not a serious plan, nor necessarily a plan which could work in real life but it is merely a plan of imagination. Hence the plan made in a day dream belongs to the world of imagination and it has no feasible execution in real life situation. The tendency to day dream is mostly found amongst introverted persons. It creates a type of transient euphoria.

Types

Psychologists attribute two kinds of day dreams:
1. *Suffering Type Day Dream*: In this type of day dream the dreamer sees a dream of suffering due to non-achievement of the desired goal. Suppose you appeared in a M.B.B.S. entrance examination and could not qualify. Then you will see the dream with open eyes that due to the febrile condition prior to the night of the entrance test you did not do well in the examination. Here you became a suffering hero.
2. *Conquering Type Day Dream*: In this type you dream with open eyes that you have became a topper in the said M.B.B.S. entrance examination and the choice lies in your decision of your joining a medical college of your preference.

Thus, day dreams give you a transient relief from anxiety and frustration. However, making it a habit may lead to maladjustment and frustration.

Dream and Day Dreams: Some Differences

An individual dreams in a state of sleep whereas he sees day dreams in an awaken state. The individual can not manipulate dreams of sleep. He just remains a witness or passive observer to it. In day dreams an individual can manipulate the theme the way he desires. In dreams during the state of sleep, the individual remains like a victim while in a day dream he can act like a hero or are authority. Hence, in day dreams, he becomes more conscious about the themes than in the dreams of sleep. Moreover, day dreams are generally connected with the future in contrast to dreams during sleep which may be associated with any time – past, present or future events.

CLINICAL APPLICATION

The importance of dreams in relation to sickness is well known to homeopathy prior to the era of Freud. The proving of various drugs has certainly brought the significance of dream, forward. Moreover, dreams are the expression of the inner man. It is ascribed to general symptoms. Case taking without considering dreams remains incomplete. But we have to remember that it is the frequency that matters. If the dream occurs frequently then it should be given priority. Students are directed to consult a repertory, especially from the Kentian school: Kent, Schroyens, Zandvoort or even Murphy (the last repertory incorporates all the concepts of Boenninghauen, Kent and Boger in an excellent manner). Now we have to look at a case in a novel way by considering dreams from above. Of course, free association and dreams analysis will be of immense value in the treatment of sickness along with our therapeutic measures.

Chapter 10

EMOTIONS

We very often talk of emotions. Emotion is related to feeling. In homeopathy the role of emotions is obvious. Till date we have been talking of emotions, but no serious effort has been taken by us to study it in depth. It has been established that emotions have a great impact on the physical health. Emotions can initiate, precipitate or aggravate an illness. It is a subjective experience which forms one of the higher hierarchies in evaluation of symptoms during case taking and repertorisation in homeopathy.

Psychologists claim that our brain has 90% of feelings and only 10 % of reasoning capacity. Since time immemorial, emotional appeal has been widely used to achieve various goals by people of various walks of life. One can move a nation with emotion alone. Leaders, business persons and other agencies of the society have to manipulate emotion to meet their self-needs and motives.

History can be summoned in the witness box to state the role of emotion from the war of Mahabharata or Trojan till today's wars. It has been observed that the root cause of all the destruction and devastation is very much related to exploitation of emotions. We should also admit that every culture and civilization has been built on some edifices of emotion. Emotion is also a binding force. It is emotion that binds us. We feel more obligated and dutiful to those people with whom we are emotionally related. It is closely related to our feelings. The relation is so close that emotion and feelings are taken as synonyms to each other. Emotions make our life infinitely varied and interesting. It is the emotions that provides us thrill, excitement and pleasure and even sets a mission to lead a life of fulfillment. Without emotion, life becomes dull, drab and monotonous. Emotional undercurrents influence our perceptions, thoughts, learning attitude, etc. But it is unfortunate that not all emotions have a positive effect. While some emotions make our life happy, others make it horribly unhappy. So, emotion has become a necessary evil for our life. Naturally, it occupies an important place in the treatment of various illnesses, at least from the homeopathic point of view, as we primarily treat the patient and secondarily the disease. The role of emotions has been well realized by Hahnemann long before the birth of scientific psychology. Anyhow, the credit goes to Kent, who has been able to elucidate it further in his repertorial work. Kent's philosophy also bears testimony in revealing the importance of emotion in relation to sickness.

DEFINITION

We say 'Rosy looks happy', 'Raja is elated'. We also comment 'Rajeswari is sad', 'Alpana is excited', 'Vandana is angry', 'Lily is jealous', etc. These expressions are termed as emotion. Despite our understanding of these emotions, it is not easy to evolve a satisfactory definition to emotion. The closer we look, the more complex these reactions seem to be. Emotion is a very complex phenomenon. Hence it invites a number of difficulties with its various facets like perception, memory, learning (except thinking and reasoning) along with various types of emotions like pleasure, jealousy, sorrow, love, hate, fear, anger, etc. which come under its purview. Various approaches have been tried for defining emotion but not a single definition gives a satisfactory answer. The definition becomes very difficult because it is concerned with subjective experience. The expression of subjective experience varies from person to person.

The word 'emotion' derived from the Latin word 'e' out, 'movere' to move. This also means 'stir up, 'excited' or to 'agitate'.

Titchener defines emotion as an affective state of the organism. Affection means an elementary process that characterizes feeling and emotion e.g., love, hate, joy and sorrow. The term 'feeling' indicates a sort of dominance over consciousness. When the characteristics of affections are added to sensation, it may becomes either pleasant or unpleasant.

According to McDougall, emotion is made up of experience that accompanies the working of an instinctive impulse. In this theory, every instinct is accompanied by a specific emotion. The fourteen emotions which accompany the fourteen instincts are known as prime emotions (see the Chapter XV, Motivation).

Let us examine another comprehensive definition of emotion given by Young. He defines emotion 'as an acutely disturbed affective process or state which originates in the psychological situation and which is revealed by marked bodily changes in smooth muscles, glands and gross behavior.

After examining the above definitions and similar definitions in the background, we can go for the definition: Emotion is a stirred up state of the organism with a disturbance (usually strong) of the whole organism, which involves physiological disturbances with subjective cognition states (i.e., personal experience) with expressive behavior (with signs of internal reactions).

From above it is clear that it embodies the following three aspects:

1. First, emotion is of psychological origin.
2. Secondly, this is a state of acute disturbance.
3. Thirdly, emotion expresses itself through physiological changes.

CHARACTERISTICS OF EMOTION

Emotions are said to be the springs of life time actions and it has got some characteristics which are narrated below:

1. Emotion causes a plethora of physiological changes:
   a. Changes in:
      - Facial expression
      - Voice
      - Body movement
   b. Heart beat increases, it may become 140-150.
   c. Breathing becomes deep and rapid; the bronchioles expand stimulating the endocrine glands and liver to release sugar into the blood stream so that the skeletal muscles may utilize the needed energy.
   d. The mouth becomes dry.

   (*The physiological changes that occur during an emotional state can be measured with reliability.*)

2. All the above conditions are related to a sensation of pleasure or displeasure, which is also a characteristic of emotion.
3. Emotion or emotional experiences are purely subjective in nature. A given situation may evoke different emotional states in different individuals. A person may become scared and run away just looking at an enemy. Another person may become angry and pick a fight.

4. Usually emotions take place abruptly and without notice. It is almost impossible for a person to enter into a state of emotion in volition.
5. Emotion is a tripolar response having affective, cognitive and conative aspects.
6. Emotions have swings. They may swing like a pendulum. Hence a particular emotion may give rise to another emotion as a complement, even though they look diametrically opposite. A common man may become angry at trifles. A saint may display empathy in a similar situation. In our day to day life we can observe this fact. You may beat your younger brother out of anger. Soon you feel sorry for the act and enter in the state of empathy (or sympathy) like a *Mezereum* patient. After some moments both the states may evaporate.
7. Emotion does not have any particular predilection for a particular age group, sex, creed, religion, society or race. Emotion may be related to one and all. Of course, the state and intensity may vary from person to person. The emotion of a child cannot be the same as that of an adult. The emotion of a child is intense, frequent and short lived in comparison to an adult.
8. Very often the cause of an emotion can be traced to non-fulfillment or blocking of a wish or goal.

Clarification of Some of its Similar Terminologies

a. Emotion vs Feeling

Very often emotion is labelled as a synonym of feeling. The reason is very simple: There exist some expressions of emotions that posses the dual quality of emotion as well as feeling. For example, anger, love, hate, fear, pleasure, gaiety, etc. can be attributed to both; emotion as well as feeling. Moreover, most of the emotions are linked with feelings. Emotions may be caused by either happiness (say happiness of parents on the return of their son from the Kargil war) or sorrow (say sorrow for parents as the son became a martyr in the Kargil war). Feelings can be pleasant or painful. Inspite of such close resemblance, emotions and feelings differ from each other to a greater extent in a various ways.

b. Emotion vs Motivation

On many occasions emotions and motivations are intimately related, which can be perceived from the following pairs:

Aggression	Fear
Sex	Lust
Maternal drive	Tenderness
Escape	Fear

Interestingly, emotional behavior itself is a strongly motivated behavior. It is the motivation that gives strength to emotion. Sometimes some motivated behavior renovates itself into an emotion. Stronger motivation instigates an emotion whereas a weaker motivation fails to yield it. Some psychologists regard emotion as merely a facet of motivation. Moreover, emotion plays a crucial part in motivational patterns.

ROLE OF LEARNING IN EMOTION

Frequently, it appears to us that emotion is innate. Let us take an example of an emotion, say fear. Fear of something strange seems to be largely innate, but maturation and knowledge are required as a background for perceiving such emotions. Watson, the founder of behavior school conducted various experiments to demonstrate the effects of learning in the development of emotion. Watson carried out an experiment with a eleven month old infant named Albert. Albert was a normal child. He was only afraid of sudden loud noises at that time. He was not afraid of white rats. Watson gradually made Albert afraid of white rats adopting conditional principles (see Chapter VI, Learning). Albert was exposed to white rats and a loud sound was made the moment Albert tried to hold the rats. Every time Albert touched the rat he was frightened by a loud sound. Thus, he became afraid of the white rats. Now the original neutral rat became a 'conditional stimulus' of fear for Albert. Not only this, later he also developed fear of white objects which closely resembled the rat in certain respects.

We can observe such examples from our day to day life. Fear of ghosts, dark places, high places, etc. are more common in childhood due to induction from various agencies, whereas imaginary or superadded fears are more frequent in adulthood and later years of life.

Now we can conclude that when a given emotional producing stimulus is associated with another neutral stimulus, the second stimulus (i.e., neutral) also gradually produces the same emotional effect that was produced by the former.

EMOTION: ROLE OF PHYSIOLOGY AND BIOCHEMISTRY

A. Role of Limbic System (Hypothalamus) in Emotion

The limbic system plays a major role in emotions. In lower animals, it forms a very large part of the brain in man. Hypothalamus is a part of the limbic system that is actively involved in emotions.

Hypothalamus plays a crucial role in emotional behavior. Various experiments on animals like, dogs and cats have been conducted. It has been observed that by taking away the hypothalamus of the animal, it became devoid of emotions. It has also been observed that the removal of any other part of the brain does not affect emotions so significantly. Any injury to the hypothalamus during accidents also confirms the stated condition. Moreover, medicines like Amytel and Metrazol, which act on the hypothalamus induce noteworthy changes in the emotional behavior of in human beings. Hypothalamus can execute primitive emotions like rage, fear, sex, etc. It has also been observed that the ventro-medial medial nuclei of the hypothalamus restrains execution of emotional behaviors. When the ventro nucleus of hypothalamus of tamed rats were plucked by surgical measures, the rats became wild and mauled iron rods relentlessly.

B. Role of Cortex in Emotion

The specific details about the role of cortex in emotion is not known. However, it is believed that the cerebral cortex is concerned with sensation, learning, speech, memory, reasoning, etc. It is also involved in current happenings and those of remote past – a process that helps us to interpret the situation and decides whether or not an emotion is to be provoked. The cerebral cortex has action over visceral activity, which is commonly associated with emotional response. When the cerebral cortex is damaged or it is under the influence of alcohol, the person becomes extremely emotional and does wrong things.

C. Role of neurotransmitters

Recent works suggest that neurotransmitters play a vital role in controlling emotion. More than 50 chemical substances have been proved to function as neurotransmitters such as Acetylcholine, Epinephrine, Nor-epinephrine, Dopamine, etc. Acetylcholine is secreted by neurons in many areas of the brain including the motor neurons that innervate the skeletal muscles. Acetylcholine is related to depression, fear and subsequent defensive behavior.

TYPES OF EMOTIONS

Two types of classification are widely accepted by most of the psychologists.

One group of psychologists classify emotions under following heads:

a. *Simple Emotions*: In simple emotional states, usually only one emotion exists, say anger, fear, love, etc.

b. *Complex Emotions*: Here more than one emotion exists at one time. Hatred is one type of complex emotion. It comprises of anger and indifference with a small amount of fear. Kindness is a complex emotion having two components – love and sympathy.

Another group of psychologists observe the following types of emotions:

a. *Egoistic*: Such type of emotions are related to self. In this type of emotion, the individual is like a pivot around which his egoistic emotions revolve. Emotions like anger, joy, fear are termed as egoistic emotions. But these emotions may result in both, promotion and demotion of self-interest.

b. *Ego-altruistic*: This emotion is related to self-satisfaction where opinion of others have a bearing. Examples are power, praise, respect, recognition, etc.

c. *Altruistic*: Such emotions are related to help others. Sympathy and empathy are under this type of emotion.

d. *Impersonal:* Ideal aspects of emotions have been included under it. Emotions like beauty, truth, benediction, etc. belong to the realm of impersonal emotions. Most emotions belonging to morality, ethics, religiousness (not parochial idea of sector religion) are incorporated under this type of emotion.

THEORIES OF EMOTION

Over the years several approaches have emerged to study emotions. You will be surprised to know that there exist as many as 50 theories of emotions. We will restrict ourselves to the following important theories of emotion only:

I. James-Lange theory of emotion.
II. Canon-Bard theory of Emotion.
III. Stanley Schachter and Jerome Singer Theory.
IV. Richard Solomon and John Corbit Theory.

Out of the above four, the first two are very important. We will discuss the following live situation with these two.

Imagine that in one of your curriculums you are supposed to present a paper in a seminar. As you proceed to the front of the dias in the seminar hall, and meet the audience including your professor and panel of judges, you become nervous, your heart beat increases, mouth becomes dry and you feel the beads of perspiration on the forehead. In short, you become terrified. What is the basis of this feeling? The answers can be pondered from below.

I. James-Lange Theory

William James is considered as the founder of Functional School of Psychology. James-Lange theory is an extended work of William James's theory of emotion that appeared in the year 1884 which has had tremendous impact on psychological thought since its formulation.

Generally we think that when we lose our fortune, say in a business, we grieve and cry. Similarly when we see a tiger, we become frightened and run away. Again, when we are offended by our enemies, we feel angry and attack. But according to James-Lange theory, *physiological changes make an emotion felt*, i.e., their theory is exactly opposite to popular belief. In other words, this theory states that *perception causes physiological or bodily changes before the individual is aware of having any emotion.*

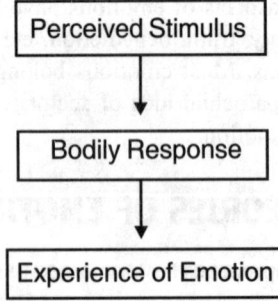

II. Canon-Bard Theory

This theory was developed by physiologist Walter B. Canon in 1927. Philip Bard, another American physiologist advanced the same view point in 1937 and hence this theory is called so .

EMOTIONS

Walter Canon was a physiologist and showed that physiological changes in many emotional states were identical.

Canon Bard's theory basically owes its origin to Sherrington's work on animal reflexes.

In 1927, Walter B. Cannon criticized James-Lange's theory of emotions under the following grounds:

1. He postulated that the physiological changes do not necessarily evoke emotion. Physiological changes can be induced by vigorous exercises or with medicines (like an injection of adrenalin) which does not produce a particular type of emotion. Therefore, he concluded that physiological changes alone cannot produce emotions.
2. Many actors do not feel the emotion when they are enacting it.
3. Again James-Lange theory fails to differentiate between evoking emotion and unproductive physical changes.
4. They also argued that emotions are often felt rapidly. We see a tiger and immediately become afraid of it. How could a viscera which reacts slowly be the basis of such sudden emotions as suggested by James-Lange. Hence the very idea that bodily response causes us to experience emotions is questionable.
5. Moreover, the James-Lange theory failed to point out the difference between emotion producing and unproductive physical changes. For example, hunger and pain in stomach cannot be attributed to emotion. Hence every bodily change cannot be subscribed to emotion.
6. They also condemned the theory stating that emotion cannot be differentiated on the basis of physiological changes. They argued that if emotion is the result of physiological changes, then we can expect different set of physiological changes for each type of emotion. On the contrary Cannon and Bard observed many of the same bodily changes occur in coincidence with different emotional states.

Canon – Bard theory of emotion came into existence as a reaction to James-Lange Theory. This theory postulates that *bodily arousal and emotional experience occur simultaneously.* In other words, Canon stated that emotional inputs were processed almost simultaneously by the thalamus and hypothalamus. Thalamus controls emotion whereas hypothalamus controls bodily responses. Let us again take the example of the tiger. You fear a tiger even if your body were totally paralyzed because fear and running are mediated by different centers in your brain.

Examples of Canon-Bard Theory of Emotion:
a. Anger is generally associated with an increase in gastric activity, whereas.
b. Fear is generally associated with an inhibition of gastric functions.

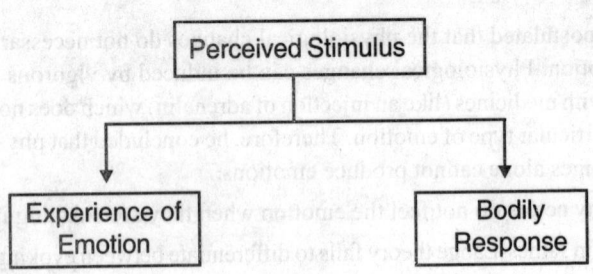

Criticism to Canon-Bard Theory

Although Canon-Bard were able to provide a more advanced theory in comparison to James-Lange, yet they are not able to free themselves from criticism. Their theory is being criticized under the following grounds:

a. Stimulation of hypothalamus is attributed to arousing emotion. But this arousal of emotion is short, less adaptive, less oriented and rather stereotyped in comparison to emotions caused in a natural way. It seems that in natural emotions, the nervous system plays a role in the causation of emotional behavior.
b. Complete removal of hypothalamus in a decorticated animal (cortex is related to adaptation of emotional behavior) has no effect on the rage action.

Which One is Superior: James-Lange or Canon-Bard?

'Until recently, most evidence seemed to favor the Canon-Bard approach: Emotion provoking events produce both physiological arousal and the subjective experience we label as emotion. Now, however, the pendulum of scientific opinion has moved towards greater acceptance of James-Lange approach – the view that we experience emotions because of our awareness of physiological reactions to various stimuli or situations. Several lines of evidence point to this conclusion. First, studies conducted with modern equipment indicate that different emotions are indeed associated with different patterns of physiological activity (Levenson, 1992). Not only do various emotions feel different, they also result from somewhat different patterns of bodily changes, including contrasting patterns of brain and muscle activity (Ekman, Davidson, & Friesen, 1990, Izard, 1991).

Second, support for the James-Lange theory is also provided by research on the *facial feedback hypothesis* (Laird, 1984; Zajonc & McIntosh, 1992). This hypothesis suggests that changes in our facial expression sometimes produce shifts in our emotional experiences. In view of such findings, the facial feedback hypothesis has been renamed the *peripheral feedback effect*, to indicate that emotions can be influenced by more than just facial expressions. While there are many complexities in examining this hypothesis, the results of several studies offer support for its accuracy (e.g., Ekman et al, 1990). These findings suggest that there may be a substantial grain of truth in the James-Lange theory (Zajonc, Murphy, & Inglehart, 1989). While subjective emotional experiences are often produced by specific external stimuli, as the Cannon-Bard view suggests, emotional reactions can also be generated by changes in and awareness of our own bodily state, as the James-Lange contends (Ekman, 1999).

(Baron, 2004)

III. Stanley Schachter and Jerome Singer Theory

This can be taken as the synthetic view of James-Lange and Canon-Bard theory of emotion. Like James and Lange, Schachter and Singer presumed that our experiences of emotion grow from the awareness of our bodily state. Like Cannon and Bard, they believed that an emotional experience requires a conscious interpretation of the event as well.

Thus Stanley Schachter proposed a two-factor theory of emotion. According to this theory, the experience of an emotion is based on a physiological change plus a cognitive interpretation of the change. Our perception, memories and their interpretations are indeed essential ingredients of emotion. The two factors are the two ingredients – physical arousal, and a cognitive label.

They observed that people do indeed interpret their emotion but not solely from bodily changes. Schachter and Singer argued that people interpret physical sensation within a specific context. Observers cannot interpret what a persons' crying means unless they know the situation to which that behavior occurs. If a man cries at a funeral, we suspect he is sad; if he cries at his daughter's wedding, we think he is crying out of happiness.

Schachter and Singer carried out an experiment with adrenalin. They took three groups for experimentation, where all subjects were informed that they were going to study and assess 'Suproxine' – a fictitious vitamin for vision (i.e., these people were not told that they were being given adrenalin actually).

Group one was informed that the 'vitamin' produced certain side effects, such as heart palpitation and tremors which are the real side effects of adrenalin.

Group two was informed about the side effects not usually associated with adrenalin, such as itching and headache.

Group three was informed that the injection had no side effects.

The first group reacted in a way similar to the physiological manifestations of adrenalin i.e., increase in heart rate, etc.

Since the other two groups were given no explanation for their physiological arousal, the researchers expected them to attribute their arousal to "emotional" factors. So, the second group while waiting for the vision test, came in contact with a group of pre-arranged and trained people who acted in a happy and frivolous manner like throwing paper aeroplanes, laughing, playing ring, etc. Similarly, the third group was also surrounded by another pre-arranged and trained group of people who acted annoyed and angry, tearing up questionnaire which they were supposed to fill up, etc.

The subjects of the last two groups, who did not expect any physiological arousal, had no way of explaining the sensations they were experiencing.

The second group expressed euphoria whereas the third group expressed anger, depending on the emotion displayed by the trained persons in contrast to group one who had expected heart palpitations and tremors. Moreover, group one did not experience the euphoria of second group or anger of third group.

Schachter – Singer Theory

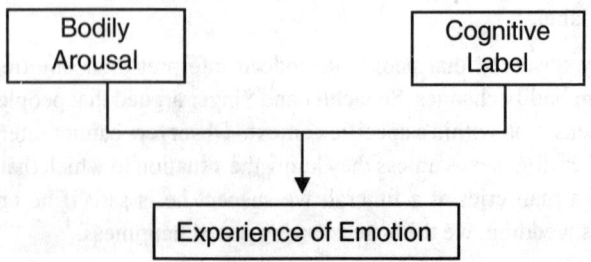

Criticism of Schachter-Singer Theory

a. Many depressant drugs affect all the three aspects of emotion:

   i.   The internal physiological responses (heart rate, muscle tone, blood pressure).

   ii. The behavior (sluggish movement, dropping facial muscles).

   iii. The subjective feelings (like feeling of depression).

   The action of depressant drugs on the autonomic nervous system produces the emotion of depression without any cognitive interpretation on the part of the individual.

b. Very often we feel emotions before thinking. It is not mandatory that emotional feelings are subject to a thinking process. Sometimes our emotions are more abrupt than our interpretations of the situation. Many of our emotional reactions are attributed to beyond our rational thinking.

c. Most of the important emotions, such as, love, elation, anger, guilt, etc. happen from our interpretations, memories and inferences.

d. Some emotional responses, especially likes, dislikes and fears do not involve conscious thinking. We may instantly fear a cockroach even though we know it is harmless.

e. Conditioned emotions cannot be easily altered by thinking (Watson's Albert experiment).

IV. Richard Solomon and John Corbit Theory (1982)

This is also known as *Opponent Process Theory of Emotion*. Very often we notice that a strong emotional reaction is followed by the opposite reaction. Is it not? Let us take the example of a common emotion, say anger. Very often extreme anger is followed by calmness. Similarly, elation is followed by let down. This relationship is the focus of the opponent theory of emotion. This theory was proposed by Richard Solomon and John Corbit in the year 1982. This theory states:

a. An emotional reaction to a stimulus is followed by an opposite reaction automatically (*Can you recall the law in physics: Every action has an equal and opposite reaction? Can you recall Organon : Primary and secondary action?*)

b. *Repeated exposure to a stimulus causes the initial reaction to weaken and the opposite reaction to strengthen.*

Canon Theory
A tragic event always makes me cry and feel sad.

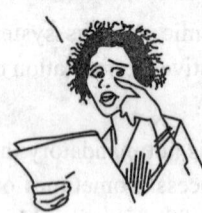

James-Lange Theory
In crying, so I'm save I must feel sad.

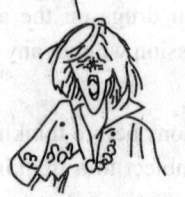

Schachter-Singer Theory
I felt strange inside and everyone around me may crying, then I started crying became I was sad

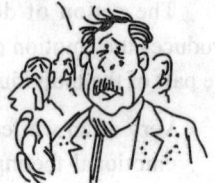

(Source: Lefton, 3rd ed.)

SOME COMMON PATTERNS OF EMOTION IMPORTANT FROM HOMEOPATHIC POINT OF VIEW

Fear

Fear is one of the most common patterns of emotions that deserve our study. It is a very common emotion in our life. It is a learned pattern of emotion. It is marked at the age of 3 and 11 at the peak. It has also been observed that girls and females are more prone to fear compared to that of their counterparts i.e., boys and males. Fear is induced by fearful stimuli or may be learned by imitation from the behavior of somebody else. Fear may also be developed from an unpleasant situation, say abnormal fear of visiting a hospital or doctor.

Children and babies may get afraid of strange persons or objects, loud noises, horrible visions of animals, dark and high places, etc. We all know the induction of fear of ghosts in children.

Psychological Approach

a. Reconditioning the child from fearful objects.
b. Acquaint the child with unfamiliar objects that he can come across in future.
c. Educate the child with a plausible and practical solution to meet a fearful situation.

d. Divert the attention of the child from fearful stimuli.
e. Advise to leave the place of source of fear.

Homeopathic Steps

Numerous rubrics sub-rubrics have been devoted for emotion in our repertories (like Kent's, Murphy's, Zandvoort's, Schroyen's, etc.) which may be used for a positive outcome.

Anger

Anger means displeasure: A strong feeling of grievance and displeasure. It is a strong feeling that comes when one has been wronged or insulted, or when one sees cruelty or injustice; the feeling that makes people want to quarrel or fight.

Anger is one of the common emotional patterns which is prevalent in all age groups, starting from infants to old people. It has a tremendous impact on the personality of an individual.

Anger is a general response to the following conditions:
a. When the behavior of an individual is blocked. If somebody (or situation) puts limits unduly on the freedom of your action, or thinking, you are apt to become irritated and express anger.
b. When an individual cannot reach the desired goal.

The anger may be expressed through screaming, kicking, crying, clenching the fist, distorting the face, etc. Boys and gents are found to be more prone to anger than girls and ladies. It has also been observed that people belonging to autocratic atmosphere become angrier in comparison to people belonging to a democratic set up. Moreover, the former express anger more in intensity and magnitude than the latter. Young children show physical movement when they get angry but the older children generally use verbal attack.

Developmental Changes in Expression of Anger

We will discuss the development under the following heads:
1. **Early Childhood:** Children express their emotion of anger by breaking things within their reach, by withdrawing from the situation in resentment, etc. There exists a three-fold expression of anger by a child:

i. *Displacing the Energy Randomly*: Anger is expressed by kicking, or screaming.

ii. *Resistance*: The children may express their anger by resisting it. They may resist without obeying what they are told to do or doing just the opposite. They may express their anger verbally or by motor resistance.

iii. *Retaliation*: Children may express their anger through motor or verbal attempts at revenge, such as biting or attacking the agent with fists or throwing away something. This is particularly seen between two to five years of age.

2. **Later Childhood:** During later childhood, anger is expressed in the form of excessive aggressive behavior directed towards something or someone.

3. **Adolescent:** Adolescents express this emotion by wearing a twisted look, wrinkled facial expression, angry eyes and running away in resentment. They generally refuse food and drink when they are angry.

Sources of Anger

The chief causes of anger are:

1. Disease state. We must not forget the miasmatic background of the child or adult. This also includes a weak state of health, fatigue, etc.
2. Deprivation of physical needs like anger, thirst or sex.
3. Obstruction in child's activity by an agent like, interference from elders and class mates.
4. When a child is being teased, being lied to, being treated unfairly, being imposed on by elder brothers and sisters or other people being bossy or sarcastic.
5. When wishes cannot be fulfilled.
6. Neglect and non-payment of attention to a child. The situation becomes worse if another child or children are paid more attention or praised.
7. Family worries also reflect in the shape of anger.
8. Frustrations beget anger.
9. Various conflicts may also result in anger when the children are asked to do routine physical habits like rising and going to bed early, washing their face, are stopped from watching cartoon shows, etc. and in case of

adolescents (and adults), when they are asked or forbidden to do some activity.

Positive Aspect of Anger

Anger is the sign of life and spirit. It is important to give a proper direction to this emotional state, so that it serves a good purpose in various situations of life. Very often it helps in letting out the pent-up energy of the individual. Expression of anger instead of repression invites the attention of parents and physician for internal disturbance of vital force (or principle). The power of anger increases the working capacity of the person who gets the challenge from the situation.

Negative Aspect of Anger

Sometimes undesirable anger is likely to complicate life, spoil happiness, and reduce efficiency rather than increasing it. It might cause digestive disorders, disorders in blood pressure, and disturbances in the internal physiological system. Anger also interferes with reasoning, and sometimes suspends rational thinking. That is why it has to be sublimated and controlled.

Anger: A Practical Approach to Meet it

We must remember that anger is mostly a pathological state. Its importance has been highlighted by our beloved masters Hahnemann and Kent. Kent has built a school imparting special focus on mental symptoms, where irritability and anger has been given higher importance. The author has been successful in treating many situations of anger with homeopathic medicines. He has got excellent results from *Chamomilla*. Moreover, medicines like *Hepar sulph.*, *Nux vomica*, *Staphysagria*, *Colocynthis* are important medicines which are required for day to day needs.

However, despite the following practical approach may prove very beneficial in preventing the state of anger in our clinic or hospital.

An individual should follow the following guidelines,

1. The exciting cause of anger must be removed.
2. The individual must be able to divert his attention somewhere else or become busy in something else so that anger can be repelled.
3. Overwork and fatigue must be restrained. It should be substituted with outdoor games, morning walk or yoga.
4. As far as possible, corporeal punishment must be avoided for children

and students. The reprimand and punishment should be done in a planned manner by an alert mind, so that the child or student may not be injured physically or mentally.

5. The child should be given due importance. His ego must not be pricked. It is a wrong notion to think that to spare the rod is to spoil the child.
6. The environment at school and other institutions should be congenial for the students.
7. Competition and ambition are the genesis of frustration and anger. Hence, education on this aspect must be imparted in a judicious manner.
8. Parents must be given health education in our clinic and hospital so that they can avoid those situations which are likely to cause anger for their off-springs.
9. Community events should be organised involving the participation of teachers, doctors and other relevant personalities for shaping out a better India.

Homeopathic Remedies

Medicines like *Chamomilla, Staphysagria, Natrium mur., etc.* can renew somebody's life. *Author considers Chamomilla as almost specific for anger. He has been able to meet the crisis of anger successfully by this medicine. Of course, your experience may differ as per your circumstance.*

Jealousy and Envy

Jealousy finds a place in the sphere of social and familial cause. A child may become jealous at the birth of a sibling. The familial rearing and preference given to a child may give rise to jealousy amongst other children of the family. Similarly, other factors like competition in class, securing a job, promotion of an individual may initiate jealousy for the rest of the competitors. It has been observed that the female gender is found to be more jealous in comparison to the male gender.

Jealousy and envy come from the feeling of insecurity and inadequacy in situations the person regards as crucial to his happiness and welfare. It keeps an individual in a state of emotional stress. Like fear, jealousy rises to the peak at the age of 3 and 11.

Jealousy and envy are separate and distinct emotional patterns, though

	Jealousy	Envy
No. of persons involved	More than two	Two
Development	Early	Late
Understanding	Cannot understand	Opposite
Anxiety	More	Less
Associated frustration	Less	More
Associated anxiety	More	Less
Expansion	Out of fear and anger	
Onset	Early childhood	Later
Feeling	As if he has been deprived of something that is rightfully his and that he is incapable of defending himself against this threat to his security.	As if immediate stimulus is a possession of another person (say a car).
Miasm	Psoric	Syphilitic

Homeopathic Remedies

Important homeopathic medicines for jealousy are *Lachesis*, *Hyoscyamus*, *Nux vomica*, etc. You can refer to various repertories to pursue an in-depth study.

Grief

This emotion results from damage to an object of one's desire. Grief ensues when our near or dear one is lost. Some important expressions of grief are:

a. Weeping.
b. Crying.
c. Sobbing.
d. Contraction of chest.
e. Running of tears from eyes
f. Catching of throat etc.

Ignatia seems to be the most important remedy for grief. Also, one should think of *Natrium mur.* and other important remedies from the repertory.

Joy

Joy is the opposite state of grief. Joy is the outcome of fulfillment of one's desire like getting a lottery or success in an examination, etc. Joy is the sign of good health. Some important expressions of joy are:

a. Smiling.
b. Laughing.
c. Jumping about.
d. Clapping.
e. Dancing.
f. Glittering eyes, etc.

Joy, pleasure, delight, etc. are needed for release of pent up emotions Although joy makes us happy and contented yet we should not exceed its limit, which may prove harmful. The important medicine for excessive joy is *Coffea*.

Love

It is a complex emotion. It is the blend of mercy, sympathy, affection and even sex. Very often emotional arousal of this kind is caused by sexual instinct. Mother's love for her child is related to her sentiment. Interestingly, two seemingly contradictory states – selfishness and selflessness are found in love. Some of the expressions of love are:

a. Kissing.
b. Embracing.
c. Cuddling.
d. Hugging.
e. Taking on the lap.
f. Caressing.
g. Sighing.
h. Thrilling, etc.

It is a positive emotion. This must be read with its rival rubrics like lewdness, shamelessness, lasciviousness, nymphomania, libertinism, naked want to be, obscene, etc. from a standard repertory.

Affections

Affections are fond or tender feelings in the direction of somebody or something .It is a positive and pleasant emotion articulated towards a person or thing. It is intended for somebody who gives us pleasure and satisfaction. A father and mother have great affection towards their only child.

Sentiments

The word owes its origin from the developed French word '*sentimentum*' (means opinion, feeling) and from the Latin word '*sentire*' which means to '*feel*'. Sentiments are a calculated appeal to feeling or emotion, especially that is in excess and beyond reasoning. It also implies refined and tender feeling expressed in work or art. It is a thought or idea based on feeling or emotion. It is a weak emotion. It generally develops in early school life. Feelings like patriotism, school spirit, etc. develop during the period of adolescence and can be attributed to sentiments.

CLINICAL APPLICATION

Emotions are salts of our life. They make our life colorful. The lack of balance in emotions may be disruptive. When an emotion becomes overpowering, the efficiency of the individual is lost. The individual may become a burden to himself as well as to the society. It seems, logic and reasoning control the society, but it is a fact that nations are swept with emoting. Repressed emotions may prove another menace to an individual's life. Let us take an example of an employer, who constantly and continually harasses one of its employees. The employee may eventually revolt and cause a havoc. Long continued worries and grief may impair the physical health of an individual. Recent work on emotion has revealed the fact it can cause various psycho-somatic illnesses, which had been postulated by Hahnemann long before the birth of scientific psychology. The importance of emotional reaction has been associated with a number of illnesses like peptic ulcers, asthma, migraine headaches, chronic fatigue, diabetes, high blood pressure, skin eruptions, etc. Again, it is obvious that long-term emotional stress can impair a person's physical and mental efficiency.

Manipulation of emotional reaction through 'lie detector' helps us detect crime. The physiological changes accompanying intense emotions are the basis for the use of the polygraph, commonly known as the 'lie detector', in checking the reliability of an individual's statements. The polygraph measures emotion by objective physiological evidence like heart rate, blood pressure, GSR (Galvanic Skin Response), etc.

In homeopathy, emotions have a special place in evaluation of symptoms. In homeopathy, emotion and its off-shoot symptoms are considered of great importance in relation to psychosomatic medicine. The author has successfully treated many cases of peptic ulcer syndrome, asthma, migraine with *Ignatia, Natrum mur., Causticum*, etc. detecting emotional disturbances like, death of near or dear ones (i.e. grief) or grief of recent or remote origin as the cause. Detection of emotion and the art of coping with it can open a new way of life for a patient. The role of placebo has become of paramount importance in our clinic, as these can be related with emotional reactions. Placebo discharges psychological influences arising from the patient's perception.

You should further consult repertories like Kent's, Murphy's, Zandvoort's, Schroyen's for rubrics of emotion so that you can help your patient in a better way.

Emotional Training

As a homeopath, we must be aware of training in emotion. This would be an adjuvant therapy for emotional sickness.

1. Sublimation.
2. Catharsis, that is, giving a free outlet to emotions.
3. Redirection.
4. Advising the patient not to lead a lethargic life. He must be exhorted to keep himself busy.
5. Adoption of co-curricular activities.
6. Creating a healthy environment.
7. Inhibition and repression.
8. Punishment, if needed.

Chapter 11

REMEMBERING (MEMORY) AND FORGETTING

Once memory was believed to be a faculty or an ability instead of the present concept of a process, a functional term. Hence, instead of the term memory, remembering is used which signifies a process, an act of remembering. The credit of experiments on remembering and forgetting goes to Hermann Ebbinghaus (1850-1909), a German psychologist. In 1885, he published his first book *"Uber das Gedachais"* on memory. Using himself as a subject, Ebinghaus memorised and recalled hundreds of nonsense syllables. The non-sense syllables were developed by combining various letters in such a way that meaningless words like, XUV, MOR, DEG, etc.

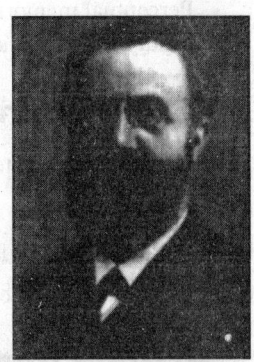

Hermann Ebbinghaus (1850-1909)

could be formed. Many of his findings about the nature of memory and forgetting have stood the test of time and are valid even today.

DEFINITION

Memory may be defined as the ability of an organism to restore information from the earlier learning.

CONTENTS OF OUR MEMORY

Contents of our memory can be broadly classified under:
I. Personal memories.
II. Generic memories.
III. Skill memories

I. Personal Memories

Personal memories pertains to personal experiences, interactions and incidents. We can recall these events through mental images like lovely days of our childhood or past events.

II. Generic Memories

Generic memories are not related to personal memories. It includes:

a. Concepts like 'love', 'faith", 'truth', etc.
b. Concepts like 'cousin', 'tree', 'sea', 'house', etc.
c. Perceptual memories like smell of rose, sweetness of chocolate, scenic beauty, color of a shirt, sensation of heat or cold, etc.

III. Skill Memories

Skill memories are related to skills like:

a. Ability of solving a problem: Numerical, puzzles, quizzes, etc.
b. Motor skills: Driving a vehicle, operating a computer, etc.
c. Remembering a phone number, bank account number, PIN, PAN, etc.

MEMORY MODELS: HOW DO WE REMEMBER?

Before understanding a memory model, first we should understand what a model is.

Usually scientists build models to meet two major goals of science, viz.,

I. Accurate description of subject matter.
II. Explanation that clarifies how the processes of an experiment are being studied or operated.

Generally, a model is proposed after a large quantity of data is gathered on a given topic or subject. The purpose of the model is to organize these research findings and to help researchers formulate predictions that can be tested in further studies. In other words, the models are miniature systems which try to explain how a system works, with all of its interrelated ingredients.

Psychology, being a science also embodies such model concepts. Hence, psychologist have developed various models for memory and forgetting, of which two most widely accepted models are given below:

Efficient learning depends upon the nature and type of materials. It is our common experience that some type of materials are easy whereas other materials are difficult to remember. It is also a common observation that logical, meaningful and familiar subjects can be easily remembered. Similarly, learning with understanding is far superior to rote memory. Again it has been found that materials of concrete and great associated value lead towards better memorisation

2. Retention

It has already been stated that memory is retained through the generation of memory traces called engrams. These engrams or memory traces or neural traces are formed out of consolidation of learning. The sum of retention depends upon the consolidation of the memory traces, which ultimately depend upon activities with which the individual is engaged during retention interval. The capacity of retention varies from person to person as it is the result of interaction of genetic endowment and hereditary predisposition. Moreover, children have relatively less power of retention due to imperfect development of nervous system. Old persons also have less power of retention due to corrosion in the nervous system.

3. Recall

By recall, the residues of learning are brought back to conscious level. When you appear for an examination, you recall all you have learnt throughout the year. You answer the question paper in the examination hall by recalling the learning what is thriving in your memory. Then you put it down in black and white. Of course, this recollection cannot be the same as that of original learning, still its contents look a lot like the original and are identical to a significant part of the previous learning. Recall becomes good if learning and retention is good.

4. Recognition

The final step in memory is recognition. Recognition means 'knowing again'. In other words, recognition means identification. Sometimes, recall appears after recognition. Hence it becomes easier to recognise a person before recalling. When you go to the railway station for receiving a friend, recall is necessary before recognition. But when you suddenly meet a long lost friend, you recognise him instantly before recalling. Moreover, recognition is easier than recall, because the object becomes evident in recognition and not assorted with some other new material. On the other hand, in recall, material is absent and has to be reproduced from memory. The process of recognition is affected by one's attitude, bias, values and other inner motives.

TYPES OF MEMORY

Psychologists have recognised various types of memories, out of which following important ones are described:

1. Sensory Memory

This type of memory helps us to recall something immediately after it is perceived. The retention time is exceedingly brief, say a fraction of a second to a few seconds. This disappears after overlapping new pieces of information. We need this type of memory while entering a hotel or lodge. We just see the number of rooms and then we do not pay much attention to it. Likewise we take the help of such type of memory while locating a seat in a theatre or movie hall, reservation coach, looking at traffic signals, while passing a traffic jam, etc.

2. Short Term Memory

This is longer than sensory memory. This may last up to 30 seconds. Usually five to nine items can be held in short term memory at any time and 11-14 items can be recalled from short term memory. Anyhow, such type of memory can be increased with tricks and manipulation.

3. Long Term Memory

In contrast to short term memory, long term memory has a seemingly limitless capacity to store information according to meaning, pattern, etc. with little or no loss. It can encode information through meaning, pattern and allied characters. For example, names of self, father, mother, date of birth, etc. come under such type of memory. Thus memory is retained for a longer period.

4. Episodic Memory

Episodic memories as these are concerned with episodes and events.

We can also call it personal memory. The memory is related to self's life and episodes. The episode that occurs in life is stored in episodic memory. You can recall an episode of an incident that has occurred recently or years back.

5. Semantic Memory

As contrast to episodic memory, semantic memory is concerned with public, that is outside personal affairs. It is connected to generalised ideas, principles, rules, etc., which are not concerned to personal memory. Semantic memories help in storing and retrieving a collection of relationships between events and association of ideas e.g., recalling capitals of various states of Indian republic, the meaning and symbol of H_2O, Kent's 12 observations, etc.

6. Photographic Memory

As the caption suggests, it stands for memories possessed by a person who can recall a scene in photographic detail.

7. Para-normal Memory

In such type of memory an individual can recall the incidents of past life. These are exceptional memory abilities gifted to very few persons.

TRAINING AND IMPROVING MEMORY

It is a debatable and controversial question whether memory can be improved and trained. Memory training cannot be compared to muscle training in a gymnasium. Psychologists claim that memory cannot be improved through any kind of exercise.

We know that the memory process consists of four stages viz., learning, retention, recall and recognition.

It is said that the capacity of retention is native and inherited and hence cannot be improved by training. Psychologists stress that steps can be taken to protect the retention ability of an individual by some measures and one can not say whether it can be improved by training.

It is also a question of doubt whether the ability of recognition can be improved as the process is prompt, unplanned and unstructured.

Learning can be improved by training, which may help in improvement of memory.

Some suggestions have been provided by psychologist to obtain the optimum ability of memorisation for which the following steps are suggested:

1. Recitation

The mental repetition of something is called recitation. It is an active way of study. Through this an individual can save time. Recitation also makes an individual's retention longer.

2. Part and Whole Method

There exist two methods of memorising a subject. One can approach the subject by reading it again and again from beginning to the end as a whole. This is called whole method of memorisation. We can also approach the subject part by part i.e., the subject is divided into some parts and each part is memorised separately.

Experiments were carried out to find out which one is superior: Whole method or part method?

These methods seem to be contradictory but not so. Both these methods have advantages as well as disadvantages. The adoption and application of one or the other method for memorisation of a subject is decided by its extent and nature in relation to the ability of the individual.

When an individual tries to learn a short poem or prose, the whole method may be preferred. But if the poem is long, then part method should be preferred. Here it is also advisable to go through the whole poem first, so that order and relation towards a unit can be comprehended or perceived. We must have the common sense of approach instead of entering the duality.

When we learn a short subject, say a drug from Allen or about a bone from anatomy or a topic like the cardiac cycle from physiology, then the whole method should be preferred. Here also due consideration must be carried out regarding the book you consult and your ability to grasp. When the subject becomes too long, the part method should be preferred. For example, when you read a drug from Farrington, then the part method should be adopted.

Very often it may so happen that both the methods in combination fetch

A. Stage model by Atkinsons and Shiffrin (1971).
B. Process model by Craick and Lokhart (1972).

A. Stage Model of Atkinsons and Shiffrin

In this model, the memory encompasses three planes:
1. First plane is sensory memory.
2. Second plane is short term memory.
3. Third plane is long term memory.

1. Sensory Memory

Sensory memory provides temporary storage of information received by us through our senses. The receptive nerve cells receive the information from the environment and retain it for a brief period; say for a second (vision) or a few seconds (hearing) until it is processed further or lost. The information in sensory memory may enter short term memory, when we pay attention to it. When we do not pay any attention to sensory memory, then it automatically fades away.

2. Short Term Memory (STM)

It has a temporary working memory having a limited capability. Here the old impressions are replaced by new impressions after the deletion of the former one. For example, the moment you pass the traffic signal in a busy schedule, you just see the face of the traffic police and the very next moment you forget it. In short term memory, the storage system lasts for only a few seconds to a few minutes.

Information in short term memory may enter to long term memory when we think about its meaning and relate it to other information already in long term memory. Short term memory fades away without any effort. We should remember that mere repetition of information silently to ourselves (called as maintaining rehearsal) does not necessarily move information from short term memory to long term memory.

3. Long Term Memory (LTM)

This provides a relatively lasting storage.

(These three memories will be again discussed in this chapter)

B. Process Model by Craik and Lokhart (1972)

In this model the memory is not accepted as the tripartite system mentioned above.

In this model, human beings are compared to computers. In computers, feeding of data is called input. The input is further processed, which is the main function of a computer. Now this information is stored in computer memory. This storage of information can be further displayed as output. Similarly, this input of computer can be compared to receiving various informations via sensory channels in a human being. Then, the received information is processed (which is the main function of our mental and cognitive activity) and stored. Later this stored information is produced as an output that becomes our behavior i.e., what we say or do. Memory is the process that is responsible for the transformation of this input into output.

PROCESS OF MEMORY

Memory forms the very basis of learning. Learning without memory is futile. It is also obvious that memory is preceded by learning. It involves four processes which are as follows:

1. Learning.
2. Retention.
3. Recall.
4. Recognition.

These divisions are only functional in nature. We cannot put each in a water tight compartment. These factors are interrelated and very often found overlapping each other. Out of these four, first two i.e., learning and retention are highly essential for memory. Recall usually follows learning but there may be no recognition. Anyhow, both recall and recognition are indispensable for complete memory. Sometimes, recall may proceed recognition but equally often the succession of the activity may be reversed.

1. Learning

This is the first step of remembering. It is natural that if learning is good, memory will also become good. What we learn leaves after effects. These effects are conserved in the form of 'engrams' composed of memory traces. Hence, efficient learning has deeper traces which in turn has a superior impact.

better results. 'For example, while reading a drug from Kent, first go through the whole chapter as a whole and then read it part by part for better memorisation.

3. Active and Passive Method

Learning a study material by utterance is called active method while mental repetition is called passive method.

Various experiments reveal that active method of memorising is superior to its counterpart, passive method. The great advantage with this method is that distraction is prevented. In passive method, the mind roams frequently here and there, which hampers the memorising process. In the active method, the subject is well understood and rhythmical grouping makes learning easier. Moreover, by reading aloud, a pattern is created and one cannot miss a sequence. By learning through the active method, relationship is established so that deeper memory traces can be generated.

However, despite the above plus points of the active method, it is still advised that while learning a new lesson, one should recite it first mentally, followed by reading it aloud for better memorisation.

4. Spaced and Unspaced Method

As the caption suggests the spaced method of memorisation is one in which there are time intervals in the memorisation and the subject is connected to memory under different sessions. On the contrary, in unspaced method, learning is carried out at one sitting at a stretch.

5. Rote and Intelligent Method

Rote implies memorising or learning a study material without understanding it. On the other hand, learning or memorising a study material with proper understanding is called the intelligent method. Hence, it is obvious that learning by intelligent method is superior to rote method because of the association between the study material and the thought processes. By this learning is strengthened.

6. Grouping and Rhythm Method

It is a commonly observed phenomenon that a poem is easily remembered than prose. Hence grouping and rhythm method is better adopted for better memorisation.

7. Association

Association plays an important role in the process of memorisation. Association of ideas, connections and systematic thinking helps in recalling various incidents and happenings.

FAVORABLE CONDITIONS IN MEMORY

To study the favorable conditions in memory, it is necessary to study the favorable conditions in learning, retention, recall and recognition. Now let us proceed accordingly.

Favorable Conditions for Learning

1. **Interest and Enthusiasm:** Interest and enthusiasm are two favorable conditions for learning. Without interest and enthusiasm, the learning will lead to a state of drudgery.
2. **Interval Study:** Psychologists suggest to learn a subject by introducing intervals in the time of study instead of uninterrupted study. Spaced learning fetches better results in comparison to unspaced learning.
3. **Help of Supporting Materials:** Learning through supporting materials like tables, graphs, pictures, over head project (OHP) materials, slides, computer graphics, etc. help the individual in learning better.
4. **Health Condition:** It is an established fact that a healthy individual can learn in a better way than a sick individual. Factors like fear, fatigue, boredom, mental exhaustion, pre-occupation, emotional tension, worried state, etc. are unfavorable conditions for learning
5. **Habit and Discipline:** Learning should be made a habit. This habit must be put in a time table and followed strictly so that learning becomes easy.

Favorable Conditions for Retention

Many experiments have been carried out on the subject of retention and many psychological and physiological conditions have proved useful. Some of the main conditions which are favorable in retention are:

1. **Nature of Material:** The following characteristics in the material to be retained help in its retention:
    i. Intensive stimuli help in better retention compared to indistinct or

weak stimuli. Clear, colorful and tidy photographs can be retained in memory for a longer period in comparison to cloudy and messy photographs.

ii. Striking and distinct stimuli like strong light, striking beauty, melodious song, etc. and alike stimuli can be retained for a longer time.

iii. Fresh experiences favor retaining memory which decreases with the passage of time.

2. **Time Period:** A stimulus which continues for a long time can be retained for a longer period whereas a stimulus of a shorter duration is usually retained for a short period.

3. **Amount of Material:** If the subject is being pursued long enough, it will be retained for a longer time, while a shorter subject will take less time to be forgotten. The amount of material to be learnt, has a suitable effect on its retention, there being two reasons for the phenomena:

   a. A man has to make less exertion in order to learn a shorter subject, while a longer subject demands more effort, and therefore, the retention is more lasting.

   b. In the longer subject, as compared to the shorter, the person finds more meaning and relates the various parts of the subject together. All this helps in retention.

4. **Amount of Learning:** The extent of retention is directly proportional to the amount of learning, that is to say, retention will be more if the amount of learning is large. A subject studied more stays longer in the mind while one studied less will remain in the mind for a shorter period. Over-learning has a favorable effect on retention. But this does not mean that retention will go on increasing to infinite with the learning because after a certain limit disinterest, fatigue and monotony set in which produce a derogatory effect on retention. Therefore, the increasing and strengthening effects of over-learning should be confined to a certain limit.

5. **Speed of Learning:** The faster the learning, the better is the retention. Thus, people learning faster seem to retain the subject for longer periods as compared to the slow learners. Actually, the speed of learning indicates the inclination and interest towards a subject and hence learning becomes faster and retained longer.

6. **Methods of Learning:** The methods of learning, too play a crucial role in the retention of a subject in memory. Learning by the whole method instead of the part method, the spaced method instead of the unspaced

method and the active method instead of the passive method result in better learning.

7. **Experience:** Freud and other psychologists assert that we retain pleasant experiences for a longer time than painful ones. Thus, feeling attached with a certain experience, has an important role to play on its retention. Similarly, meaningful experiences favor retention for a longer period in comparison to meaningless experiences. Again the retention will be more if the experience is great.
8. **Attention:** It is obvious that attention and distraction promote and demote retention respectively.
9. **Sleep:** It is believed by some psychologists that sleep helps in better retention. They claim that lessons learnt before sleep can be retained better because the memory traces are settled down during sleep. Anyhow, some psychologists do not agree with it. However, lack of sleep definitely has an adverse effect on retention.
10. **Review of Materials Learnt:** Making another study facilitates the retention power to a greater degree.
11. **Mental Set:** A person retains those things for a longer period that suit his mental setup. A student having a mental set for history will have a better retention power in history in comparison to other subjects, where he lacks mental set say, mathematics.
12. **Apperception:** Apperception means the process of understanding something perceived in terms of previous experience. A subject learnt in terms of previous experience makes the retention of a newly learnt subject better in comparison to new learning not based on previous experience.
13. **Purpose of Learning:** If a subject is learn with a given purpose, it can be retained better in comparison to learning that lacks a purpose.
14. **Condition of mind and body:** Retention is comparatively easy when the mind and the body are healthy and fresh. Ill-health and sickness hinder recall.

Favorable Conditions for Recall

By and large, the factors which favor retention also hold good for recall. If the retention is better, the recall will also be better. There are some factors which favor the recall of experience over and above the factors favorable to retention. The major ones are as follows:

1. **Role of Hints and Clues:** Many a time we resort to recall with the help of hints and clues. Hints and clues are the replicates of recall. To take an example, if we learn a drug from the Materia Medica, we cannot recall it without the help of the title, the first line or the hints or clues to some part of it. Hence, hints and clues are considered favorable factors for recall.
2. **Mental Set:** The mental set of the individual too, affects recall. If your mental set is attuned better in Anatomy, then you can recall the information regarding various muscles, bones, etc. instantly. Similarly, whose mental set is attuned to Organon of Medicine, will reproduce the themes and meaning of various aphorisms easily and instantly. In general, in life, a sensuous person finds it easy to remember things associated with sex, while a religious person can recall religious subjects easily.
3. **Background Knowledge:** Recall is facilitated by its background knowledge. While writing an essay, or even in conversation, things pertinent to the background knowledge keep on flowing to the focus of attention. The recall of the subject matter due to the background knowledge unfolds like a chain of linked thoughts and experiences.
4. **Drives and Needs:** Drives and needs favor recall. When a person is under the influence of a drive or need, he can display a better retention capacity.
5. **Feeling:** Recall is modulated by feelings of pleasure and pain. According to Freud, pleasurable occurrences can be recalled with no trouble.
6. **Effort:** This has a very significant effect on recall. Recall generally increases with the effort.
7. **Elimination of Inhibition:** Various factors of inhibition like shyness, nervousness, reticence, etc. block the process of recall. It is a common experience with all of us that nervousness paralyses recall during examination. Hence, elimination of such type of inhibition can promote the process of recall. Of course, medicines like *Anacardium, Medorrhinum, Gelsemium, Argentum nitricum*, etc. can help immensely in meeting such type of inhibition.

Favorable Conditions for Recognition

As a general rule, the conditions found favorable for retention and recall are equally favorable for recognition. Additionally, *favorable mental set* and *self-confidence* are two prime conditions that favor recognition.

SIGNS OF GOOD MEMORY

Following aspects are judged as the signs of good memory:
1. Recalling a past experience with rapidity.
2. Recalling a past experience with accuracy.
3. Having reasonable length of time in retaining and recalling.
4. Revival of past experience in detail.
5. Recalling a right thing at the right time.

FORGETTING

Memory is the basic process in understanding behavior because it forms the very basis of all learning. It has two aspects:
a. Positive aspect called remembering.
b. Negative aspect called forgetting.

Forgetting is the opposite of remembering and is a basic failure in recalling or recognising or reviving an idea, an experience or something that had been learnt.

Very often we blame ourselves for bad memory. Generally, we think that forgetting is a curse for us. But that is not always correct. Forgetting has two aspects:
a. Positive.
b. Negative.

From a positive aspect, forgetting is a great boon for us. Life would have become wretched and miserable if all painful and agonising events had been stored in memory. Hence the process of forgetting is a blessing in disguise for all of us.

From the negative aspect, it can cause a lot of problems in facing interviews, examination and even day to day living.

There is a curve of forgetting. We forget various things in a proportion, which can be represented with the help of a graph. This is called the *Curve of Learning*, which was first postulated by Ebbinghaus.

Ebbinghaus's Curve of Forgetting

Ebbinghaus was the first psychologist who carried out various serious studies on memory. He carried out an experiment and observed the phenomena of forgetting and described his findings by plotting a graph (see figure).

As a subject of his own experiment, Ebbinghaus memorised a list of nonsense syllables and tested himself at a given interval and brought out the result as follows:

No.	Time Elapsed	Amount of Forgetting
1st interval	20 minutes	47%
2nd interval	One day	66%
3rd interval	Two days	72%
4th interval	Six days	75%
5th interval	Thirty one day	79%

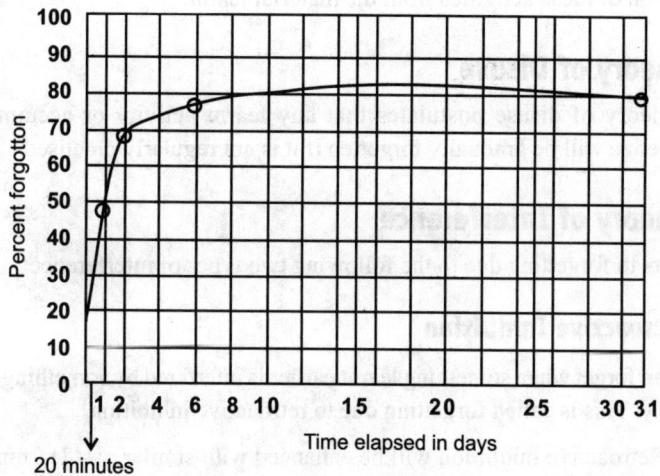

Ebbinghaus's Curve of Forgetting

From the above graph, Ebbinghaus reached the conclusion that:

a. The amount of learnt material forgotten rests upon the time expired after learning.
b. The rate of forgetting is very rapid at first and gradually dropped proportionally as the interval extends.

Why do We Forget?

Many theories about causes of forgetting have been subscribed, out of which the following are very important:
1. Theory of interpolated activities.
2. Theory of disuse.
3. Theory of interference.
4. Psycho-analytical theory.
5. Miscellaneous factors.

1. Theory of Interpolated Activities

Interpolated activities means activities that alter or corrupt inserting as new or foreign matter. According to this theory, it is the interpolated activity after learning which causes forgetting. The extent of forgetting depends upon the deviation of these activities from the material learnt.

2. Theory of Disuse

The theory of disuse postulates that any learnt activity or accumulated knowledge will be gradually forgotten if it is not regularly practised.

3. Theory of Interference

It refers to forgetting due to the following two types of interference:

a. Retroactive Inhibition

One can forget when something learnt earlier is interfered by something learnt recently. This is called forgetting due to retroactive inhibition.

i. Retroactive inhibition will be enhanced with similar past learning and interpolated activities.
ii. Retroactive inhibition will be more if the quantities of interpolated learning dominate the past learning. Naturally, if the interpolated learning is less than the hindrance, it will also be less.
iii. If the interpolated activities take place soon after the previous learning, the hindrance will be accentuated.
iv. Retroactive inhibition may decrease with increase of age.
v. Retroactive inhibition is reduced with intelligence of the learner.

b. Proactive Inhibition

Forgetting can occur when something learnt recently is interfered by something learnt in the past. This is called forgetting due to proactive inhibition.

4. Psycho-analytical Theory

The school of psycho-analysis attributes repression as the chief cause of forgetting. Repression means pushing the experience or thoughts into the unconscious mind. Freud maintains that it is natural in human beings to repress unacceptable, antisocial, sorrowful and unpleasant thoughts because of the pain they cause. It is a common observation with us that certain activities that we do not like to perform, are being forgotten by us. Similarly, we forget frequently the names that we do not like. Anyhow, this theory is an important theory but cannot explain all the phenomena that are related to forgetting.

5. Miscellaneous Factors

i. Factors Affecting Learning

All the factors which affect learning also affect forgetting because forgetting is the unlearning of a learnt subject. The major factors are:

a. *Method of Learning*: As a general rule, it can be said that forgetting is less in the case:
   i. of whole learning in contrast to part learning;
   ii. of spaced learning in contrast to unspaced learning;
   iii. of active learning in contrast to passive learning;
   iv. intelligent learning in contrast to unintelligent learning.
b. *Speed of Learning*: Rapid learning ensures retention while sluggish learning is forgotten relatively quicker.

ii. No Repetition

Lack of mental thinking and repetition of learning enhances forgetting.

iii. Disease

Various diseases, especially chronic diseases, brain injury, accidents etc. definitely play a role in forgetting.

iv. Use of Drugs

Use of stimulants, narcotics, substance abuse and other drugs enhance forgetting.

We should also note down that in addition to the causes mentioned above, factors which affect retention and recall may also affect forgetting.

Forgetting and its Remedial Measures to Enhance Memory

1. It is a common observation that *a weaker learning leads to a weaker memory*. In weaker learning, the neural tracts formed are fainter which lead to weaker memory power. But it does not mean that stronger learning can increase retention to infinity. Anyhow, psychologists suggest preferring over-learning to under-learning.
2. It has also been observed that meaningful and rhythmic study of a given subject helps retain the matter for a relatively longer period.
3. Psychologists also advise one to associate a topic with nonsense syllables. Of course a strong positive relation findings has a better edge for learning, retention and production in memory form.
4. Perceptual motor activities have a better edge over verbal learning in retention of memory.
5. Peculiar, uncommon and unusual experiences or events are better retained in memory.
6. Memory counsellors advise people to learn a lesson part by part instead of learning the whole at a time to have a better memory.
7. It has also been commonly observed and proved experimentally that we have a better retentive power in remembering pleasant experiences, than unpleasant events. For example, unpleasant experiences like death of near ones, suspension from a job, and failure in examination are easily forgotten than to that of romantic days of life or visiting a scenic beauty of Manali or Kashmir.
8. Followings are important determinants of learning and memory:
    a. **Learning Material:** Learning material is a decisive factor in retention of memory. Some materials are difficult in memorising whereas others are easy. Memory also depends on the type of material. Visual presentations are better retained in comparison to verbal presentations.
    b. **Motivation:** Perhaps the biggest force in this universe is motivation. This motivation leads a Buddha to have Nirvana and a person like Nathuram to kill a Mahatma like Gandhiji. Motivation has wonderful power in learning and memory.
    c. **Interest and Desire to Learn:** Today you may not like Anatomy

or Organon of medicine. You put these subjects under the categorisation of boring subjects. But take a little interest and see the miracle. Soon your interest will make the subject interesting.

In fact, excellency comes from desire and interest in learning.

9. Rapid learning has a better edge over gradual or slow learning. Rapid learning is inversely proportional to forgetfulness.

CLINICAL APPLICATION

Memory is the most recognized cognitive function of a human being. It is extremely sensitive and easily influenced by emotion, day to day problems, psychiatric disturbances, sleep deprivation, over-work, fatigue, consumption of intoxicants, drugs, head injury, etc. So when a patient comes to us for memory disturbances we should examine his background, which may require an etiological prescription. Moreover, the background may also form the totality of symptoms.

In your clinical practice you shall come across many patients having minor memory disturbance to very severe memory disturbances like Korsakoff's syndrome where the patient may even forget his name, or to which place he belongs. He may go from one place to another and have total loss of memory of the incident. Here the brain cells in the area of hippocampus are destroyed. Your role here becomes crucial.

In memory loss due to aging, the individual sometimes may remember everything of the past, but is unable to form new memories. Here we have a great role to play. Medicines like *Graphites*, *Sulphur*, etc. are useful here.

Retrograde amnesia in epilepsy is another point that is needed for consideration in a clinical setup. Here the seizure and other physical symptoms are considered in a special way.

Traumatic amnesia also bears great clinical importance for us. We have a better edge than other modes of treatment. We can do miracles with medicines like *Arnica*, *Natrium sulph.*, etc. in such cases.

Emotional amnesia, a type of psychogenic disorder is also important for clinical practice. For this we need medicines like *Ignatia*, *Natrium mur.*, etc. Of course, aphorisms 210-230 are our guidelines that must not be forgotten.

Memory problems are very common amongst students. High anxiety states in students during examination impairs retention. They may need *Gelsemium*, *Argentum nit.*, *Anacardium*, *Kalium phos.*, *Picricum acidicum*, etc. Children with below average intelligence also have memory problems. Similarly, poor memory is reported in children with attention deficit disorders. They may need *Aethusa*, *Baryta carb.*, etc.

All the medicines suggested above are mere suggestions. This must corroborate the totality of symptoms.

Psychological Strategies

Psychological strategies are used for the enhancement of memory for rehabilitation purposes. It has three components:

a. Encoding.
b. Storage.
c. Retrieval.

In encoding, the information is instilled in the patient. The information should be simple. The amount of information must be reasonable. Excessive amounts of information may not be received by the patient. The information can be better encoded if the help of association is fixed. The instillation of information should be repeated frequently, so that the engrams can be memorised better.

Encoding i.e. supplying the information is not enough for its retention in memory. The memory may be decayed in course of time. Hence, rehearsal, test, and retest should be done at a suitable interval with objective assessment of forgetfulness.

Retrieval becomes better in context where the patient is learning, so that he can be instructed to go the situation in which retrieval is required. For example, he may be encouraged to retrieve the events or lessons by prompting the first letter or sentence, allowing him for alphabetical search. He may be also injected glimpses of some events for the retrieval.

Along with the above we must be able to take the help of technical supports like labels, sign posts, color coding along with the use of diaries, plans, lists and other curing devices.

The role of memory pertains to the higher state of mind in homeopathy. It has been given due importance in our science. We have to go a long way to understand its ultimate nature and implications. But the role of miasm and allied factors in relation to memory cannot be neglected. It is quite possible that the overlapping of miasm over memory might exist on a great chunk of humanity. Hence, removal of the noxious cover over memory can be done by anti-miasmatic treatment. This may help us restore memory better. Moreover, the role of psychological strategy seems to be impotent when the health condition is deteriorating. Hence, restoration of general health is of paramount importance to have better memory. The role of yoga should also be examined here.

Chapter 12

INTELLIGENCE

Can you define God?
Can you define love?
Can you define education?
Can you define woman?

No! We are still in search of a comprehensive and satisfactory definition for the above terms. Similarly, it is also difficult to define intelligence. Intelligence is like one of the above concepts which are easy to recognize but difficult to define.

The term 'intelligence' owes its origin to the Latin word 'intellegere', which means perceive, discern (i.e., to *inter* 'between' + *legere* 'choose, read').

The term was coined by Cicero to translate a Greek word used by Aristotle to include all cognitive processes. This cognitive process is otherwise termed as intelligence which is innate and general in nature.

DEFINITION

There exist innumerable definitions on intelligence and as indicated above, there prevails controversy about its total acceptance. However, there hardly exists a satisfactory definition of it. Anyhow, let us explore a few of them:

Intelligence is the capacity in an individual to reason well to judge well, and to be self-critical *(Alfred Binet 1904).*

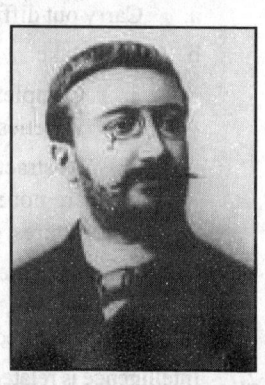

Alfred Binet (1857-1911)

Intelligent may be defined as the power of good responses from the point of view of truth or fact (*Thorndike*, 1914).

Intelligence is the capacity to learn and adjust to relatively new and changing conditions (*Wagnon*, 1937).

Intelligence is the global capacity of an individual to act purposefully, to think rationally and to deal effectively with his environment (*Weschler*, 1944).

Intelligence is the ability to adapt to one's surroundings (*Jean Piaget*, 1952).

After examining the above and some other definitions, the following definition is suggested for an easy comprehension:

The term intelligence refers to an individual's ability to understand complex ideas, to adapt effectively to the environment, to learn from experience, to engage in various forms of reasoning and to overcome obstacles by careful thought (*Neisser et al in Baron, 2004*).

After examining the above and alike definitions, we can safely state that intelligence encompasses the following three aspects:

a. Adjustment or adoption of the individual to his environment.
b. Ability to learn.
c. Ability to undertake abstract thinking.

CHARACTERISTICS OF INTELLIGENCE

1. Intelligence is characterised by a person's capacity to:
   a. Carry out difficult assignments.
   b. Undertake:
      i. Complex activities i.e., to take responsibilities of different varieties of different degrees of difficulty.
      ii. Abstract thinking i.e., pertaining to ideas and things which are not real. Abstract is related to words, numbers, letters, figures, etc.
      iii. Activities that are characterised by 'economy'. Here economy implies to the rate at which the activity with accuracy is executed.
2. **Intelligence is related to adaptiveness for an objective i.e., what intelligent action is directed towards a goal or purpose.**

3. Intelligence is also an attribute to creating something new and different i.e., creativity is another aspect of intelligence.

CLASSIFICATION OF INTELLIGENCE

E.A. Thorndike has classified intelligence into three categories, which are mentioned below :

I. Concrete intelligence.
II. Abstract intelligence.
III. Social intelligence.

Let us explore them further, step by step.

I. Concrete Intelligence

Concrete connotes a real form that can be seen or felt. Hence we generally say concrete achievements or concrete actions. Obviously, intelligence is concerned with concrete material that comes under this category. It is the ability of an individual to handle the actual situation and respond to it effectively. Suppose you are in a market place and all of a sudden a group of terrorists started spraying bullets at a nearby shop. Now what you are going to do in such a situation? Here comes the role of concrete intelligence. It is your concrete intelligence that will make you appraise your surroundings and help you in running to or hiding in a safer place so that you can save your life. Concrete intelligence is used by all of us in day to day life in various ways.

II. Abstract Intelligence

Contrary to above, abstract means which is not real; relating to ideas and things which are not real. Intelligence concerned with ability to respond to words, numbers, letters, symbols, etc. falls under this category. Abstract intelligence is required in normal academic subjects in schools, such as reading, writing, etc. Anyhow, academicians, philosophers, mathematician, etc. necessitate the highest level of abstract intelligence.

III. Social intelligence

We are of the society, by the society and for the society. Social well-being is also an integral part of our health. Social intelligence means the ability of an individual to respond to social circumstances in day to day life in a harmonious way. Social intelligence does not allow us to give a practical shape to an individual's personal feelings or emotions that would be detrimental to society. Social intelligence also does not take account of the feelings or emotions aroused in us by other people. Social intelligence helps us to understand others in a better way. It helps us to respond in such a way towards them that the desired goal is accomplished. High social intelligence is possessed by those who are able to handle people well. Rama, Krishna, Buddha, Christ, etc. belong to the highest state of intelligence. Fitness or adequate adjustment in social situations with positive intention and positive outcome is the indicator of social intelligence.

THEORIES OF INTELLIGENCE

I. *Factor Theories of Intelligence:*
1. Unitary or Monarchic theory.
2. Anarchic or Multi-factoral theory.
3. Spearman's two factor theory.
4. Group factor theory.
5. Thompson's sampling theory.
6. Vernon's hierarchical theory.
7. Guilford's theory involving a model of intellect.

II. *Cognitive Theories of Intelligence:*
1. Cattell and Horn's theory of intelligence.
2. Jenson's theory of intelligence.
3. Campion and Brown's theory of intelligence.

III. *Cognitive-Contextual Theories of Intelligence : The Recent Trend*
1. Gardener's theory of human intelligence.
2. Sternberg's theory of intelligence.

I. Factor Theories of Intelligence

1. Unitary Theory or Monarchic Theory

This is the oldest theory and even today a lot of laymen believe in this theory. This theory states that intelligence consists of a single factor, a stock of intellect proficiency, which is common to all actions of the individual. Accordingly, the source of all action has only one source of intelligence; say weight lifting to chess playing to performing a mathematical equations.

Criticism

The theory does not hold good in real life situations. For example, one of you may not be good in Organon of medicine despite your genuine interest and diligence in it; whereas you may excel in Anatomy even though you have a little interest in the subject. This proves that intelligence is not just a unitary factor and hence this theory cannot be accepted.

2. Anarchic or Multifactor Theory

This theory was postulated by the famous psychologist Thorndike. It is also known as Atomistic theory of intelligence. It asserts that intelligence is a blend of several separate elements, each being a minute element representing one ability. It rejects the theory of general intelligence.

Criticism

We cannot hold that good intelligence is a passport of success in every sphere of human life. So also we cannot assume that with certain specific types of abilities, an individual would be absolutely successful in a given area and utterly unsuccessful in other areas. Here it fails to evolve a common factor that is necessary for evaluation of all tasks.

3. Spearman's Two Factor Theory

The limitations of above have their own problems and hence another theory called Two-factor theory was developed by an English psychologist, Charles Spearman in 1904. He proposed that intellectual abilities comprised of two factors:

i. General ability or common ability known as 'g' factor and,
ii. Group of specific abilities known as 's' factors.

Characteristics of 'g'

i. It is a universal, inborn ability.
ii. It is general mental energy.
iii. It is constant in a given individual.
iv. The amount of 'g' is not equal for all individuals.
v. It is used in all life's activities.
vi. 'g' determines the success of a given individual in life. Greater the 'g' in an individual, greater the success in life.

Characteristics of 's'

i. It is learnt or acquired from the environment.
ii. It differs from activity to activity in the given individual.
iii. The amount of 's' ability varies from individual to individual.

Spearman asserted that there was a general ability employed by people while adjusting with different types of intellectual tasks. He wisely refused to identify 'g' with intelligence or any other quality that may lead to wide criticism or controversy. He suggested that this 'g' or general factor depends on mental energy with which each one of us is endowed.

His theory can be expressed with the following equation.

$$A = g + S1 + S2 + S3 + \ldots$$

Criticism

The two factor theory of Spearman has been subjected to criticism on the following grounds:

i. Spearman talked of two factors, whereas we possess several factors (g, S1, S2, S3…) in this respect.
ii. According to Spearman each job needs some specific ability. This view cannot be accepted as it is supposed that nothing is common to various jobs except a general factor. In medical profession, individuals like doctors, nurses, pharmacists etc. are attached. But they cannot be put in one group although all of them have a general factor. Moreover, factors like S1, S2, S3... are not mutually exclusive. Very often, they overlap and generate some common factors.

4. Group Factor Theory

As mentioned above, the overlapping and grouping of intelligence could not satisfy the psychologists. Hence they were compelled to think deeper and at last L.L. Thurston, an eminent psychologist from America brought out the Group Factor theory, which is an off shoot of overlapping and grouping of intelligence. This theory is the intermediate of Thorndike's multi-factor and Spearman's two factor theory.

Thurston along with his associates developed 'Test of Primary Mental Ability' (PMA). He carried 56 tests on 240 college students and resolved their factor analysis.

He postulated that some mental operations have a common 'Primary' factor, which gives them psychological and functional unity and which differentiates them from other mental operations. These mental operations constitute a group factor. So there are a number of groups of mental abilities (the number being not determined so far) each of which has its primary factor, giving the group a functional unity and cohesiveness. Each of these primary factors is said to be relatively independent of each other. Thurston and his colleagues have identified nine such factors:

1. *The Number Factor* (N): This factor is related to the ability to carry out numerical calculations accurately and rapidly.
2. *The Verbal Factor* (V): This factor is concerned with comprehension and verbal relations, words and ideas.
3. *The Space Factor* (S): This factor is involved in any task in which the subject manipulates an object imaginably in space.
4. *The Rote Memory Factor* (M): This factor is related to the ability to memorise quickly.
5. *The Deductive Reasoning Factor* (RD): Is the ability to make use of generalised results (i.e., to reach generalisation from particulars).
6. *The Inductive Reasoning Factor* (RI): Concerned with the ability to draw inferences or conclusions on the basis of specific instances (to reach at the particulars from generals).
7. *The Perceptual Factor* (P): It is concerned with the ability to perceive objectives accurately
8. *The Problem Solving Factor* (PS): It is the ability to solve problems with independent effort.
9. *The Word Fluency Factor* (W): It is involved whenever the subject is asked to think of isolated words at a rapid rate.

As per this theory, the group factors were suggested for factors not common to all intellectual abilities but to certain activities comprising a group.

Criticism

This theory discarded the concept of common factor. This fact was later realised by Thurston. Hence he included a general factor later to the above.

5. Thompson's Sampling Theory (1939)

This theory was explained by G.H.Thompson, a British psychologist. According to this theory, mind comprises of several independent elements. A given action is the outcome of the amalgamation of some of the elements.

6. Vernon's Hierarchical Theory (1950)

British psychologist P.E. Vernon recommended a hierarchical organisation of intelligence from extensive research which is based on empirical data, which may be conceived from the figure below.

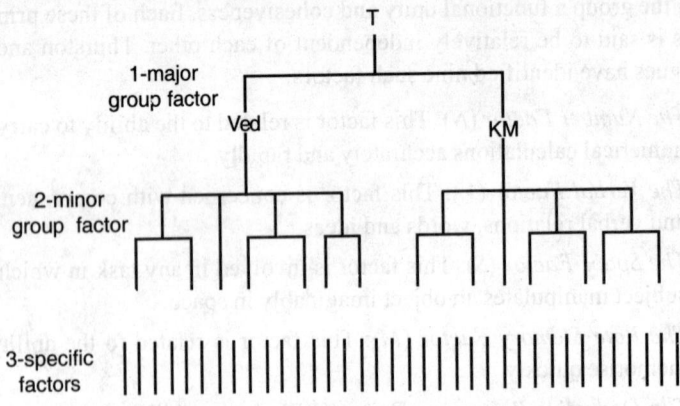

Vernon's Hierarchical Structure of Human Intelligence

According to Vernon, mind is a type of hierarchical order in which 'G' is the most prominent mental ability i.e., by and large factor measured through intelligence tests. Under 'G', we have two major group factors which are :

i. Ved : Verbal, numerical and educational.
ii. KM : Practical, mechanical, spatial and physical.

These two major factors can be further divided into minor group factors like, mechanical, manual etc., and eventually these minor factors are again sub-divided into different specific factors related to minute specific mental abilities.

7. Guilford's Theory of Intelligence (1961)

Guilford and his associates, while working in the psychological laboratory at the University of Southern California, developed a model of intelligence on the basis of factor analysis. They explained that mental process or intellectual activity can be depicted in terms of three different basic dimensions or parameters known as:

i.   *Operation*, the act of thinking.
ii. *Content*, the term in which we think of words or symbols.
iii. *The product*, the idea we come up with.

Operation

- Evaluation (E)
- Convergent thinking (N)

Parameters =
1. Operation
2. Product
3. Content

Operation
1. Evaluation (E)
2. Convergent (N)
3. Divergent (D)
4. Memory (M)
5. Cognitory (C)

Product
1. Units (U)
2. Classes (C)
3. Relations (R)
4. System (S)
5. Transformation (T)
6. Implications (I)

Content
1. Behavioural (B)
2. Figural factors (F) i.e. perception of concrete materials
3. Semantic factors (M) i.e. related to verbal meaning of ideas
4. Symbolic factors (S) i.e. related to sign and symbols

Through above Guilford expanded his cube shaped model of the structure of intellect to include 120 factors (5X6X4) that constituted human intelligence. His cube model is given below for an easy understanding

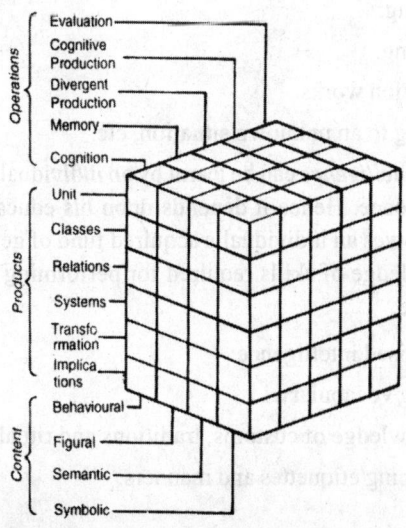

II. Cognitive Theories of Intelligence

1. Cattell and Horn's Theory of Fluid and Crystallised Intelligence

Cattell (1965) and Horn (1978) suggested a theory of intelligence consisting of two types:

1. Fluid intelligence.
2. Crystal intelligence.

Although these look contradictory, yet in reality they are complementary to one another and interact to produce overall intelligence.

Fluid intelligence is the mental ability of an individual used for learning and solving problems. It is put to use when a person faces an unknown and strange situation. Role of fluid intelligence is of paramount importance for adaptation, comprehension, reasoning, problem solving identifying relationships, etc.

Fluid intelligence is said to be innate in nature which depends on the development of the nervous system which is guided by genetic configuration and biological growth. This intelligence is not guided by training, experience or culture.

Example of fluid intelligence:
  i. Thinking.
  ii. Imagining.
  iii. Reasoning.
  iv. Abstraction works.
  v. Adapting to an unknown situation, etc.

Crystallised intelligence can be learnt by an individual through exercise, training and experience. Hence it depends upon his education and cultural background. It involves an individual's acquired fund of general information consisting of knowledge of skills required for performing different tasks in one's day to day life.

Example of crystallised intelligence:
  i. Learning vocabulary.
  ii. The knowledge of customs, traditions and rituals.
  iii. Maintaining etiquettes and manners.

iv. Facing interviews/ board.
v. Behaving in society.
vi. Handling of machines and tools, craftsmanship and art.
vii. Computing, doing calculations, keeping accounts etc.
viii. General knowledge of world affairs.
ix. Playing various games, etc.

2. Jensen's Theory of Intelligence (i.e. Mental Functioning)

Arthur Jensen (1969) suggested another theory of intelligence. According to him, the functioning of one's mind depends upon the type and degree of intelligence one possess. He further asserts that intelligence consists of two types of mental abilities:

a. Conceptual abilities.
b. Associative abilities.

a. Conceptual Abilities

Conceptual abilities involve one's ability to carry out a higher order of:

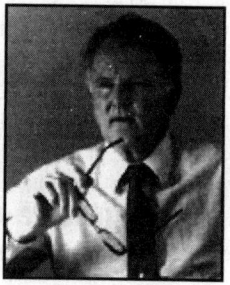

Jensen

i. Thinking and divergent thinking.
ii. Reasoning.
iii. Analysing.
iv. Synthesising.
v. Capacity to solve a problem.
vi. Abstract reasoning.

b. Associative Abilities

Associative intelligence can be measured by means of intelligence tests. Following items are attributed to associative abilities.

i. Remembering.
ii. Reproducing.
iii. Identifying.
iv. Discriminating.
v. Synthesizing.
vi. Associating.
vii. Assimilating (not pertaining to digestive system).

viii. Transferring.
ix. Applying.
x. Recalling.
xi. Recognising.
xii. Serial learning.
xiii. Free and controlled associative learning.
xiv. Selecting and discriminating, etc.

As maintained by Jensen, associative abilities are linked to biological developments and show no disparity amongst social classes and races.

3. Campion and Brown's Theory of Intelligence

Joe Campion and Ann Brown developed this theory and stated that intelligence has a two systems:

a. Architectural system, which has a biological base.
b. Executive system which is influenced by the environment.

The architectural system is the basis of an individual's intellectual functioning whereas the executive system works as a store house of knowledge, information and cognitive abilities.

III. Cognitive-Contextual Theories of Intelligence: The recent trend

One of the recent developments in the theory of intelligence has been cognitive-contextual theories advocated separately by Howard Gardener and Robert Sternberg, both being American psychologists.

Cognitive-contextual theories deal with the way cognitive processes operate in various environmental contexts.

1. Gardener's Theory of Multiple Intelligence

In 1983, Howard Gardner of Harvard University proposed a theory that he called "multiple intelligences", which was a revolutionary concept.

Gardner equipped his list of intelligences from a variety of sources: Studies of cognitive processing, of brain damage, of exceptional individuals, and of cognition across cultures. Gardner proposed that most concepts of intelligence had been ethnocentric and culturally biased representing a parochial approach whereas his was universal, based upon biologic and cross-cultural data as well as upon data derived from the cognitive performance of a wide assortment of people.

Gardener challenged the existing theories of general intelligence 'g' and its basis. He went a step further and rejected the single intelligence theory. He postulated that the intelligences are pluralistic and independent in nature and exist in seven types which are as follows as:

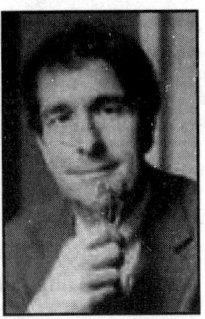

Howard Gardener

a. **Linguistic Intelligence:** This form of intelligence dominants professions like lecturers, writers, lyricists, etc. It is answerable to all kinds of linguistic competence abilities. It is concerned with written, verbal and understanding skills.

b. **Logico-mathematical:** This sort of intelligence is related to logical reasoning (inductive as well as deductive), mathematics, scientific thinking, etc. Professionals like mathematicians, philosophers, physicists rely upon such form of intelligence.

c. **Spatial Intelligence:** Spatial is related to space: Relating to, occupying or happening in space. Professionals like sculpturists, artists, cartoonists, painters, engineers, mechanics, etc. are found to display such type of intelligence.

d. **Musical Intelligence:** Abilities, talents and skills pertaining to the field of music belong to musical intelligence. Hence musicians, music directors and composers heavily rely on musical intelligence.

e. **Bodily- kinaesthetic Intelligence:** This type of intelligence is related to abilities, talents and skills involved in using one's body and its various parts to perform skilful and purposeful movements like dancing, performing a feat, etc. Dancers, athelets, surgeons, etc. are guided by this intelligence.

f. **Intra-personal Intelligence:** This kind of intelligence enables an individual to know about his self: Understanding his cognitive abilities, styles and mental functioning, emotions and skill to use his fund of knowledge in practical situations. This type of intelligence is found amongst Yogis, Zen masters and people who regularly practice meditation.

g. **Inter-personal Intelligence:** This kind of intelligence enables an individual to understand individuals who are outside the self. This intelligence gives the ability to act productively, based on the perceptions of others. Teachers, sales persons, politicians, psychotherapists rely heavily on this form of intelligence.

2. Sternberg's Theory of Intelligence

In the year 1985, Sternberg propounded the theory of intelligence as information process. Later in 1995 he along with his colleagues modified the theory, which is known as Triacrchic theory, where the earlier theory was merged and augmented.

A. Information Processing Theory

It was introduced in the year 1985. It explains the individual's cognitive or problem solving behavior. This theory states that the individual proceeds to perform mental tasks or solve a problem from the moment he receives the information till the task comes to an end. This explains an individual's cognitive and problem solving behavior. Accordingly, as mentioned, this theory divides the various basic skills that people,

- use to receive information,
- process it,
- derive reasoning behind it and,
- then use in problem solving

Sternberg terms two types of components in relation to information processing, viz.,

i. *Information Processing Component:* Components are the steps to solve a problem.

ii. *Information processing metal components:* Metal components are the basic knowledge that one has to know to solve a problem.

Sternberg suggests the following steps for processing information:

i. *Encoding*: First the individual identifies the relevant information in the mind called *encoding*.

ii. *Inferring*: Secondly, he derives the necessary inferences called, *inferring*.

iii. *Mapping*: Thirdly, identify the relationship between a previous situation and the present situation. This is called *mapping*.

iv. *Application*: Fourthly, apply the inferred relationship, this is called *application*.

v. *Justifying*: Fifth, justifying the analysed solution to the problem is called *justification*.

vi. *Response*: Sixth, providing the best solution for the problem is called *response*.

B. Triarchic Theory of Intelligence

In the year 1995, an advanced version of the theory of intelligence was provided by Sternberg and his associates called the "Triarchic" theory of human intelligence.

Sternberg agreed with Gardner that conventional notions of intelligence are too limited. However, he did not agree that abilities such as musical and bodily-kinaesthetic ones are talents rather than intelligences. He also differed from Gardener's notion on multiple intelligence, which are separate and independent.

According to Sternberg, intelligence has three aspects, which are integrated and interdependent. These aspects of intelligence relate–

a. to what goes on internally within a person.
b. to what goes on in the external world.
c. to integration of the above two i.e., to experience the internal and external worlds.

   i. The first aspect consists of the cognitive processes and representations that form the core of all thought. Sternberg subscribes three kinds of processes that are involved in this type of intelligence:
   - What to do and later in deciding
   - How well it was done, and those involved in doing
   - What one had decided to do

   ii. The second aspect consists of the application of these processes to the external world. According to Sternberg, mental processes serve three functions in the everyday world:
   - Adjustment to existing environments
   - Shaping of existing environments into new ones
   - Change to new environments when old ones prove disappointing

The theory holds that more intelligent people are not those who can execute many cognitive processes quickly and correctly. Their greater intelligence is reflected in knowing their strengths and weaknesses. These intelligent people can manipulate nicely with these strengths. They can also find the means and ways for compensating their weaknesses. Thus, they can capitalize both of their strengths and weaknesses and find a place or position from where they can operate most efficiently.

iii. The third aspect of Sternberg's triarchic theory is the integration of the internal and external worlds through experience. One aspect of intelligence is the ability to cope with relatively new situations. For example, intelligence can be measured by transferring someone from a familiar position (to which he is well accustomed) an unfamiliar situation, in order to assess his ability to cope with the new situation.

The Triarchic theory further elucidates 3 types of intelligences:

Type I – This is called Componental or Analytical intelligence. This ability makes an individual think critically and analytically. People possessing high dimension in this respect usually excel academically.

Type II – This is called Experiential or Creative intelligence. This intelligence makes an individual formulate new ideas. Great people like Einstein, Newton, Freud, C.V. Raman, etc. possessed such intelligence.

Type III – This type of intelligence is called Practical intelligence, which is with most of us. This intelligence is used in solving day to day problems.

NATURE OF INTELLIGENCE

Proper understanding of the true nature of intelligence demands appreciation of three important aspects which are described below:

a. Meaning and definition of intelligence.
b. Various theories of intelligence.
c. Characteristics and function of intelligence along with its concomitants.

We have already discussed the first two points. Now let us discuss the third point.

1. Existence of individual differences in intelligence

There are many individual differences amongst individuals in respect to intelligence. No two individuals (even twins) possess an equal amount of intelligence. This fact has been proved by assessments of intelligence. Intelligence oscillates from circumstance to circumstance, and age to age in the given individual.

2. Distribution of intelligence

The distribution of intelligence is also not equal amongst all human beings. It is an observable fact that a majority of people are average, a few are very bright and a few are dull.

3. Age factor in intelligence

Various experiments suggest that intelligence grows as the child grows. But, it has not been ascertained when the growth of intelligence comes to a halt. This varies from person to person. Psychologists have found that intelligence tends to stabilize at the age of 10 and fully stabilizes during adolescence. Sometimes it has been observed that intelligence reaches its peak between the age of 16 to 20. It is said that intelligence is basically a function of the nervous system. Hence, development of intelligence goes hand in hand with the development or deterioration of the nervous system.

4. Race, Culture, Religion, geographical distribution and intelligence

Various races, cultures, religions and geographical distribution may claim superior intelligence, which does not seem correct. It has been established that intelligence is not the monopoly of any race, state, religion or culture. The 'bright' and 'dull' can be found everywhere irrespective of the above factors.

5. Low Socio-economic status and environmental factors

These factors play a crucial role in relation to intelligence. Very often people belonging to a lower strata of life, having a poor economic background and deleterious effect of environment have lesser intelligence. However, we also find great people of high intelligence in this strata.

6. Miasmatic State (and Consideration of Constitution)

Psychology has not given due importance to this factor because of its non-extension of knowledge to homeopathy. We, the homeopaths have observed that intelligence can be developed to the fullest under anti-miasmatic (a part of constitution) treatment because miasms act as a veil for the development of premier intelligence. We need a joint venture of psychology and homeopathy in this respect.

DETERMINANTS OF INTELLIGENCE

1. Hereditary factors

Newman, Freeman and Holzinger (1937) adopted 19 pairs of like twins for experimental purpose. The twins were nurtured separately in different foster houses. Newman et al discovered that intelligence scoring of alike twins (who were nurtured separately) were almost as similar as two scores achieved by the same person at different times. Hence, they concluded that dominion of identical heredity was a factor operating systematically to determine the development of identical intelligence.

Shields also carried out another study in a different fashion for the same purpose to evaluate the role of heredity in relation to intelligence. He experimented with 88 pairs of alike twins, out of which 50 % were nurtured together and the remaining 50% were separate in different homes. The correlation between their intelligence test scores were .77 for those nurtured together and .76 for those, who were brought up separately. This proves the role of heredity in the development of intelligence.

Teasdale and Owen (1984) also subscribe similar views. They took full siblings, half siblings and unrelated children. They studied these children with rearing together and apart. Ultimately they confirmed a very high correlation in the I.Q. scores of full siblings (whether they were raised together or apart), and less correlation amongst half siblings and no correlation amongst those unrelated.

The study of Bouchard et al (1990) reveals the following closer genetic relationship:

Relationship	Correlation
Parents & natural children	.40
Parents & adopted children	.31
Dizygotic twins	.60
Monozygotic twin	
a. Reared together	.86
b. Reared apart	.72
Cousins	.15

2. Environmental Factors

Some studies were also carried out to determine the role of environment in the evaluation of intelligence.

It has also been observed that children from large families tend to have lower I.Q. scores than those from small families.

Order of birth also has a role in relation to intelligence. The first born child has better I.Q. in comparison to his fellow siblings.

The author has served the state government as a medical officer and has worked in remote areas of the state. He has observed that people who are unprivileged and residing in remote hilly areas score less due to lack of schooling and language training.

It has also been observed that when children are provided with a conducive environment, their scoring rate increases.

Conclusion

From above it is obvious that a group of psychologists are in support of heredity and the rest for environment. Both have their own reasons to justify. These studies are empirical in nature and we can move to either side like a pendulum and fix ourselves. The reality is that both heredity and environment are so interlinked that it is difficult to disconnect one from the other and both play a crucial role for the development and provision of intelligence.

MEASUREMENT AND ASSESSMENT OF INTELLIGENCE

Although everybody has two legs, two ears, two eyes, etc. in common, yet we differ from each other in many respects. Primitive men largely employed crude methods of measuring intelligence by means of physical strength and solving puzzles. With the advancement of civilization and advent of scientific inquiry, the method for measuring intelligence has advanced significantly.

We can observe the intelligence of an individual through various intelligence tests. The term 'assessment' should be preferred instead of 'measurement' in relation to test of intelligence because intelligence belongs to the domain of abstract and it cannot be measured like weight, height or temperature of the body.

Before exploring the above aspects of intelligence, let us take a glance at *Intelligence Quotient* through which intelligence is assessed.

Intelligence Quotient

Intelligence is assessed through various tests, which is expressed in the terms of I.Q. William Stern, a German psychologist, first coined this term.

We use the word I.Q. in everyday life. I.Q. is the ratio of Mental age divided by Chronological age. The percentage is calculated as per the following formula:

$$I.Q. = \frac{MA}{CA} \times 100$$

Mental age concept was introduced by Alfred Binet, a French psychologist. The Chronological age is determined from the date of birth whereas the mental age is determined by intelligence tests. We have to remember that the mental age increases with the chronological age.

I. Q. reveals the mental ability of the individual based on which he can be directed about the future.

I. Q. is not the quantity of a person's intelligence. Also, different tests yield different results. Even when a person is exposed to the same test from time to time, the results differs. Hence a test difference of 4 to 5 points has been allowed in Stanford-Binet and Wechsler–Bellevus test of intelligence. Hence, we have to be careful in assessing in I.Q. while interpreting. Interestingly, the I.Q. changes every 3 years. Again, I.Q. does not start with zero as every individual is born with some I.Q. I.Q. is the result of both heredity and environment. Hence, a conducive environment shows a better I.Q.

Garret's Classification of I.Q.

Garret has classified people as per to their I.Q., which follows as:

I.Q.	Classification	Percentage
140 and above	Very superior	1.5
120-139	Superior	11
110-119	Bright	18
90-109	Average or normal	48
80-89	Dull or backward	14
70- 79	Very dull	5
0-69	Feeble minded	2.5

We must remember that the level of I.Q. in directly proportion to the socio-economic conditions and health. It has generally been observed that the I.Q. remains constant from 5-24 years.

Assessment of Intelligence

Assessment of intelligence is done under the following heads:

I. Verbal:

A. Verbal individual intelligence tests.

B. Verbal group intelligence tests.

II. Non-verbal:

C. Non-verbal individual intelligence tests.

D. Non-verbal group intelligence tests.

In verbal tests, the subjects use language in which they are instructed in words, written, oral or both. Tests like vocabulary, memory tests, comprehensive tests, reasoning tests, etc. are included in this.

In non-verbal tests, language is not used except for giving directions. The test materials provided are in the form of objects. The candidate's responses are assessed on the basis of his reaction instead of his verbal expression or writings.

A. Verbal Individual Intelligence Tests

We will discuss these verbal tests under three heads:
1. Pre-Binet period.
2. Binet period.
3. Post-Binet period.

1. Pre-Binet Period

Galton's Tests

Sir Francis Galton (1822-1911) was the first psychologist who carried out studies to know whether individual characteristics are inherited. He took great interest in studying individual differences. His main focus of study was in measuring the sensory discrimination, sensory perception and sensory acuity.

Wundt's Introspection

We have already read that the first laboratory of experimental psychology was established by Wundt in 1879 in Leipzig. Wundt, mainly employed physiological methods and introspection as the major method to study vision, hearing, reaction-time and other sensory-motor activities.

Tests of Ebbinghaus

In the year 1880, Ebbinghaus arranged many tests measuring the differences in the intelligence of various individuals.

Test by Cattell

James McKeen Cattell, an American psychologist, was the first person in the world of psychology who used the word 'mental test'. He had studied in Europe and was very much influenced by Galton's ideas. Cattell accepted the idea of Galton, that intellectual functions can best be measured through tests of reaction-time and sensory discrimination. In 1890, Cattel worked out some mental tests, through which he was able to measure the individual differences among various individuals pertaining to memory, speed of reaction, sensory acuity and some other mental activities.

Drawbacks of Pre-Binet Period

a. Tests failed to evaluate the nature of intelligence.
b. Intelligence was interpreted as the acuity of senses.
c. Tests were too simple and too limited, which could not be utilised for the real assessment of intelligence.

d. Complex functions like judgement, reasoning, etc. could neither be assessed nor measured.
e. Fine mental abilities were not assessed with the help of physical sensory tests.

2. Binet Period

Prior to advent of Binet, tests of sensory discrimination, speed of motor responses and similar types were taken as tests of intelligence. Binet and Simon dramatically changed the scenario and explained various tests of more complex mental functions like judgment, reasoning, memory, etc. Binet and Simon decided upon a novel way of arranging or grouping their test items which was of great practical importance. In giving their tests to children of different ages, they were able to categorize the items. For example, a given item might be correctly responded to by most eight year olds. By arranging the items in terms of age-level, an age scale was developed. Furthermore, if the assumption is made that the average 8 year-old child functions intellectually at a level commensurating with his chronological age (CA), the age scale can be viewed as a mental age scale and judgments can be made concerning the intellectual level of an individual expressed in terms of mental age. If an individual, regardless of age, can satisfactorily pass items on the 12 year-old level, he can be presumed to have the ability of the average 12 year-old or in other words, a mental age of 12 years. The mental age scale and the concept of mental age were Binet's great contributions to the field of intelligence testing.

Introduction

In the beginning of the twentieth century in France, most of the students did not do well in various examinations. As a result, teachers blamed students and students blamed teachers. The superintendent of Public Instruction appointed Binet and Simon for curbing this menace. Binet and Simon studied the situation and developed a variety of test items which were not only concerned with intelligence testing but also psychological movement that stood supreme and unparallel.

The first scale was produced by Binet and Simon in 1905. The 1905 scale consisted of thirty items in order of increasing difficulty. The scale however was rudimentary and faltering. The scale was not differentiated from the angle of age.

In 1908, Binet and Simon rectified the defects and raised the items up to fifty nine. Moreover, two new concepts were added to the tests i.e.,

i. The age range extended higher and there was a specific group of items for each age.
   ii. The concept of mental age was added for the first time.

The 1908, revision produced interest among psychologists of USA, England, Switzerland, etc. They adopted the scale in their countries and gave valuable suggestions for the improvement of the scale.

The scale was again revised in 1911 as a correction measure suggested by psychologist of Europe and America. Unfortunately in the same year i.e., in 1911 Binet died. His work was further augmented by L.M. Terman and others.

1905 Binet –Simon Scale

The 1905 scale has 30 items, out of which we will discuss only a few.

1. Visual coordination, movement of head and eyes when a lighted match is moved slowly before the subject's eyes.
2. Comprehension.
3. Recognition of food.
5. Seeking food: The subject is given food in a wrap and it is seen how the subject gets the food.
7. Verbal knowledge of objects like parts of the body.
17. Recalling picture of a familiar object.
18. Drawing from memory.
26. Devising a sentence.
30. Giving definition and differences between a paired abstract word.

1908 Binet-Simon Scale

Age of 3 years:
1. Points to nose, eyes, mouth, etc.
2. Repeats two digits 3, 5.
3. Gives family name, etc.

Age of 8 years:
1. Reads a passage and recalls two items.
2. Adds up the value of 5 coins.
3. Can differentiate between two objects, etc.

1911 Binet-Simon Scale

Age of 6 years:
1. Make a distinction between morning and afternoon.
2. Define names of familiar objects in terms of application.
3. Copies a diamond figure from a book.
4. Counts one to thirteen.
5. Distinguishes between pictures of ugly and pretty faces.

Age of 8 years:
1. Gives differences between two objects.
2. Counts backward from 20 to 0.
3. Point out omissions from unfinished pictures.
4. States the date of the day.
5. Repeats the digits.

Age of 10 years:
1. Arranges five blocks in order of weight.
2. Reproduces two geometric designs from memory.
3. Criticizes stupid statements.
4. Uses three given words in two sentences, etc.

Salient Features of Binet Scale

First, they are scales, which was very different from the earlier works. The items and tasks are shaped on the basis of their difficulty beginning with easy items.

Secondly, the revised Binet's scales are related to a general global measure of intelligence instead of an investigation of separate special abilities.

Thirdly, they are grouped by age levels and measure mental growth of the subject.

The fourth characteristic is that the tests are carried out by skilled examiners for a subject for evaluation or assessment.

3. Post-Binet Period (Stanford Revision of Binet's Scale)

In 1916, L. M. Terman of Stanford University revised and refined the original Binet-Simon scale in America according to the needs of American culture without changing any principle. His focus of research was related to normal, defective and superior children and adults.

The 1916 scale includes 90 items, ranging from 3 years to 14 years of age. Some items of the 1916 Stanford scale are as follows:

1916 Stanford Scale

Age of 3 years:
1. Points to parts of body like nose, eye, mouth.
2. Names familiar objects.
3. Name objects in pictures.
4. Gives his/her sex.
5. Gives last name.
6. Repeats six to seven syllables.

(A1) Repeats three digits.

Age of 7 years:
1. Knows numbers of fingers on each and both hands.
2. Narrates pictures.
3. Repeats 5 digits.
4. Gives differences between paired objects.
5. Copies a diamond figure from a book.

(A1)1. Names days of week in correct order.
(A1)2. Repeats 3 digits backwards.

The Stanford revision (1916) was again revised in 1937 and 1960. It remains one of the most popular tests of its kind. The latest re-standardised version of the S.B. scale was introduced in the year 1972, with some minor changes.

Binet test has also been accepted in India. Such an attempt was made by C.H. Rice in 1922 in his book 'Hindustani Binet Performance Point Scale'.

B. Verbal Group Intelligence Tests

These tests are designed to test the intelligence of a group of individuals. All the people in the group have to follow a common pattern of direction and activities.

Some of the verbal group intelligence tests are narrated below:

1. Army Alpha Tests

These tests were evolved during the 1st world war. The tests were adopted for recruitment of American soldiers. The aim of this test was to discriminate between the soldiers who are feeble-minded and who are skilled specialists.

2. Naval and Army General Classification Tests

These tests were evolved during World War II. It is said that one billion people were tested by the military general classification tests during the years 1941 to 1946. The test included vocabulary mathematics and numerical tests for the selection of candidates.

3. Sohan Lal's Intelligence Test

From the Indian scenario, Dr. Sohanlal's intelligence test in this direction is praiseworthy. Sohanlal's test is recommended for 11 to 15 year old children. The Uttar Pradesh State Bureau of Psychology employs this test.

Demerits of Verbal Group Intelligence Tests

In conduction of verbal group intelligence tests, some defects have been observed:

a. One of the major defects of such tests is that it is difficult to discern whether the examinee is performing the test out of compulsion or not.

b. In these tests, it is difficult to determine whether the physical and emotional balance of the examinees are even or disturbed.

c. Malpractice like copying from the neighbor is another negative aspect of such tests.

C. Non-verbal Individual Intelligence Test

1. Pintner-Paterson Tests

It was evolved by Pintner and Paterson in 1917. This test consists of 15 types of tests, of which 4 are form boards, 6 are picture completion, memory span and the rest picture puzzles and imitation. This is a popular scale in the U.S.A. This was mainly devised for use by deaf and linguistically backward children of ages between the 4 – 14. The test incorporates picture puzzle tests, Seguin form board tests, Five figure tests (five geometric figures are cut into two or three parts and the subject has to construct them and fix into appropriate places), two figure tests (identical to five figure test), triangle test (four triangular pieces are to be fitted in the form board), diagonal tests (five different shaped sections are to be put into rectangle spaces), feature tests (wooden parts of a man's head are to be put together), a ship test (scattered parts of ship are joined to form a ship), etc.

2. Merrill-Palmer Block Building Tests

One of the most important of performance tests for children is Merrill-Palmer Block Building Test. In the following figure, a girl of four years is building a structure by means of blocks as demonstrated by the instructor who sits beside her.

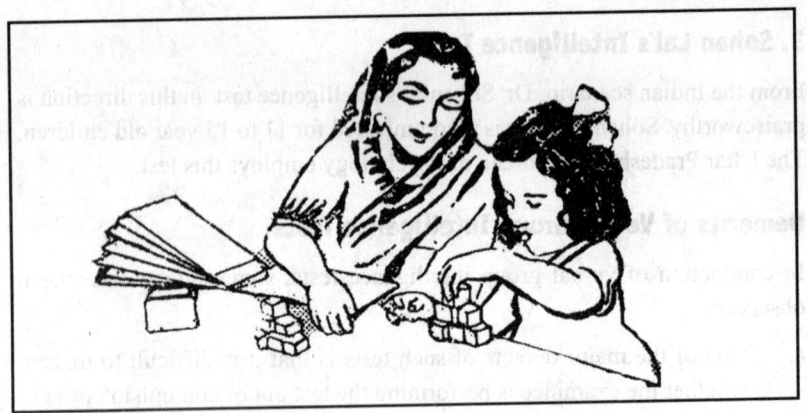

Merrill-Palmer Block Building Test

3. Porteus Maze Test

Porteus maze test is considered as an important test in the assessment of non-verbal individual intelligence test. The following figure is called a maze. Maze means a complicated system of passages which people try to find their way through for amusement. The tests consist of a series of mazes of ascending difficulty each printed on individual sheets. For these tests, Porteus created mazes for children from 3 to 14 years. These tests designed by Porteus not only measure the intelligence, but also

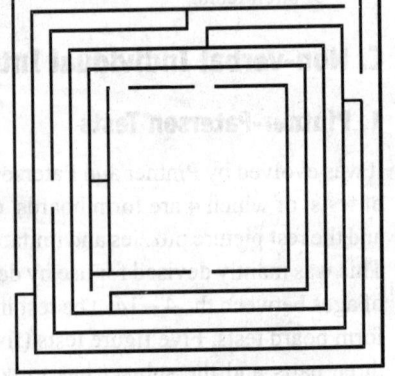

Proteus Maze Test

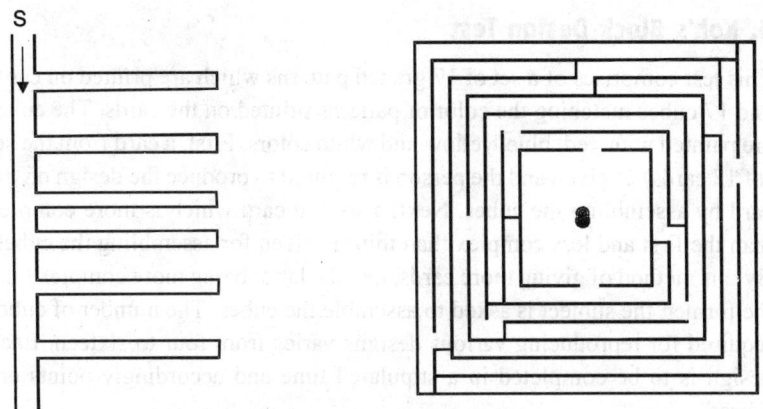

A Simple and a Complex Maze from the Porteus Maze Test

replicate the temperament of the individual. It evaluates some aspects of intelligence that are not met by the criteria of Stanford-Binet tests.

4. Form Board Test

Out of various form board tests, test of Seguin deserves special attention. In this form board test, there are ten blocks and a board in which there are apertures corresponding to this block. The instructor removes the blocks from the apertures and directs the subject to fit the blocks in the appropriate aperture.

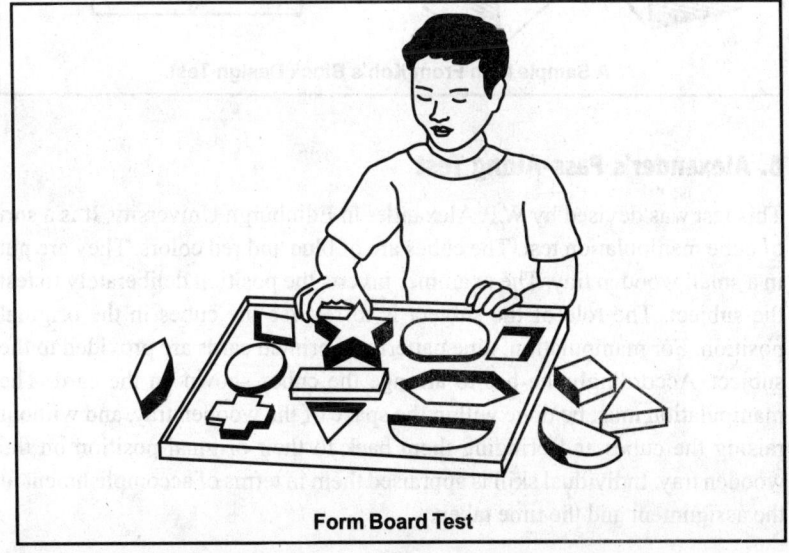

Form Board Test

5. Koh's Block Design Test

This test comprises of a set of 17 graded patterns which are printed on cards and 17 cubes matching the color of patterns printed on the cards. The cubes are painted with red, blue, yellow and white colors. First, a card from the set (of 17 cards) is given and the person is required to produce the design on the card by assembling the cubes. Next, a second card which is more complex than the first and less complex than third is given for assembling the cubes. By this method of giving more cards, i.e., the latter being more complex than the former, the subject is asked to assemble the cubes. The number of cubes required for reproducing various designs varies from four to sixteen. Each design is to be completed in a stipulated time and accordingly points are scored.

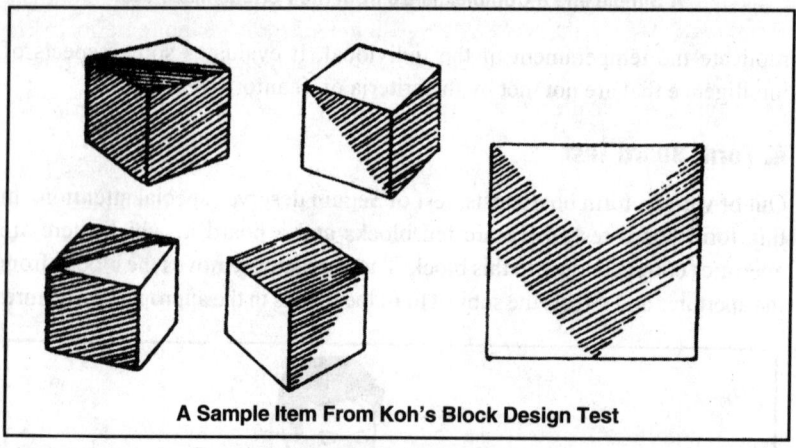

A Sample Item From Koh's Block Design Test

6. Alexander's Pass-Along Test

This test was devised by W.P. Alexander in Edinburgh University. It is a sort of cube manipulation test. The cubes are of blue and red colors. They are put in a small wooden tray. The examiner inverts the position deliberately to test the subject. The role of the subject is to reverse the cubes in the original position. For manipulation, nine patterns of printed cards are provided to the subject. Accordingly, he has to arrange the cubes shown on the card. The manipulation must be done within the space of the wooden tray, and without raising the cubes and bringing them back to their original position on the wooden tray. Individual skill is appraised them in terms of accomplishment in the assignment and the time taken.

7. Bhatia's Battery of Performance Tests

This test was devised by Dr. Chandra Mohan Bhatia, who was the former director of Uttar Pradesh Manovigyanshala. It comprises of the following sub-tests:

a. **Block Design:** Koh's block test as mentioned above.
b. **Alexander's Pass-Along Test:** as mentioned above.
c. **Pattern Drawing Test:** This test consists of eight cards of a particular form. The subject is asked to draw a particular figure or pattern after observing the forms.
d. **Immediate Memory Test:** Some digits are recited by the examiner. The subject has to repeat those digits immediately in the same order. This activity is an indicator of the immediate memory of the subject.
e. **Picture Construction Test:** In this sub-test, five scattered pictures of rural life of India are given to the subject and he has to complete the test by jotting down those pictures in a correct way.

The test items are arranged in an ascending complexity. The scores on these five tests depends upon the time taken for the completion of the task successfully. Then these scores are added to reach the final score. Finally the scores are converted into the mental age with reference to norms for different age groups. The I.Q. is calculated using the following formula:

$$\frac{Mental\ Age}{Chronological\ Age} \times 100$$

8. Wechsler-Bellevue Test (1939)

The Stanford-Binet (1937) scale was widely accepted by various parts of the globe. But it could not cater to the needs of adults or old people. The test was only standardized for people up to 18 years of age. Hence, there was a need of another alternative that could be utilised for a higher age group. Thus, the Wechsler-Bellevue scale came to light in 1939 as a compliment to the Stanford-Binet test. The scale was revised in 1955 and called as WAIS (Wechsler Adult Intelligence Test). With this method we can go for intelligence test, for 16 to 60 years of age. In modern clinics, it is used along with Binet test. This test affords not only an index to mental abilities but also a profile of abilities.

This scale is available in two forms i.e.:

a. WISC for children.
b. WAIS for adults.

The scale consists of the following sub-tests which fall into two broad categories:

i. Verbal tests which comprises of six tests:
   - Test of vocabulary
   - Test of general information
   - Test of arithmetic reasoning
   - Test of comprehension
   - Test of discrimination between similarities
   - Test of digit span

ii. Non-verbal performance tests which comprise of five tests:
   - Bock design test
   - Picture completion test
   - Picture arrangement test
   - Object assembly test
   - Digit symbol test

Salient Differentiating Points Between Stanford-Binet and WAIS Test

i. First, Stanford-Binet is a mental age scale whereas WAIS is a point scale. In WAIS, points are given for evaluation of responses. This test is not concerned with the mental age group.

ii. Secondly, in Stanford-Binet scale, types of test-items are meant for different age-levels whereas in WAIS test, items of alike types are set together for sub-tests.

iii. Thirdly, in the Stanford-Binet, all individuals above the age of 18 are treated in a similar fashion in terms of computing I.Q. On the other hand, WAIS has separate age-norms for adults. The mental age beyond 14 cannot be interpreted in the same simple and straight forward manner as those below 14.

iv. WAIS consists of verbal scale (6 tests) and performance scale (5 tests) which differs considerably, from the Stanford-Binet scale

Other tests are Arthur's Point Scale, Chicago Non-verbal Tests, Ravet's Progressive Matrices Tests, C.I.E. Non- verbal Tests, etc.

INTELLIGENCE

D. Non-verbal Group Intelligence Tests

Verbal intelligence tests are meant only for literate subjects. It is for this reason that the non-verbal group intelligence tests have been developed so that a test can be conducted while making minimum use of language and performing many activities.

Examples of the non-verbal intelligence tests are:

1. Army beta tests developed in the 1st World war.
2. Catell's culture free test and the N.I.I.P. test.
3. Chicago non-verbal test.
4. Raven's progressive matrices test.
5. C.I.E. non-verbal group test of intelligence.

Some examples of non-verbal group intelligence tests are:

a. Which one of the figures does not belong to the other four:

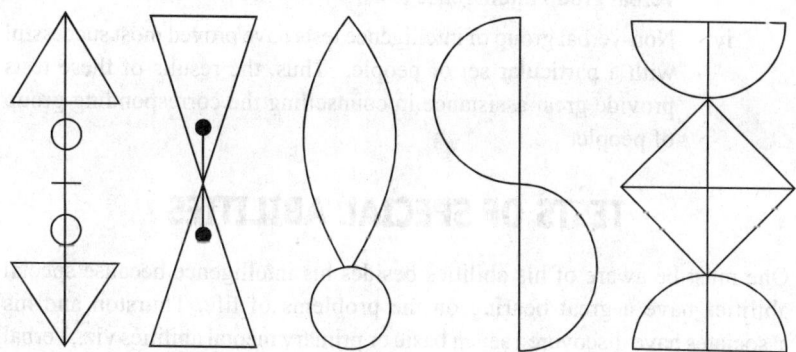

Figure

b. The following circles have an arrow following a pattern. Fill up the next figure of this series in the question mark.

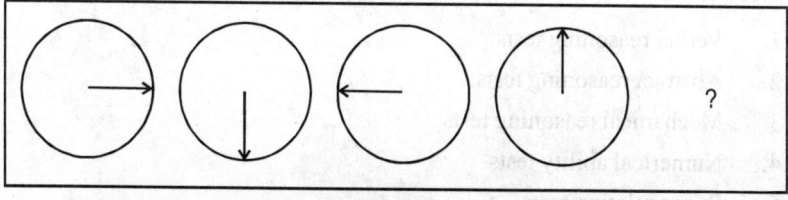

Figure

c. Find the odd figure among the following:

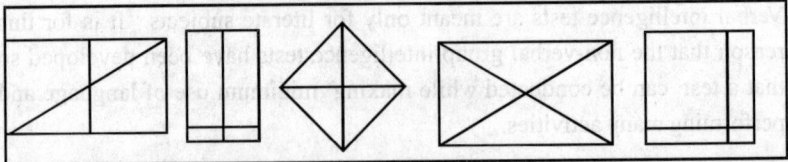

Figure

We need non-verbal group of intelligence test for the following reasons:

i. Difference of language is the first obstacle in the comparison of human groups, which can be permeated through the non-verbal group intelligence tests.

ii. The linguistic ability is very low in the case of children and therefore, intelligence testing of children is conducted through employing non-verbal group intelligence tests.

iii. Potentialities of illiterate solders are assessed by utilizing the non-verbal group intelligence tests.

iv. Non-verbal group of intelligence tests have proved most successful with a particular set of people. Thus, the results of these tests provide great assistance in counselling the corresponding group of people.

TESTS OF SPECIAL ABILITIES

One must be aware of his abilities besides his intelligence because special abilities have a great bearing on the problems of life. Thurston and his associates have discovered seven basic or primary mental abilities viz., verbal expression, numerals, reasoning or logic, memory, etc. Mental ability tests have been geared upon the foundation of these mental abilities. The Psychological Corporation of America and some other agencies around the globe conduct a test battery for selection of candidates based on the following seven tests:

1. Verbal reasoning tests.
2. Abstract reasoning tests.
3. Mechanical reasoning tests.
4. Numerical ability tests.
5. Space relation tests.

6. Clerical speed and accuracy tests.
7. Language tests.

Other Important Tests for Different Abilities

1. *Mechanical Ability Tests* are used in discovering the mechanical ability of the individuals.
2. *Motor Dexterity Tests* are used to determine the motor dexterity of fingers and hands of the candidate.
3. *Clerical Tests* are used to determine the clerical ability of the subject.
4. *Artistic or Ability Tests* are used to discover the artistic or aesthetic ability of the contender.
5. *Spatial Ability Tests* are used to verify the individual's skill regarding forms and space.
6. *The Sea Shore Measure of Musical Talent Test* is used to test the musical ability of an individual.
7. *Meier's Art Judgment Test* is applied to test the aesthetic judgment of a candidate.

CLINICAL APPLICATIONS

Mental sub-normality must be suspected from delay in motor milestones in the first few months of life. Here the role of medicines likes *Calcarea phos.* and *Natrium mur.* prove immensely helpful not only for restoration of mental functions but also for restoration of normal milestones in life.

Understanding of intellectual functions is highly necessary for us to understand intelligence. Through this we can evaluate sub-normality or very superior intelligence of an individual. In some diseases like epilepsy, various psychiatric disorders (including neuropsychiatry), some form of endocrine disorders, the assessment of intelligence is of great assistance in their management.

You should also know that distressing physical symptoms or mental symptoms like anxiety, bereavement, sadness, etc. may impair mental functioning, which can be prevented with homeopathic medicines and psychotherapy.

Again, you should know that very often an organic disease can affect the functioning of the brain that is likely to impair intellectual performance.

Here, you may resort to homeopathic medicines or you may refer the case to a neuro-surgeon.

In clinical practice, you may come across feeble minded individuals who seek treatment. Generally, these type of patients come to you for other problems. It is your knack to discover and add it in your totality. Feebleminded people possess less than average intelligence. These individuals cannot manage their own life without the supervision of others. Feeble minded individuals come under the following three categories.

Idiots: In common language we call such type of individuals stupid. These are people with very low intelligence, who cannot think or behave normally. These individuals cannot save themselves from even common dangers like crossing a road or lighting a fire. They are dirty people who, do not care about cleanliness. Moreover, these individuals depend on others for food and clothing.

Imbeciles: These individuals are superior in intelligence to idiots. They are quite capable of preventing themselves from common dangers like crossing a road or lighting a fire. They can talk but cannot write. These individuals can be trained for eating, bathing, putting on clothes, etc.

Morons: These individuals are superior to the above two catagories. They can perform jobs like eating, putting on clothes, etc. They can also carry out day to day routine jobs. However, they cannot earn a livelihood without somebody's help. They can be engaged as assistants in jobs like tailoring, carpentry, etc.

From the above it is clear that the assessment of an individual's intellectual abilities is of immense value for our clinical life where psychological problems may be arising in an educational or vocational context. Moreover, as a homeopath we possess a rich armament of medicines to treat such patients. In most cases, we can restore their physical and mental condition in toto.

You must posses the knowledge of intellectual functioning as a student now. You will need this in the future as a clinician and as a teacher for imparting education to students.

Chapter 13

THINKING

Why did you pick up this book (or chapter) for reading? You thought of something: May be the caption of the book or it may be related to your syllabus or it may be your general interest. In fact, it is the thinking (rather the process of thinking) that helps us to find the solution every moment of our problematic life. It is the higher level of thinking that differentiates us from lower animals. Psychologists admit that thinking is the most complex of all psychological processes.

THINKING: WHAT IT IS NOT?

The term 'thinking' is often used indiscriminately in day to day life. If you examine scrupulously the beginning of this book, you will discover that the word 'thinking' has been used inappropriately. If you ask somebody what he is doing right now in the evening by the seashore, the answer may be that he is thinking of his yester moments of life that have been happily spent with his wife. Similarly, if you ask another person in the vicinity of your campus during the admission session, the person may say that he is thinking of taking admission into B.H.M.S. course. Another may answer to your analogous question by saying that he is thinking of a home where he can lead a happy life.

Infact, none of the above instances can be attributed to the realm of thinking. In the first instance, may be the old man, was just collecting past events. In the second instance, he be a young aspirant, who was deciding about his career with a conflict. Similarly, in the third instance, she may be a young lady, who was imagining a beautiful house.

We should know that recollection is a process by which situations or events are recreated by the person concerned and recognized by him as coming from the past.

We should also know that imagination creates objects without the help of sense organs. These twin processes of recollection and imagination are parts of 'perception' and are not attributed to thinking.

Again, psychology of thinking should not be confused with logic. Logic is concerned with correct reasoning. Logic explains whether a given statement is correct or not by the process of analysis.

THINKING: WHAT IS IT?

Thinking is a very intricate mental process, usually associated with learning, memorizing, imagining, etc. From above, we have to admit that thinking is an incredibly complex process and cannot be separated easily from learning, memory (remembering), imagination, etc.

Thinking has been described in different ways by different psychologists on the basis of characteristics such as mental exploration, symbolic process, cognitive activity, problem solving behavior, mental or implicit trial and above all thinking.

Let us explore some of these definitions:

Thinking is a mental activity in its cognitive aspect or mental activity with regard to a psychological object (*Ross*, 1965).

Thinking is behavior which is often implicit and hidden, in which symbols (image, ideas, concepts) are ordinarily employed (*Garrett*, 1968).

Thinking is a problem solving activity in which we use ideas or symbols in place over activity (*Glimer*, 1970).

Thinking is an activity concerning ideas. It is symbolic in character initiated by a problem or task which the individual is facing, involving some trial or error but under the directing influence of that problem and ultimately leading to a conclusion or solution of the problem (*Waren*).

From above, it is obvious that psychologists view thinking under two aspects:

a. Some psychologist view thinking is an internal process.
b. Rest view it as a problem solving behavior.

Hence, on fusing these two aspects we can define thinking as an internal depiction of exterior actions, belonging to the precedent, current or upcoming, and may even relate a thing or an event which is not being actually observed or experienced by the thinker, whose goal is directed towards the solution of some specific, purposeful problem.

NATURE OF THINKING

Sometimes we exhort our friends by advising them not to think aimlessly. By saying so, we are not doing justice. Aimless thinking is a misnomer. No one can think in an aimless way. Thinking pre-supposes an aim with a reason. Secondly, it is a cognitive activity where signs, symbols, images, etc. are used, as thinking is a symbolic activity. In thinking, the problem is resolved mentally by the use of signs, symbols and mental images. Finally, thinking is a cognitive process where mental effort (along with a little motor activity) is involved.

TOOLS OR BASIC ELEMENTS OF THINKING/STAGES OF THINKING

Thinking involves assistance of six important elements:

1. Images

Thinking involves the use of images. There exist two contradictory views in this regard. Wurzberg school asserts that it is impossible to think without an image, while Binet, Kulpe and Woodworth state that one can think even without images. Let us synthesize both the views.

Image is a type of symbol which includes the faint recollection of perceptions. They are the mental pictures having personal experiences of persons, objects including scenes (or pictures or sights) seen, heard or felt. The mental images symbolize actual objects, experiences and activities. While thinking, we manouver the images rather than the actual objects, experiences or activities. Past experience of an individual moves around in the form of images in his mind. Images may be recalled through a conscious effort but they also flash on the mind involuntarily.

Anyhow, images are important ingredients of thinking but it does not mean that images are everything for thinking. Various experiments have pointed out that images are not fairly as necessary to thinking as they were regarded earlier. A singer or a philosopher uses less or no mode of images. They make better use of words than images. Similarly, subjects like arithmetic hardly use any images.

Finally, we can conclude that images may not be a need for abstract thinking, while in ordinary thinking we cannot evade images.

2. Concepts

Concept means a general idea that represents universal class and stands for the common attributes of all objects or events of this general class. In other words, the symbolic process in thinking, consists of images and implicit muscular activities. When symbols do not stand for a particular object (image) but for classes of objects it is called a concept. When you say a flower, it becomes generalization, but when you say 'a rose', this becomes a particular. In the previous point (i.e. flower) we are not referring to any particular flower but to all flowers, flowers as a class and in the latter case (i.e. rose) we are at once reminded not only about the nature and qualities of a rose as a class but also its individuality as a rose that is related to our own experiences and understanding of rose as a whole that appear in our consciousness to stimulate our thinking at that time.

The concept may be simple and objective (dog, elephant, flower) or abstract (God, life, vital force or principle), etc.

3. Symbols and Signs

During thinking one has to use symbols and signs as basic elements of thought. This can be compared to a chess board. Over a chess board, real kings or soldiers (pawn) are not used. Some icons are used for kings, soldiers, etc. Similarly, while thinking, an individual does not need the display of an item. He has to resort to symbols for thinking. Suppose you want to write an article on Kent's contribution to homeopathy, then a real Kent is not needed. You can employ Kent's portrait as a symbol for the article. The mental icon of Kent is essential for your thinking. While moving in traffic you might be well accustomed with the signals like red, which makes you stop, yellow that makes you to get ready and green to start. These are all symbols that represent a particular type of activity.

4. Language

Language is another resourceful and developed medium used for thinking. We use language in reading, listening, writing, etc. During this process we also adhere to thinking.

5. Muscle Activities

During thinking the role of various muscles is greatly reduced. Still a positive correlation has been established between muscle activity and thinking.

6. Function of Mind

Thinking is pre-eminently a function of mind. We also know that mind's primary function is to think. Without mind, we cannot think at all. We think most of the things by:

a. Perception.
b. Concept building.

a. Perception

It is the process of using the senses to acquire information about the surrounding environment or situation. When we listen to something or see something we are simulated to think. Hence, percepts are essential factors in thinking.

b. Concept Building

Concepts are understanding or grasping – the most basic understanding of something.

The mental portraits or images can be accumulated, created, renovated or put to use by our mind. These are the results of our mental functions.

THEORIES OF THINKING

In comparison to other branches of experimental psychology, research in psychology of thinking has been insufficient. Most of the works are empirical in nature. Here some important theories of thinking have been presented in a concise form:

1. Watson's Peripheral or Motor Theory

This theory states that we think not with our mind or brain alone but with the whole body. Watson, the founder of behaviorist school maintains that thinking is the function of the whole body.

2. Behaviorist Learning Theory

The chief exponents of this behavioristic school are Pavlov, Watson and B.F. Skinner. This school views thinking as that personal behavior which is guided by stimulus control and reinforcement in the same way as overt behavior.

According to this theory, the psychology of thinking is learnt or acquired. The behavior is associated with S-R mechanism, which has been described in the learning chapter. For example, movement of one's tongue or vocal cord is associated with one's thought. Thus a stimulus generated the process of thinking. The theory further asserts that a specific stimuli generates corresponding specific type of thinking, which has been conditioned.

3. Piaget's Development Theory

Piaget; the swiss postulated another type of explanation for the development of thinking. He interpreted his theory as per the successive stages of cognitive development, which consists of the following stages:

a. Sensory-motor stage.
b. Pre-operational stage.
c. Concrete operational stage.
d. Formal operational stage.

a. Sensory-motor Stage

This stage is attributed to the first two years of life from birth. In this stage the child is restricted to direct sensory and motor interaction with the environment. In this stage language is not used.

b. Pre-operational Stage

This stage lasts from two to seven year of age. In this stage, the child acquires himself with words, symbols and images. His thinking process becomes egoistic and not in a position to understand other's point of view.

c. Concrete Operational Stage

This stage starts at the age of seven and ends at about eleven years of age. During this period the child learns to think in a logical and concrete form. He is also able to understand cognitive concepts such as number, classification,

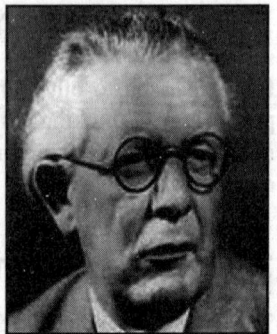

Jean Piaget (1896-1980)

conversation, etc. Anyhow, in this stage the child cannot comprehend the abstract type of thinking.

d. Formal Operational Stage

This stage starts at the age of 12 and lasts up to 15 years of age. In this stage the individual is able to think in abstract form. This is characterized by most advanced functioning of the cognitive system. Now he can engage himself in scientific thinking, problem solving, etc.

4. Bruner's Theory of Cognitive Development

Jerome Bruner, the American psychologist reckons cognitive development under 3 stages:

a. Enactive Representative Stage

This stage is characterized by the child's depiction of things and events in terms of appropriate motor responses and activities.

b. Iconic Representation Stage

This stage is characterized by the child's representation of things and events in terms of sensory and mental pictures.

c. Symbolic Representation Stage

This stage is characterized by depiction in the form of words, symbols and other imaginary and abstract things.

5. Sullivan's Basic Modes Theory

Sullivan postulated 3 basic developmental stages referred as modes of thought processes for explaining cognitive development. There are 3 modes which are mentioned below:
a. Prototaxic mode.
b. Parataxic mode.
c. Syntaxic mode.

a. Prototaxic Mode

This mode operates from birth. In this phase, there does not exist any distinct organization of thought process of the individual. The organism seeks pleasure by sucking the nipple and gets scared when separated from the mother.

b. Parataxic Mode

This mode is related to the childhood period. The child begins to differentiate between self and the world. But the thinking in this stage is in a rudimentary form. Usually such thoughts do not pertain to logical thinking.

c. Syntaxic Mode

In this mode, the development of logical thought processes including symbolic process and abstract reasoning is developed.

6. The Gestalt and Holistic Theory

This theory accentuates the magnitude of the organization of the perceptual ground in the development of thinking leading to problem solving behaviors. This pre-supposes that the psychology of thinking is always purposeful and goal oriented. Thinking is a holistic approach because, while thinking, we sort out and rearrange the perceived field to bring forth the finest solution for the given problem. Such acts of sorting out and rearranging of the perceptual field belong to the process and product of thinking.

7. Freud's Psycho-analytic Theory of Thinking

According to this theory the psychology of thinking is operated by two factors:

a. Internal desire for gratification of sex.
b. Role of unconscious moulding and shaping of one's behavior.

In the process of development of thinking, the infant does not show any activity by thinking. During this period the infant is dominated by Id principle. The principle of Id always seeks pleasure. As the child grows older, Ego comes into play in his personality. Then he begins to pay attention to people and his surroundings in order to be able to cope with them effectively. Now he begins to operate according to the reality principle and his thinking process becomes more rational and logical. In due course, Super Ego enters into his personality and it modifies thinking in accordance with morals, values and ideals of the society. Thinking becomes more objective. Hence it is the Super Ego that is instrumental in bringing creative thinking and abstract thinking together.

8. The Information Processing Theory

As the caption suggests here the information is processed for thinking. First the individual has to process the information by recording the current information and next to retrieve the relevant material involved in this information from memory. Then both the informations are subjected to thinking from various facets to solve the given purpose.

CLASSIFICATION OF THINKING

Thinking is a mental process which can be classified into:

I. Direct thinking, which is further classified into:
   1. Perceptual thinking.
   2. Conceptual thinking.
   3. Reflective thinking.
   4. Creative thinking.
II. Associative thinking.

I. Direct Thinking

1. Perceptual or Concrete Thinking

This is the simplest form of thinking. In this thinking only the actual objects and events are perceived. It is a very superficial way of thinking. Problems cannot be solved through such type of thinking.

2. Conceptual Thinking

It is a deeper form of thinking in comparison to perceptual form of thinking. In abstract thinking, an individual uses concepts, language and generalized ideas. It helps us in understanding and solving a problem.

3. Reflective Thinking

It is a higher form of thinking in comparison to perceptual and conceptual type of thinking. Such type of thinking is needed for solving complex problems. The relevant information is neatly collected, arranged in a logical order and treated with judicious thinking with a view to solve the complex problem. It pre-supposes that the thinker reorganizes his relevant experiences and the findings in a novel way in order to tackle the situation. Reflective thinking demands cognitive approaches instead of simple association of experiences or ideas. Reflective thinking shuns mechanical or trial and error method of solving problems. As a homeopath we need such thinking in meeting chronic cases of multi-miasmatic nature. We badly need reflective thinking during repertorisation of a given case to bring out the simillimum among many similar medicines.

4. Creative Thinking

This type of thinking is essentially intended to create something new. It examines new links and associations for describing events or situations.

Creative thinking has four stages:

i. Preparation.
ii. Incubation.
iii. Illumination.
iv. Verification.

In the phase of *preparation*, facts relating to the problem are collected. Relevant information is processed. The relevant and important aspects of the subject preserved. Superfluous and unnecessary materials are pruned and thrown away, like the process of separating chaff from grain.

In the *incubation period*, the above facts are given a thought to evolve a disciplined and distinct pattern of thinking. During this period, serious type of contemplation is carried out. One has to meditate a lot to present a plausible presentation.

In the *illumination phase*, inspiration is drawn from living or non-living media. Although in general, inspiration comes from a given source it may be related to motivation. The author was illuminated to write this book after realising the importance of role of the psychology in homeopathy and his desire to share his knowledge with other homeopaths.

In the *verification stage* the future presenting materials are verified. This is very important for scientific thesis or discovery.

II. Associative Thinking

See Day dreaming from the chapter 'Dreams'.

STRATEGIES INVOLVED IN PROBLEM SOLVING

1. Awareness and Identification of the Problem

First, an individual should be aware of the problem. He must perceive the problem in a right way. Moreover, it should be a well defined one. A problem ill understood may not lead to a plausible solution, Moreover, the problem must be an important one and he should be interested to solve it for an immediate need.

2. Understanding of the Problem

In this step, the problem is analysed and synthesised for understanding the real nature of the problem. The individual must be able to discover the modes and means to solve the problem along with anticipating possible impediments in the course of action.

3. Collection of Relevant Information

This step involves to collection of all the information regarding the problem including data and knowledge in relation to the problem. Own experience, knowledge from books or other alike sources may prove beneficial in exploring the relevant information for the given problem.

4. Formulation of Hypothesis for a Possible Solution

Hypothesis means a theory needing investigation, a tentative explanation for a phenomenon, used as a basis for further investigation. This step pre-supposes that the individual successfully identifies and understands at the same time collects information regarding the solution. Now he must make certain assumptions regarding the end result. The problem is moved in the right perspective for fulfilling these assumptions.

5. Evaluation and Selection of the Correct Solution

This step requires examination and scrutinization of the hypothesis against the solution obtained. The individual should also evaluate the negative aspect which may cast any doubt upon the conclusion. The thesis may be discarded and resorted to another alternative if the hypothesis failed to yield a solution.

6. Verification of the concluded solution or hypothesis

When the solution of the problem is arrived at, it must be further verified by applying it as the solution of various identical problems. By this we reach a general aspect from a particular aspect. Such solutions may be very useful for future similar problems.

Although in above, the strategies in relation to problem solving behavior are delineated, we must guard ourselves about factors like frustration, stress and rigidity; that can influence solving behavior.

ESSENTIAL ELEMENTS IN THINKING

We must remember two fundamental things about thinking. Good thinking means:
1. Adoption of correct thinking.
2. Ination of faulty methods of thinking.

Let us discuss what the essential elements in thinking are:

A. Interest and Attention

Interest and attention are very essential elements of thinking. Both favor thinking. It is a common observation that when we are interested in something then that something becomes a source of pleasure. On the contrary, when we are not interested in anything, then thinking becomes difficult. Interest facilitates attention for better thinking.

B. Motivation

Motivation is one of the important factors required for valid thinking. Motivation facilitates organized and controlled thinking. Motivation creates enthusiasm and wipes out fatigue by which one can adopt deep and sensible thinking.

C. Alertness and Flexibility

Alertness serves to keep away external faults and this helps us in proper thinking. It also checks errors and myths from sneaking into thinking.

Flexibility also keeps away traditional and blind believes. Flexibilities also open new arenas for judicious thinking. An alert person has novel methods and ways which promote favorable thinking. Alertness prevents occurrences of mistakes and omission of details in the process of thinking. Alertness and flexibility are of immense use for thinking.

D. Time Factor

For a successful thinking, time factor plays a crucial role. Hasty decision taken due to shortage of time or for other reasons may lead to premature thinking and failure. Moreover, too much time consumption may also have a deleterious effect on the assignment undertaken. Hence, a reasonable amount of time is needed for successful thinking.

E. Knowledge Factor

Knowledge is a very powerful factor for thinking as knowledge gives insight and right direction for thinking. The role of this factor is very decisive in professional achievements.

F. Incubation Factor

Very often we may find ourselves amidst a labyrinth of problems. We try again and again to think and yet do not get any solution. Then we lay aside the problem and engross ourself for some time in another alternative. One day, all of a sudden, we find the solution. This happens so, because of the incubation of thinking. During incubation period, that is, during the period when we laid aside the problem, our mind kept pondering for the solution and ultimately became successful in solving the problem. But we must remember that incubation does not mean the avoidance of the problem. Incubation can only occur if a good effort is attempted for the solution of the problem.

G. Miscellaneous

We must know that thinking must be free from prejudice, belief and emotion. One must guard oneself from various advices while thinking as a wrong advice may lead us astray while the right one may provide us rich dividends. The conclusion must be drawn with the help of logical steps.

HOW TO THINK CORRECTLY

Education and science provide a factual background which the individual needs in his thinking, where as, psychology provides knowledge about the actual thinking process and the causes of faulty thinking. The fundamental problem of applied psychology of thinking is to enhance the ability. Thinking does not seem to be an ordinary process and there is no simple or easy substitute for it. But the best can be obtained if it becomes spontaneous or natural. Again if you enjoy it like playing, thinking becomes easy and leads to the right way of thinking.

Good and correct thinking depends upon the following factors:
1. **Motivation:** Motivation is the prime factor for thinking, which can be employed during powerful thinking for the given problem in hand.
2. **Interest and Enthusiasm:** Interest and enthusiasm favors insight thinking.
3. **Knowledge:** Knowledge factor in relation to a given problem facilitates the right manner of thinking so that one can have the right solution.
4. **Incubation Factor:** It is not easy to have the advantage of incubation factor. Think hard and honestly to find a solution for the given problem. If you cannot reach a plausible solution, lay the problem aside. Then there is maximum chance that you will find the solution out of the blue. Even if you obtain an average solution to the problem from the blue, the next attempt at thinking may fetch the perfect answer to your problem.
5. **Other Factors:** Other factors like logical pattern of reasoning along with burning zeal help in correct thinking. Too rigid and too short a time for thinking may prove detrimental. Of course, the time schedule may not be fixed for thinking if the problem is interesting, whereas time must be fixed for thinking for an interesting problem.

CLINICAL APPLICATION

After the advent of computer, a new programme called 'decision tree' has been developed which is used largely in clinical decision making in relation to diagnosis, treatment, management, prognosis, etc. The decision is taken on the answer of patients to various questions that relate to signs, pathological finding, etc.

Disorder of thinking is also attributed to schizophrenia, and neurological disorders like dementia, delirium, conflicting ideas, delusions, etc.

We can adopt cognitive therapy as an adjuvant means to treat conditions like pessimism and allied negative and harmful thinking.

We can also encourage patients to think in a proper way, so that life will become easier. Sometimes many patients refrain to undergo surgery. In such cases, making the patient think in the right way is important.

From homeopathic treatment point of view, thinking comes under perversion of understanding which is given higher order in evaluation of symptoms.

Chapter 14
PERSONALITY

People very often talk of personality. Generally we think personality as the external appearance of an individual. Personality is also taken as reputation or physical appeal of an individual. Philosophers use this term for designating self.

In psychology, personality implies something more than these fixations. The word personality comes from the Latin word '*persona*' which means 'mask'. Mask is used by actors to represent a specific character in a drama However, generally speaking, the personality of an individual is judged by conduct, behavior, activities, movements, etc.

We must understand something more about this concept. When we take birth, our state can be compared to a blank board. Here our parents write our name as "Amar" or "Akbar" or "Anthony". Similarly, we are told that we belong to a particular religion say Hinduism or Islam or Christianity. Events after events are written on this blank board. Hence we convert to a personality from an individual. Despite all these inscriptions, on our board, we are individuals and this can be attributed as our personality.

DEFINITION

One of the earliest definitions given by Watson (1930), the Father of Behaviorism is:

Personality is the sum of activities that can be discovered by actual observations over a long enough period of time to give reliable information.

A better definition of personality is given by another contemporary psychologist, Morton Prince (1930), which is widely accepted by various psychologists:

Personality is the sum total of all the biological innate dispositions, impulses, tendencies, appetites and instincts of the individual and the disposition and tendencies acquired by experience.

This definition has a broader base which includes environment and heredity factors in constituting what is termed as personality. However, some later psychologists criticized this definition stating that it lacks the integral and organizational view of personality. Moreover, they argue that personality cannot be a mere summing up of the various elements, which can be compared to a house being a mere collection of bricks.

Gordon W. Allport of Harvard University (1948), after dissecting, analyzing and synthesizing 50 such definitions, presented a beautiful definition, which is accepted by most of the contemporary and modern psychologists. It is presented below:

Personality is a dynamic organization within the individual of those psycho-physical systems that determine his unique adjustment to his environment.

The above definition can be better comprehended if its key words are further discussed.

Dynamic refers to the regular evolvement of the nature of personality. The individual's structural, physical, psychological characters develop from time to time which are neither fundamental nor everlasting, hence dynamic.

Organization means the patterning of the independent parts of the individual towards a whole. These parts are not aimless or scattered congregations. These may exist in different traits but has a special relation to the whole.

Psychophysical system is composed of habits, attitudes, emotional states, sentiments, motives and beliefs, all of which are psychological in nature having a physical basis in the individual's nervous, endocrine including bodily states.

Determine emphasizes the motivational role of the psycho-physical systems. Once attitude, belief, habit, sentiment, etc. of psychophysical system have been aroused by a stimulus may it be from the environment or within the individual, it provokes.

CHARACTERISTICS OF PERSONALITY

1. Personality is unique and specific. Each and every individual possess his own self or characteristic personality.

2. Personality depicts dynamic bearings of an organism to the environment. It is not given readymade at birth. Basic structures and characteristics of personality interact with each other. Some of them change in course of their development. Except the basic physical structure and native ability, all traits are acquired.
3. Personality is the product of heredity and environment.
4. Personality refers to persistent qualities of an individual. Most of the characteristics remain relatively persistent and permanent.
5. Personality is greatly influenced by social interaction. After birth, the neonate comes in contact with other people for the fulfilment of the basic necessities of life. In course of contact he develops interaction with surroundings and its people, that influence his personality development.
6. Personality represents a unique organisation of persistent dynamic and social predispositions.
7. Personality by itself is an unique organisation and remains as a whole. Each personality has many dimensions: Physical, mental, intellectual, emotional, social, etc. But these dimensions are not scattered or disorganised or isolated components of personality. They are interrelated with each other in cohesion. All these traits operate as a whole, as a totality. Personality is not just a conglomeration of some traits or characteristics but a psycho-physical arrangement which functions like an integrated whole.
8. Personality expresses itself in three ways:
   a. The explicit act related to muscular activities.
   b. The verbal and communicative activities. Hence we often say a neonate or infant or an animal does not have a personality.
   c. The thought and other internal subjective activities that is emotions, impulses, etc. Some of these can be expressed along with language. Same word uttered in different accent will connote different meanings.
9. Personality can be assessed (and even measured).
10. Personality should not be confused with terms like character, temperament or ego. We must know that character is an ethical concept and it is the moral value of a person. Temperament is a system of emotional disposition. Ego means 'I' and it is a part of personality.

11. Personality may also disintegrate under stress, severe anxiety, prolonged illness, grief, traumatic experiences, and brain and nerve affections. The disintegration may lead to serious conditions.

TYPES OF PERSONALITIES

I. Type approach :
   The exponents of this theory are:
   1. Hippocrates.
   2. Kretschmer.
   3. Sheldon.
   4. Jung.
II. Trait approach:
   The view point subscribed is:
   1. Allport.
   2. Catell.
III. Type cum trait approach:
   1. Eysenck.
IV. Psycho-analytical approach:
   1. Freud.
   2. Adler.
   3. Jung.
V. Humanistic approach:
   1. Carl Roger.
   2. Maslow.
VI. Learning approach:
   1. Dollard and Millers.
   2. Bandura and Walter.

I. Type Approach

The exponents of this theory are Hippocrates, Kretschmer, Sheldon and Jung.

1. Hippocrates's Classification of Personality (460 BC- 377)

(*Hippocrates is traditionally regarded as the father of medicine. You are aware of Hippocratic Oath (not written by him), which in modified form is still often required to be taken by medical students on graduating.*)

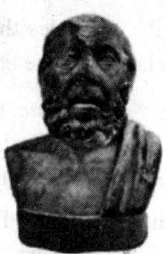

Hippcrates (460 BC-377)

Types of Personality	Dominance of Fluid type in the body	Temperamental Characteristics
Sanguine	Blood	• Optimistic • Happy • Light hearted • Adjusting
Phlegmatic	Phlegm (mucus)	• Calm • Cold • Sluggish • Indifferent
Choleric	Yellow bile	• Irritable and angry • Passionate
Melancholic	Black bile	• Pessimistic • Dejected • Sad • Bad tempered

2. Kretschmer's Classification of Personality

Types of personality are illustrated by E. Kretschmer in his book "*Physique and Character*". Kretschmer has classified people into two classes according to their physical structure:

a. *Cycloid*: These people are obese, sociable and happy, and possess an independent temperament.

b. *Schizoid*: People belonging to the schizoid group are thin and tall. They are temperamentally self-centred, emotional, reserved and peaceful, and seek solitude.

Besides these two types, Kretschmer has mentioned some more sub-classes on the basis of physical structure, some of the main ones being:

i. *Asthenic*: People of this group are short and thin. They are self-centred, emotional, dreamy and intellectual. Such people possess peace and solitude, and have a loving temperament.

ii. *Athletic*: People of this type have broad shoulders and a slim waist. They are energetic, active, optimistic and highly adjustable people.

iii. *Pyknic*: These people are obese. Their tummy has a round look. They are jolly, happy, good natured, sociable and easy going people.

3. Sheldon's Classification of Personality

W.H. Sheldon mentions the following types of personality in his book *'The Varieties of Temperament'*. On the basis of shape and size, Sheldon classified people into these groups:

a. *Endomorphic*: This type of personality is also called *Viscerotonia*. People belonging to thus group of personality have highly developed viscera with weak somatic structures. The body of these type of people has a tendency towards roundness and softness. They are fond of eating delicious food. They suffer from apprehension and insecurity. They are friendly, amiable and social people who obey the rules of social conventions. The endomorphic type of personality greatly resembles Kretschmer's asthenic type.

b. *Mesomorphic*: This type of personality is also known as *Somatotonia* personality. In this type of personality, the individual possesses balanced development of viscera and somatic structure. There is predominant development of muscular and bony growths. These are adventurous people. They can do strenuous exercise and can withstand various kinds of physical pains easily. Kretschmer's athletic type of personality greatly resembles this type of personality.

c. *Ectomorphic*: This personality is weak in somatic structure with underdeveloped viscera. Their bones are long and soft while the physical structure is weak. They are social, amiable people who do not like taking exercise (*Capsicum*). They are over-sensitive to pain. This type of personality coincides with Kretschmer's pyknic type of personality

4. Jung's Classification of Personality

(See chapter "8" Neo-Freudian Psychodynamics)

II. Trait Approach

The chief exponents of this view are Allport and Cattell.

1. Allport's Approach

Allport views personality from the particularisation point of view instead of generalisation as far as investigation of its behavior is concerned. Hence he adheres to the synthetic approach instead of analytical approach. This made him differ from his predecessors, who had tried to categorise personality in sectoral approach.

Allport stood with three types of traits:

a. Cardinal trait.
b. Central trait.
c. Secondary trait.

a. Cardinal Trait

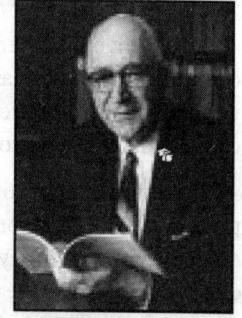

Gordon Allport
(1897-1967)

Cardinal traits are limited to one or two in number. These are relatively permanent manifestation in behavior. This can be compared to a prism through which every aspect of one's behavior is modulated. If a person's cardinal trait is argument, then he will fetch argument in all circumstances irrespective of its need or no need. This cardinal train outshines other traits.

Once a senior lady teacher in the subject of Materia Medica in a homeopathic institution was asked by the principal to submit the percentage and mark sheets of students in a test examination. She submitted the mark sheet and attendance of a student in Materia Medica for a student who had died in a rail accident six months prior to the conduction of the examination. 'When the principal asked for an explanation regarding this, the lady teacher, instead of apologising, retorted that this is not her problem but is the principal's outlook and she is not responsible for this lapse. Here, the teacher's cardinal trait is argument, which has been observed on many instances. Myrill's *Thematic Repertory* seems to have a great resemblance with this concept. *In homeopathy, any symptom that is predominant, persistent and permanent is taken into account for a prescription.*

Similarly, if a person's cardinal trait is a marked sense of humor then he will display a sense of humor in almost all circumstances irrespective of its need in a given situation. The cardinal trait dominates the whole personality of an individual along with other traits.

b. Central Traits

Central traits are those few characteristic tendencies which are generally used to describe a person. For example, a person may be honest or kind or benevolent or philanthropic.

c. Secondary Traits

Secondary traits appear on fewer occasions and are generally not noticed.

We have to remember that a cardinal trait is like a pivot around which central traits revolve and form a personality. Other common traits are not very significant and are found in almost all individuals. These common traits cannot attribute a personality.

Allport's vision of equilibrium between common trait and individual is praiseworthy. His theory evidently delineates that an individual differs from others in many ways, yet possesses common traits with them. He attributes cultural fixation as the involvement of common traits. *This concept remains identical with our concomitant symptom/s of a given disease condition.*

Initially Allport selected 18,000 terms out of which he selected 450 psychological traits for describing human behavior. Regarding development of personality, he has contributed a novel view. He divides 3 steps of growth and development:

i. Childhood.
ii. Adolescence.
iii. Adulthood.

According to his view, this growth pattern is neither linear nor continuous from childhood to adulthood. Rather, it is discrete and irregular. He further points out that what matters during childhood certainly differs from values during adolescence and adulthood. Allport further maintains that the adult's or adolescent's functioning is not constrained by his past. Only the relevant aspects of present are collected for the future and reflected in behavior manifestation and development of personality.

Criticism to Allport's Views

Despite of plus points of Allport's theory, he is still not free from criticism.

a. His theory of personality lacks a feasible proposal to study the growth pattern and development from conception to old age.
b. His assertion of personality which is not continuous between childhood, period of adolescence and adulthood. Naturally, here rises the question how the continuation of childhood, adolescent, adulthood, etc. can be detached from the past or future.
c. Again his uniqueness of one's personality did not convey existence and utility of specific trait concept.
d. The reason that the trait theory seems to be confusion.

2. Catell's Approach

The full name is Raymond Bernard Cattell, British-born, American psychologist, who is considered to be one of the world's leading personality theorists. He was born on March 20th, 1905 at Staffordshire, England. Cattell was educated at the University of London, receiving a B.S. in 1924 and a Ph.D. in 1929. He taught at various universities of the globe like Atthe University, Clarke University and Harvard University at various capacities. He was appointed research professor of psychology at the University of Illinois in Urbana (1945), a position he held until becoming Emeritus Professor in 1974. He died on February 2nd, 1998, in Honolulu, Hawaii, U.S.

Cattell is one of the chief exponents of trait theory. According to him traits are the structures of the personality inferred from study of behavior under various situations. He classifies traits under four heads:

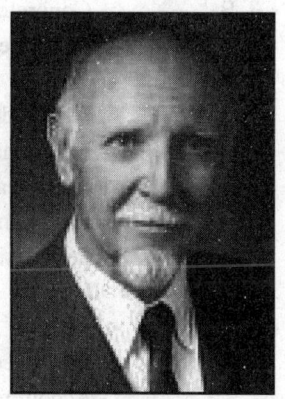

Raymond Cattell (1905-1998)

a. *Common Traits*: Traits like honesty, aggression, cooperation come under common traits which are distributed widely among the general population.
b. *Unique Traits*: These traits are found among selected groups of people like temperament traits, emotional traits, etc.
c. *Surface Traits*: These are observed as overt behavior such as curiosity, integrity, tactfulness, dependability, etc.
d. *Source Traits*: These are the underlying structures or sources that determine behavior such as dominance, submission, etc. (see below).

Cattell and his associates started with a list over 4500 adjectives applicable to human behavior. Later, they adopted a simpler version of 170 adjectives, which were the essence of those 4500 adjectives. Then those adjectives were given to college students to describe their acquaintances with those adjectives. The result was treated with statistical analysis to identify groupings or factors among the items. Out of these 170 adjectives, 16 factors were identified by Cattell to reflect key characteristics or source traits of human personality. These 16 factors are bipolar in nature which are given below.

Symbols	Traits	Name of the Factors
A	Cool	Warm
	Reserved	Outgoing
	Impersonal	Kindly
	Detached	Easy going
	Formal	Participating
	Aloof	Likes people
B	Concrete Thinking	Abstract Thinking
	Less Intelligent	More intelligent
		Bright
C	Affected by feeling	Emotionally stable
	Emotionally less stable	Mature
	Faces reality	Calm
	Easily annoyed	
E	Submissive	Dominant
	Humble	Assertive
	Mild	Aggressive
	Easily led	Stubborn
	Accommodating	Competitive
		Bossy
F	Sober	Enthusiastic
	Restrained	Impulsive
	Prudent	Heedless
	Taciturn	Expressive
	Serious	Cheerful
G	Expedient	Conscientious
	Disregards rules	Persistent
	Self-indulgent	Moralistic
		Staid
		Rule bound

H	Shy	Bold
	Threat sensitive	Venturesome
	Timid	Uninhibited
	Hesitant	Can take stress
	Intimidated	
I	Tough minded	Tender-minded
	Self-reliant	Sensitive
	No nonsense	Over-protected
	Rough	Intuitive
	Realistic	Refined
L	Trusting	Suspicious
	Accepting conditions	Hard to fool
	Easy to get on with	Distrustful
		Sceptical
M	Practical	Imaginative
	Concerned with "down to earth" issues	Absent-minded Absorbed in thoughts
	Steady	Impractical
N	Forthright	Shrewd
	Unpretentious	Polished
	Open	Socially aware
	Genuine	Diplomatic
	Artless	Calculating
O	Self-assured	Apprehensive
	Secure	Self-blaming
	Feels free of guilt	Guilt prone
	Untroubled	Insecure
	Self-satisfied	Worrying
Q1	Conservative	Experimenting
	Respecting traditional ideas	Liberal Critical
		Open to change
Q2	Group oriented	Self-sufficient
	A "joiner" and sound follower listens to others	Resourceful Prefers own decision
Q3	Undisciplined self-conflict	Controlled
	Lax	Self-respecting
	Careless of social rules	Socially precise
		Compulsive

Q4	Relaxed	Tense
	Tranquil	Frustrated
	Composed	Over-wrought
	Has low drive	Has a high drive
	Unfrustrated	

III. Type Cum Trait Approach: Eysenck

Catell's main approach was to give an explanation about personality by using the factor analysis technique. Hans Jurgen Eysenck was a German-born British psychologist, who goes further, and complements catell's factor analysis technique by extracting second order factors and grouping traits into special personality traits.

Eysenck divided 4 levels of behavioral organizations:

1. Specific response.
2. Habitual response.
3. Organizational response.
4. Organization of the above acts into traits.

Let us take an example of a lady, who blushes (1st Phase) on the slightest cause and examine through Eysenck's approach. After blushing, she gets embarassed and she avoids people. However, sooner or later she will meet an acquaintance. Now she will either avoid friendship or deal with the habitual response (IInd phase). Later, in a similar situation in a group trait express shyness (IIIrd phase). At the IV the level the lady may become introvert and shun the world.

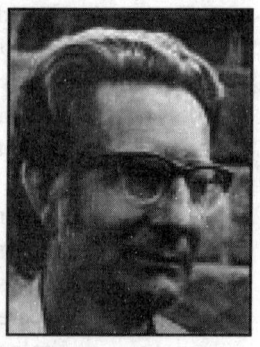

H.J. Eysenck (1916-1997)

IV. Psycho-analytical Approach

Freud, Adler, Jung (See Freud and Neo-Freudians).

V. Humanistic Approach

Under this we will study carl Rogers and Maslow.

1. Carl Rogers

The full name of Carl Rogers is Carl Ransom Rogers. He was an American psychologist, born on January 8th, 1902. He died on February 4th, 1987 at La Jolla, California. He was the creator of the non-directive or client-centred approach to psychotherapy, emphasizing a person-to-person relationship between the therapist and the client. He prefers the word client for patient. From this he evolved his 'theory of self'. In fact, his ambition was to be a minister, but he was destined for something else that is what we obtain today.

Rogers criticises learning theory of personality as mechanical. He rejected that behavior is not based on primary or physiological needs, drives or avoidances but on higher driving forces within the human being which compel him towards complex personality patterns.

Rogers does not attribute any fixation of stage of personality like Freud. Carl Rogers explained personality as a process of growth. He asserted that every individual endeavors to develop his self continuously. He propounded the symbolization of personality. Symbolization means formation of concept of self in an individual. The concept of self is formed by introducing the external factors or stuff that fits into his conscious world and discards those that do not.

Rogers also attributes creativity as the outcome of an individual's flexibility in the development of a personality. The flexibility helps in solving various problems and initiates greater creativity and productivity.

Structure of Personality

Carl Roger's divides structure of personality under:

a. Organism.
b. Self.

Rogers stresses that the individual is the centre of all experiences which are taking place within the individual in a given time. The totality of experience is called 'phenomenal field'. It develops a person's sole outlook.

The self: In addition to the present self, there is also an ideal self, the self, the person would like to be i.e., the projected self.

Trouble occurs when there is non-coherence of the present self and projected self. Self is the inner world in the form of natural impulses which interacts with our entire range of experience which is acquired from the environment. For example, when somebody is told that he is brave or she is beautiful, then the individual accepts and includes it in his self. Such acceptances and inclusions are a continuous process based on one's own needs than on reality.

The ideal self is the projected self. The important fact of development is how the person projects himself and elevates his worth at a particular time.

As per Carl Rogers, each of us has the potential for self-actualization. For him self-actualization means a set of guiding principles which are the bridge between the present self and the projected self. But one must be aware of his potential. Potential requires further care and nurture. According to him behavior is basically the goal oriented efforts of the organism to satisfy needs as experienced in the field.

Dynamics of Personality

Carl Rogers stressed that an individual frequently strives to build up and expand himself. Motivation is focussed on striving to one's goal of self-actualization. In order to have a self-actualization, following conditions have been attributed by Carl Rogers:

a. The person must respect and have confidence in himself.
b. He must be aware of his potential.
c. He must have the abilities of achieving that goal.
d. He must be able to clearly perceive his choices. Being unaware of choices leads to impediment of self-growth.
e. The choices must be clearly symbolised. He should be thorough with alternatives or choices with full understanding of each of the choices.
f. The individual must be loved and respected by others.

2. Maslow

Abraham Harold Maslow was an American psychologist and philosopher best known for his self-actualization theory of psychology, which argued that the primary goal of psychotherapy should be the integration of the self (see the next chapter for details).

VI. Learning Approach

Under this caption we will study:

1. Dollard and Miller.
2. Bandura and Walter.

1. Dollard and Miller

John Dollard and Neil Miller postulated a new theory on the theory of personality in the year 1950. Their approach was the synthesis of psychology of learning with psycho-analytic theory. Their theory postulated that personality is the outcome of the following three factors:

i. The pleasure principle with the principle of reinforcement.
ii. The concept of ego with the concept of learnt drive and learnt skills.
iii. The concept of conflict with fighting reinforcement.

2. Bandura and Walter

Albert Bandura and Richard Walter developed a new type of theory called observational learning in relation to personality. This is also known as social learning theory. Its various aspects are highlighted below:

i. It is the cognition, i.e., the role of observational learning that is responsible for the development of personality. They categorically rejected the SR connection of personality.
ii. Bandura and Walter firmly rejected the psycho-analytical approach as it appeared fragmentary and incomplete.
iii. They also criticized the personality theory of Dollard and Miller, which synthesises concepts of Freud and Neo-Freudians, because they do not subscribe Freud and others.

Basic Principles of Social Learning

According to Bandura and Walter, the most fundamental and significant principle of social learning is principle of reinforcement in relation to a model. They argued that when an individual comes to the world, he is exposed to various agencies, and stimuli and his interaction with them develops the personality.

Social learning involves real as well as symbolic models. Hence the development of personality takes place through social learning, which is a continuous process of structuring and restructuring as a process of social learning. Real life models may develop their personality from parents, teachers, friends, sports personalities or film heroes or other celebrities, who have gained success in society or in the immediate environment. Symbolic models include verbal, pictorial, book, magazines, etc. Two to three decades ago it was the film personalities who modified the personality of thousands of youths. The hair style, the style of speaking and dressings of the most popular hero was in vogue among many youths. Today cricket and other sport stars have taken a major chunk of popularity. Models influence an individual through self-reinforcement which operates in observational and social learning. An individual, especially children and young adults tend to adopt such standards through reinforcement which matches the standard of models. The more the stimuli between the model and the individual, the more the imitations occur. This observation learning is guided by attention, retention, motor reproductive skills and the role of reinforcement.

Criticism of Type Theories

The above theories of classifying personalities are not accepted in modern psychology. On this subject, the following criticism is given:

a. Experience and observation make it obvious that most people cannot be fitted into any one type.

b. The 'type' raises doubts on the subject of cause and effect. It would be incorrect to assert that a certain individual loves solitude because he is an introvert.

c. Type cannot be established by measurement. Only the different qualities of personality can be measured. It is not essential that these qualities will remain the same in a person all the time.

Thus, the attempt to classify people into groups seems to be neither feasible not practical.

ASSESSMENT OF PERSONALITY

Personality is assessed and not measured for the following important reasons:

a. The personality of an individual cannot be measured as it belongs to the domain of a complex character.

b. Secondly, personality is a not a thing that can be measured. It is related to an abstract idea.

c. Thirdly, personality is dynamic and not static. Hence it cannot be measured.

d. Finally, the process of measurement requires appropriate tools and units. Hence measurement of personality is impossible.

In olden days, the personality of an individual was assessed by astrology, palmistry, looking at the temporal region of the head, etc. Also the position of various planets at the time of birth was considered for the assessment of a personality. These things are still in vogue in India and some other parts of the world.

Modern day psychologists assess the personality of an individual through various procedures out of which a few have been produced which are modern, more acceptable and recognized by various sectors of state:

1. Case history method.
2. Questionnaire method.
3. Performance method.
4. Interview method.
5. Situation test.
6. Psycho-analytic techniques.
7. Projective methods.

1. Case History Method

In this method, the facts in relation to the life of the subject are evolved. This method enables the examiner to assess and perceive the factors concerning and environment of the subject.

As a homeopath we are well versed with these type of case histories. In homeopathy 'life situation' is judged so that a proper anamnesis can be evolved for a successful prescription.

2. Questionnaire Method

In this method a list of carefully and judiciously selected questions are prepared for the investigation of the personality of the subject. He has to answer all the questions in terms of "Yes" and "No". The questions are generally set in relation to traits like self-confidence, sociability, introversion or extroversion, tendency to dominate or be dominated, etc.

In this method, some cautions must be adopted. First, the questions should be selected very carefully. Secondly, the subject must be honest and answer the questions accurately after thinking. Thirdly and lastly, the subject should not conceal anything.

As a homeopath we are well versed with these methods. Our beloved Hahnemann has facilitated the way in the *Organon*. We can use this method after collecting all the information or after taking the case. Moreover, we can use negative leading questions for a confirmation. Instead of double choice, multiple choices may be successfully given for better results.

3. Performance Method

The performance method was conceived by May and Hartshorne. In this method the subject is given a variety of specific jobs to be performed to examine his personality.

4. Interview Method

The interview method is the most normal of all the methods for the study of a personality. In this method, the subject and the examiner sit face to face. The examiner asks various questions to assess the personality of the subject and the subject answers various queries made by the examiner. We have to remember that this is not a mere session of questions and answers alone. Rather, the examiner judges the various attitudes, expressions, mode of answering, etc. Interview method depends as much on the examiner as it does on the subject. Generally it is of three types:

a. *Free interview*, where any question under the sky is asked.
b. *Non-directive interview*, where a conducive atmosphere is created to encourage the subject to express the facts of his behavior and the truth about his attitude, conflicts and allied problems. *This type of interview is very essential for our case taking.*
c. *Standardized interview,* where standardized interview techniques are adopted to obtain reliable information in order to assess the personality.

In homeopathy, this is not new for us. A homeopath is well attuned to such interviews. Our Master Hahnemann has given all the details in Organon of Medicine from Aphorism 83 to 104.

5. Situation Test

In this method, the subject is placed in some specific situations and the qualities of his personality are ascertained.

6. Psycho-Analytic Method

In the psycho-analytic method of investigation of personality, the following two techniques are employed and the personality of the individual is assessed:

i. Free association.
ii. Dream analysis.

(see the Chapter VII, Freud and Psycho-analysis)

7. Projective Method

This is the most popular method for the assessment of personality of the an individual. This method is meant for the observation of some specific thing in some thing or an action according to one's personality and mental state. Let us take the example of Konark temple. A group of people may denounce its carvings stating that these can mislead the present youths, whereas another group may take a positive way and comment that a man must go above these petty things prior to meditation. Hence, different people deduce different aspects of the same thing which exposes the peculiarities in their personalities. Here an individual does not observe a material object alone as it is, but also projects the specialties of his own personality upon it.

There exist so many types of projective methods like Rorschach Ink Blot test, Murray's Thematic Apperception Test (TAT), Children Apperception Test (CAT), BG Test, Mosaic Tests, Psycho-drama, Szondi Test, etc. out of which we will discuss a few here:

A. Rorschach's Ink Blot Test

This test was conceived by the Swiss scientist Hermann Rorschach in 1921. He used 10 bilaterally symmetrical ink blots on separate cards of 11X 9 inches.

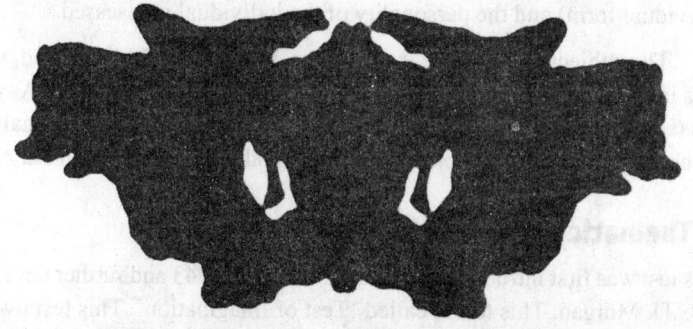

Rorschach's Ink Blot Test

These ink blots do not contain any picture. Five of these are black, two black and red and the other three multi-colored. These cards are produced before the subject. Then he is asked to describe everything he sees in the blot. The procedure is repeated for the second time and he is asked to point out the location of whatever he has seen on the blot.

The psychologist analyses the responses under the following four features:

a. Location in which the subject may react.
   i. To whole blot (W).
   ii. Major detail (D).
   iii. Small detail (d).
   iv. Unusual detail (Dd).
   v. White space (s).
b. Determinants:
   i. Form (F).
   ii. Color (C).
   iii. Combination of the two (FC).
c. Content:
   i. Animal (A).
   ii. Human being (H).
   iii. Natural objectives like river, green fields, etc. (N).
   iv. Inanimate objects like lamp shade, pot, etc. (O).
d. Originality
   i. Original responses (O).
   ii. Popular responses (P).

All the above factors are treated holistically (and not in a separate and individual form) and the personality of the individual is assessed.

The subjective response is one of the drawbacks of this method, which fails in evolving the correct personality peculiarities of the subject. Anyhow, this test still forms one of the most important tests to asses the personality by psychologists. Even as a homeopath we can take its advantage in our clinic.

B. Thematic Apperception Test

This test was first introduced by Henry Murray in 1943 and further developed by C.D. Morgan. This test is called 'Test of Imagination'. This test owes its origin to the research programme at the Harvard Psychological Clinic.

The test material consists of 31 cards out of which 1 is blank. The remaining 30 have pictures which show human beings in diverse real life situations. Ten of these cards are assigned for males, ten for females and the remaining are common for both the genders. The highest number of cards used for any subject is twenty. The test is carried out in two sessions.

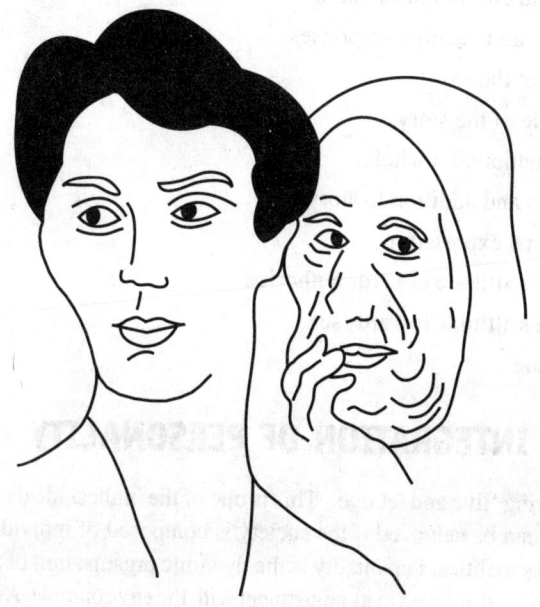

Thematic Apperception Test
(Source: Lefton, 3rd ed.)

First the psychologist (or physician or experimenter) should make an amicable rapport with the subject so that the experiment can conducted under natural and conducive conditions. Secondly, the experimenter must not reveal his real intention before the subject. The subject should be told emphatically that this was a test of creative imagination. The experimenter should ask the subject to build an imaginary story on seeing the cards while taking no tension about the of outcome. The subject is expected to make a story with each card within the stipulated period of time. The subject must be directed to build the story in relation to past, present and future, i.e., he should answer what is happening in the picture (present state), what had led to this happening (past happening) and what is likely to occur in such a state (future state).

Here the subject is bound to create a story spontaneously in the stipulated period of time. By this he does not have time to think and therefore the stories will manifest his own natural life's wishes, complexes and conflicts in relation to his personality.

The stories of TAT are scored under the following aspects:

a. Hero of the story in relation to his personality.
b. Need and conflict of the hero.
c. Unusual and peculiar responses.
d. Theme of the story.
e. The style of the story.
f. Test situation as a whole.
g. Deletion and addition to story.
h. Emotional expression.
i. Subject's attitude towards authority.
j. Subject's attitude towards sex.
k. Outcome.

INTEGRATION OF PERSONALITY

There is a saying 'live and let live'. This is one of the highest ideals of a healthy society. This can be achieved if the society is composed of individuals having integrated personalities. Personality is the dynamic organisation of the psycho-physical qualities, displayed in its adjustment with the environment. Any deviation in the organisation of psycho-physical qualities will result in personality adjustments to the environment. Such a personality will be called disintegrated.

A man having an integrated personality is basically a social man. He works for himself as well as for the welfare of the society. He is able to deal with other people and is also capable of maintaining an amicable relationship with them. He can also efficiently meet day to day problems of life that arise during the interaction.

A disintegrated personality is not only a problem unto himself but to the society as a whole. We find disintegration of personality among unsocial elements of society. An unsocial man finds it difficult to meet people. Interacting with the same people daily, is also difficult, hence, dealing with day to day problems also becomes a matter of concern. A father having a disintegrated personality is likely to induce various abnormal behavioral patterns to his off-springs. Even the neighbourhood and the society as a whole are affected by him. Disintegration of personality may lead a person to undergo depression, schizophrenia, adopting criminal activities, etc.

Sometimes disintegration of personality is found amongst great people. This may not deter or hamper their greatness, but it makes the lives of these people and of those associated with them miserable. They may even disrupt the peace of other people or of surroundings. In history, people like Genghis Khan, Timur and Hitler seem to have disintegrated personalities.

The integration of personality is the integration of all the psycho-physical qualities of personality and is of paramount importance for complete adjustment to the environment. Adjustment will be natural and easy if this integration is well-built.

We have already discussed the three elements of personality as postulated by Freud: Id, Ego and Super Ego (see Chapter VII). Id embraces the person's animal desires, instincts, etc. Super Ego is the representative of moral principle and ideal social norm which helps socialization of an individual. Super Ego exercises social control over the person. Ego incorporates the tendencies, which work for the existence and sustenance of life. Thus, the Super Ego comes in conflict with the Id or the Ego. The disintegration of personality is the disintegration of the mental adjustment of these three elements of personality.

Now let us take a glance over the salient features of an integrated personality so that we can help people with disintegrated personalities.

Characteristics of Integrated Personality

1. A personality does not undergo any conflict of irreversible character. He may have conflicts but that does not interfere with his normal of life.
2. The individual works in an organised way. His mind and emotions, desires and determination, and other mental activities work in a harmonious way in an organised manner. An integrated personality is flexible, strong and organised, besides being balanced.
3. An individual's emotions cannot sweep him away or his mind, i.e. the individual has full control over his emotions.
4. The individual is a social man. He posses all the qualities of sociability, which is an essential quality in the adaptation to society. Sociability makes an individual and other people's life happy and peaceful.

Thus psychologists and their various strategies aim at helping the individual in building integration so that he can lead a normal life and help the society. Moreover, as a homeopath, we can help the individual in a better way by removing the blocking factor of miasms. By psychotherapy and homeopathy we can evolve an ideal society, as taught by Hahnemann in aphorism 9 of Organon of Medicine.

CLINICAL IMPORTANCE

1. We know that no two persons are equal. We can hardly use the same medicine for the same nosological diseases. Understanding the personality is of prime importance for us for the selection of a simillimum.

2. An extrovert and an introvert may react differently to an inimical agent or medicine. When a *Staphysagria* patient is insulted, he does not react outward but suffers inside, whereas in a similar situation, a *Pulsatilla* patient weeps or sobs, a *Causticum* patient fights for justice for the victim, etc. These are the outcomes of particular personality traits.

3. Introverts are more prone to depression, anxiety, schizophrenia, whereas extroverts are more prone to disorders like somatoform and hypomania.

4. It seems that sex difference plays a significant role in relation to personality. It has been found that introvert boys and extrovert girls generally perform better in their academic performances.

5. An understanding of the patient's personality can help the physicians in providing specific treatment strategies.

6. Some knowledge of a person's 'normal' or 'previous' personality can provide valuable information to detect changes which may have occurred as a consequence of disease – either organic or psychological – and also to assess the degree of recovery or cure from the concerned illness.

7. An individual's personality will also 'color' the clinical picture of any psychiatric disorder that he develops, so that it is not identical with that of another patient. Master Hahnemann illustrated long before psychologists like Eysenck, the personality type determines the nature of illness. Hahnemann has clearly illustrated in the following example:

   People who grow too rapidly, are slender, fair, delicate, fine blonde or red haired, who are quick to perceive, very sensitive to external impressions, light noises, odors, having sanguine, bilious, irritable, temperament, chilly, are likely to be *Phosphorus* patients. Moreover, recent studies co-relate personality patterns of individuals with disorders such as irritable bowel syndrome.

8. There are, some people whose personalities depart, in various ways, from the norm to such an extent that they experience difficulties themselves, resulting in anxiety or depression, or cause difficulties to others in their attempts to cope with the normal pressures and responsibilities of life; they may therefore be diagnosed as having a personality disorder. Here we can instill a new life in the patient.

Chapter 15

MOTIVATION

In day to day life we perform activities like eating, roaming, selecting a career, etc. But why do we do so? Why do we select a particular activity whereas there exist a galore of alternatives? Again,

Why do we want to be attractive?

Why do we want to help others?

Why do we run on seeing a tiger or bear?

The answer to all the above is that behind all this scenario there is one motivational force which compels us to do so.

It is the motivation that can do wonders for you. Heraclites, the Greek philosopher said that you can drag a horse to a river but you cannot compel it to drink water. But had Heraclites been aware of the various facets of motivation, he might have changed his view. It may be the battle of Mahabharata or Ramayan or War of Trojan or even the recent wars around the globe, it is the motivation that plays the key role. Moreover, motivation is an integral part of health education. Hence, this topic is of prime concern for us.

DEFINITION

The word motivation has been derived from the Latin word 'moveers' which means "to move". So roughly, we can say that motivation is the arousing movement in an organism.

A motive may be defined as a readiness or disposition to respond in some ways and not others to a variety of situations.

Motivation may also be defined as an internal process that provides energy for behavior and direction towards a goal.

Motivation is a process that both energizes and directs goal-oriented behavior.

ACTIVATING FACTORS FOR MOTIVATION

Psychologists attribute the following factors for motivation:

1. **Needs:** Needs are general wants and desires. We have biological needs like air, water, food, sex, etc. We can also include needs like sleep, rest, regular elimination of waste products like stool, urine, sweat, etc. under needs. We also have socio-psychogenic needs which include freedom, security, achievement, recognition, self-assertion, expression, company, etc.

2. **Drives:** Arousal awareness in an individual is termed as drive. The strength of drive depends upon the stimuli formed by the concerned need. We have primary drives like the above that are biological drives like hunger, thirst, sex, escape from pain and secondary drives like fear of anxiety, desire for approval, struggle for achievement, aggression, etc.

3. **Motives:** Motive may be defined as an inclination or impulse that generates an action caused by drives and needs with a direction for achieving a goal and is hunted till its attainment. There exist many types of motives like, hunger, thirst, sex, aggression, achievements along with maternal affiliation, etc. Maternal motives implies behavior involving the care and protection of an offspring by the female species, whereas affiliation motives spring from affiliation needs, i.e., to be with other people.

CLASSIFICATION OF HUMAN NEEDS AND MOTIVES

Motivation has been classified in various ways by various psychologists with different view points, out of which the following selected clippings have been presented for an easy comprehension:

1. Biogenic:
    i. Physiological needs:
        a. Homeostasis.
        b. Regulation of temperature.
        c. Sleep.

MOTIVATION

        d. Hunger.
        e. Thirst.
   ii. Psychological needs:
        a. Sex.
        b. Maternal behavior.
   iii. General needs:
        a. Escape (i.e., flight due to action of adrenalin).
        b. Combat (i.e., fight due to action of adrenalin).
        c. Curiosity.
        d. Play humor.

2. Sociogenic:
   i. Praise and blame.
   ii. Mastery motive.
   iii. Aggressiveness.
   iv. Self-submission.
   v. Gregariousness.
   vi. Imitation.
   vii. Sympathy.

3. Innate and acquired.
4. Personal and social.
5. Woodworth's classification.
   i. Organic needs : Hunger, thirst, etc.
   ii. Emergency motives: Motive to escape.
   iii. Objective motives: The objective of this type of motive is attributed to impressive behavior with demand of environment and people.
      (**Note:** Words like needs, propensities, etc. are also used as synonyms for motive)

6. Primary and secondary.
7. Prescott's classification:
   a. Physiological (needs for essential materials and conditions, for a certain rhythm of activity and rest, and for sexual activity.
   b. Social (need for affection, belonging and likeness to others).
   c. Ego-integrative (need for contact with reality, harmony with reality,

progressive symbolization, increasing self-direction, a fair balance between success and failure, and attainment of selfhood).

8. Edwards's classification of human needs and motives:
   a. **Achievement:** To do one's best, to be successful, to accomplish to be a recognized authority, etc.
   b. **Dependence:** To get a suggestion from others, to find out what others think, to follow instructions and do what is expected, to praise others, to accept leadership of others, to conform to custom.
   c. **Order:** To keep things neat and orderly, to make advance plans, to organize details of work, to have things arranged so that they run smoothly and without changes.
   d. **Exhibition:** To say clever and witty things, to have others notice and comment upon one's appearance, to say things just to see the effect upon others, to talk about personal achievement.
   e. **Autonomy:** To be able to come and go as desired, to do things without regard to what others may think, etc.
   f. **Affiliation:** To be loyal to friends, to participate in friendly groups, to form strong attachments, to share things with friends, etc.
   g. **Interception:** To analyze one's motives and feelings, to predict the behavior of others, etc.
   h. **Succorance:** To help others when in trouble, to seek encouragement from others, etc.
   i. **Dominance:** To argue for one's point of view, to be a leader in groups to which one belongs, to persuade and influence others, etc.
   j. **Abasement:** To feel guilty when one does something wrong, to accept blame when things do not go right, to feel timid and inferior, etc.
   k. **Nurturance:** To help friends when they are in trouble, to treat others with kindness and sympathy, etc.
   l. **Change:** To do new and different things, to travel, to meet new people, to participate in new fads and fashions, etc.
   m. **Endurance:** To keep at a job until it is finished, to work hard at a task, to stick to a problem even though no apparent progress has been made, etc.
   n. **Hetero-sexuality:** To be interested in the opposite sex, to be regarded as physically attractive by those of the opposite sex.

o. **Aggression:** To attack the contrary point of view, to avenge insults, to blame and criticize others when things go wrong.

THEORIES OF MOTIVATION

There exist more than two dozen theories of motivation, exploration of which is neither desirable not feasible for our purpose. Hence, only the salient, prominent, widely accepted and relevant theories in a synthetic mode are given below:

1. Pawn theory.
2. Physiological theory.
3. Energy theory.
4. Behaviorists learning theories of motivation.
5. McDougall's instinct theory.
6. Psycho-analytical theory of motivation.
7. Maslow's self-actualization theory.
8. Social theory of motivation.

1. Pawn Theory

The word pawn expresses two things, first : One that can be used to further the purpose of another, two : One of the chessmen of least value in the chess board that represents soldier. According to this theory, we are a 'pawn' or a 'puppet' in the hands of Nature or God. We do not act, rather we cannot act. We feel free, but we are free to the end of our chain only. We are free to think what we will, but we are not free to will what we will. This can be compared to a hackney-carriage, where the horse is under an invisible force which controls the reins in the direction he likes.

2. Physiological Theory

In the laboratories now, there are attempts to construct a physiological theory of motivation. Rutherford, William James, Zangwill, Lashley, Beach, Morgan, etc. are the exponents of this theory. Among them, Morgan deserves special attention. He propounded that there is a central motive state (CMS) and this is the pivot of all activities. Hence, behavior can be explained in the terms of CMS. He mentions the following four characteristics of central motive state:

a. There exists an arousal central motive state, which remains persistent and does not fade because it does not require any backing from internal or external stimuli.
b. The motivated individual has enthusiastic physical activity.
c. A central motive state results in selectivity of reaction to stimuli
d. It prompts the individual to adopt a fitting behavior.

Psychologists have carried out experiments with rats and have justified the above. Olds and Milners took rats for experimentation. The area in the brain that controls the pleasure sensation of rats was identified and fixed to electrodes. The terminals of electrodes were exposed outside the skull. Then the exposed electrodes were connected to low voltage current in such a manner that the current flow was actuated when the exposed terminals electrodes touch the bar. It has been observed that the rats touch the bars for an innumerable times within a minute for seeking the pleasure sensation. Such experiments fortify the physiological theory of motivation. Similar experiments have been carried out in the U.S.A. with the help of electric waves for de-motivating frantic bulls. It is claimed that such experiments have become successful and have given a valid buttress to this theory.

3. Energy Theory

According to this theory, the basis of motivation is energy. Physical energy comes from food. Accordingly our motives are guided by energy. This theory stresses that without energy there cannot be any genesis of motivation. It simply substitutes the word 'motivation' by the word 'energy'.

4. Behaviorists Learning Theories of Motivation

Psychologist belonging to behavior school observe that an individual's behavior in a particular manner is the outcome of his early learning or training. Accordingly, an individual's behavior is guided through:
a. the mechanisms of classical conditioning (Pavlov) or,
b. a simple stimulus response mechanism (Thorndike) or,
c. operant conditioning as advocated by (B.F. Skinner). See Chapter VI.

5. McDougall's Theory of Instinct

It was William James who propounded the concept of instinct to explain behavior, but it was McDougall who developed it into a full fledged theory. William McDougall was a British-born, U.S. psychologist. He was the author of 'An Introduction to Social Psychology' (1908, 30th edition in 1960) where he states, "The human mind has certain innate or inherited tendencies which are the essential springs or motive powers of all thoughts and actions, whether individual or collective, and are the bases from which the character and will of individuals and of notions are gradually developed under the guidance of the intellectual faculties". According to this theory, an individual's instincts are the springboards of his behavior. These instincts are subscribed to the mind, which may be innate or acquired. These tendencies are the crucial springs or motive powers. All thoughts and actions are the bases from where character, will and notions of an individual gradually grow under the control of intellectual faculties. McDougall explains all human behavior on the basis of some instinct. He justifies his maxim by supplementing a list of 14 instincts (which was initially 12 and later extended to 18), each one is accompanied by a specific emotional disposition. McDougall's list of instincts with its counterpart emotional response are given below:

	Instinct	Emotional Response
a.	Combat or Pugnacity	Anger
b.	Anger	Repulsion, disgust
c.	Curiosity	Wonder, surprise
d.	Submission	Negative self–feeling
e.	Food-seeking	Appetite, hunger
f.	Sex	Lust
g.	Parental	Tender emotion
h.	Gregariousness	Loneliness, solitude
i.	Escape	Fear
j.	Appeal	Distress
k.	Self- assertion	Positive self-feeling
l.	Constructiveness	Feeling of creativity
m.	Acquisitiveness	Feeling of ownership
n.	Laughter	Amusement

According to him, as we grow up, these instincts, under the influence of education, become organized into sentiments, or attachments to people and principles. These sentiments or attachments bring order, integration and continuity into our emotional life and make our behavior consistent or predictable. Now the source of motivation is within the man and no longer above the man.

The instinct to escape, for example, is accompanied by the emotion of fear, the instinct of combat (pugnacity) by anger, the instinct of repulsion by the emotion of disgust, and so on. McDougall further claimed that all behavioral acts are essentially instinctive. He attaches the following three aspects to instinctive behavior :

a. *Cognition or Knowing:* The individual perceives and pays attention to certain objectives or situations
b. *Affection or Feeling or Experiencing an Emotion*: The subject experiences positive or negative emotional excitement on perceiving them.
c. *Conation or Doing or Striving:* Acting upon above, the individual takes steps to preserve himself. Let us take an example, when a child sees a cockroach; approaching him, he undergoes the above three stages. First, along with an instinctive behavior (as mentioned above) he sees the cockroach; second, he experiences an emotion of fear and; third, he tries to run away. Thus, according to McDougall, what we do and how we do it, can all be explained through our instinctive behavior which is governed by our instincts accompanied by our emotional experience.

The theory of instinct proposed by McDougall has been a subject of great controversy and criticism by later psychologists on the following grounds:

a. After the advent of the above theory, the later psychologists developed their own list of instincts. The number of instincts rose up to 849; which led to utter confusion because other instincts could not evoke the said motivation.
b. Innate instincts are usually found among children and not in adults. Adult behavior is affected by learning.
c. It has also been observed that most of the innate tendencies in children have been acquired in early life. Naturally, this has raised doubt regarding all other innate behaviors.
d. In a peculiar experiment, another psychologist called Kuo has been able to demonstrate that kittens and rats together fondled each other.

e. Studies in anthropology reveal that human behavior is modified by culture factor and not by instincts.
f. It is a general observation that an individual during his life time acquires new motives which are self-motivating and autonomous and not derivatives of any inherited tendencies.
g. American psychologists severely criticize it stating that it tends to substitute abstract tendencies for concrete causes, which is blind to the evidence of learning, development and adjustment.

Despite of the above criticism, the instinct theory is still a burning topic in comparative psychology. It is not yet dead and seems to have some ingredients of truth in relation to motivational behavior.

6. Psycho-analytic Theory of Motivation

Freud ushered a new era in rejecting the traditional view of intellectual attribution to motivation. His psycho-analytic theory of motivation is centred around the following concepts:

a. Instincts and,
b. The unconscious.

In Freud's view, human behavior is motivated by two biologically energized instincts, respectively termed *Eros*, the life instinct and the *Thanatos*, the death instinct. The life instinct was considered to be the basis of sexual motivation while the death instinct underlay aggressive motivation; the desire to destroy even to the extent of destroying oneself are the ultimate sources of motivation. When the life instinct ceases to operate, the death instinct takes over. Freud maintained that from birth onwards human beings experience sexual gratification and the sex motive, therefore, is quite an important motive that activates human behavior.

He subscribed that motivations are the spring actions of unconscious mind besides the life and death instinct and sexual urges. According to him, unconscious mind is a great determinant and activating force for the cause and operation of one's behavior. The unconscious forms $9/10^{th}$ of one's mind. According to Freud, unconscious mind is dark, ruthless, very powerful, illogical and remains hidden and usually inaccessible. It consists of one's unfulfilled desires, wishes, ideas, feelings, repressed sentiments, etc. Man, as Freud maintains, is but a puppet in the hands of the mighty unconscious mind and thus he has to behave in the way and manner in which his unconscious mind dictates. Hence, techniques like free association, dream analysis, etc.

are adopted to explore the unconscious mind. Prior to that one cannot open the gateway of motivations guided by the unconscious mind. Of course, the unconscious mind guides our conscious mind through defence mechanisms like identification, regression, repression, etc. (see Chapter VII). Anyhow this theory has to undergo the criticism of post-Freudians. According to senior Neo-Freudian like Adler and Jung, the unconscious mind is attitude and unrealized potentiality respectively. Post-Freudians like Karen Horney, Sullivan, Maslow, Rogers, Erich Fromm, etc. differ from Adler and Jung and even themselves. Their criticism can be bundled under the following points:

1. Structure of unconscious mind is doubtful.
2. Unconscious mind is not all sex and aggression.
3. Factors like social environment are neglected in building the concept.
4. Ezriel's group therapy opposes the individual psycho-analysis.

7. Maslow's Self-actualization Theory

The full name is Abraham Harold Maslow. He was born on April 1st, 1908 in New York and died in June 8th, 1970 at Menlo Park, California 1970. He was an American psychologist and philosopher, best recognized for his self-actualization theory of psychology, which insists that the primary goal of psychotherapy should be the integration of the self. In 1951 he became head of the psychology department at Brandeis University (Waltham, Massachusetts), where he remained until 1969. He was the chief contributor in the United States to humanistic psychology, which is sometimes called the "third force."

In 1954, Abraham Maslow proposed a hierarchical order of needs from physiological aspects to self–actualization. He also asserted that those needs are also multi-motivated. Human needs, according to Maslow, arrange themselves in hierarchies of pre-potency. The appearance of one need generally depends on the satisfaction of the others. They are closely related to one another and may be arranged from the lowest to the highest development of the personality. The order of needs starts from basic survival called lower order of needs to higher order of needs. The proposed five sets of basic needs can be arranged in a definite hierarchical order for understanding human motivation as shown in the figure below:

a. Physiological needs.
b. Safety needs.

c. Belongingness and love needs.
d. The esteem needs.
e. Self-actualization needs.

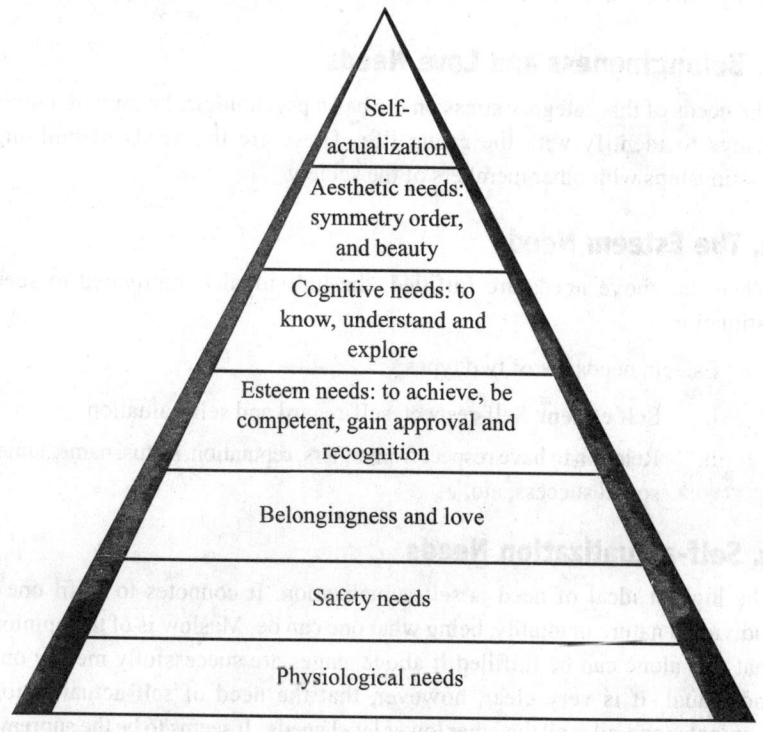

a. Physiological Needs

The most powerful needs of all the needs, yet the least significant for self-actualizing persons are the physiological needs. Maslow maintains that other needs can only appear if these needs are fulfilled. We can think of the other needs only when the need for food and alike basic physiological needs are gratified. A hungry person cannot think of casting his vote during elections. He cannot also engage himself in participating in social service nor make an attempt at attaining salvation by remembering God. Deprivation of physiological needs blocks other needs for appearance.

b. Safety Needs

After the fulfilment of physiological needs, there appears the need of safety.

Accordingly, when an individual is able to meet physiological needs successfully like hunger, thirst, sex, etc. he wants safety concerns like having a good house, depositing money in a bank, etc. One who is insecure or unsafe may hardly be motivated to gratify his needs for love or esteem.

c. Belongingness and Love Needs

The needs of this category stress on the basic psychological nature of human beings to identify with the group life. These are the needs of building relationships with other members of the society.

d. The Esteem Needs

When the above needs are fulfilled, the individual is motivated to seek estimation.

Esteem needs are of two types:

i. Self esteem: Self-respect, self-regard and self-valuation.

ii. Relation to have respect from others, reputation, status, name, fame, social success, etc.

e. Self-actualization Needs

The highest ideal of need is self-actualization. It connotes to fulfil one's individual nature in totality, being what one can be. Maslow is of the opinion that this alone can be fulfilled if above stages are successfully met by one individual. It is very clear, however, that the need of self-actualization dominates and rules all the other lower level needs. It seems to be the supreme mission of human life and is termed as the master motive for motivating human behavior. In the words of Maslow, "A musician must make music, an artist must paint, a poet must write poetry, if he is to be ultimately at peace with himself. What a man can be, he must be. He must be true to his own nature. This need we may call self-actualization". Judging orthodox behaviorism and psycho-analysis to be too rigidly theoretical and concerned with illness, he developed a theory of motivation describing the process by which an individual progresses from basic needs such as food and sex to the highest needs of what he called self-actualization—the fulfilment of one's greatest human potential.

Maslow attributes the following fifteen characteristics to a self-actualized person:

i. Self-actualized persons identify and live in close proximity with Nature.

ii. They involve themselves with little guilt or anxiety.
iii. They display spontaneity in both their thought and behavior.
iv. They are the people who stand and execute themselves for broad social problems as a mission of life. They first think of society instead of self.
v. Sometimes they prefer privacy and solitude, and are capable of looking at life from a detached, objective point of view.
vi. They are relatively independent of their culture and environment but do not exhibit convention just for the sake of being different.
vii. They are capable of deep appreciation of the basic experiences of life, even if things they have done or seen many times before.
viii. Many of them are likely to undergo mystic experiences with a conviction that some momentous things had happened to them.
ix. They take genuine interest in social milieu and identity in an understanding with mankind as a whole.
x. They maintain an amiable and deep satisfying, inter-personal relation with others.
xi. They show respect for all with an egalitarian attitude.
xii. They can evidently discern between means and ends. They take pleasure in the means towards their ends with patience and pleasure.
xiii. They possess a good sense of humor.
xiv. They are highly creative with their own individuality.
xv. They fit in their culture but are resistant to enculturation i.e., they are not prejudiced people. They do not blindly comply with all its demands.

It seems that Maslow's spirits of self-actualization is a part of Hahnemann's higher sense of living as elucidated in aphorism 9 of Organon of Medicine but Maslow fails in execution due to failure in taking account of health factor.

Criticism to Maslow's Theory of Self-actualization

The history of mankind may point to countless heroes, saints and other great people who always stood up for their ideals, and religious or social values without caring for the satisfaction of their biological or other lower needs.

a. It appears that the effects of gratification of a need are more stimulating and important than the effects of deprivation. Gratification of needs of the lower order motivates an individual to strive for satisfaction of needs of the higher order. An individual, as Maslow emphasized, can actualize his potential as a human being only after fulfilling the higher level needs like love and esteem.

b. There may be exceptions to the hierarchical order. One may be more motivated for the satisfaction of one's needs at the cost of another and therefore a person can reach the top without caring for the satisfaction of needs of the lower order.

c. The fulfillment of self-actualization is thus a must for an individual as he will feel discontented and restless unless he strives for what he or she is fitted for.

8. Social Theory

This theory explains the causes of social behavior in the social environment for the genesis of motivation. There exist two main theories:

a. *Culture-pattern theory*, which highlights the impact of the culture pattern for the development of motivation.

b. *Field theory*, which puts stress on the immediate social field in respect of the individual who is very much in the field.

a. Culture Pattern

Margaret Mead is the main exponent of this theory. Mead (1901-78) was an eminent anthropologist of U.S.A. She is well known for her various studies concerning primitive people with their culture and psychology. She lays emphasis on the cultural conditioning of an individual that develops motivation and personality. In her book *'Sex and Temperament in Three Primitive Societies'* (1935; reprinted, 1968), she narrates differences in sexual behavior and aggression among the inhabitants of Mundugumor, Arapesh and Tchamubli. She brings to light that these differences are mostly due to the different customs, standards, expectations and institutions of the three societies. According to this view point, an individual is the outcome of culture in such a way that he can be taken as a representative of the given culture. Different cultures would, therefore, produce different types of personalities. Her theory is further fortified and explained by Linton who points out that every individual posseses two types of personalities:

i. Basic personality and,

ii. Numerous 'status personalities' which are generated by the various sub-groups (or culture) to which he belongs.

b. Field Theory

The field theory states that behavior is a function of interaction between a person and his environment. This theory also considers that the individuality of the individual is also an important factor which is related to his past. Therefore, the past of an individual cannot be ignored in the present context of generation of motivation. Kurt Lewin, the chief exponent of field theory, insists that behavior is to be explained by reference to a person-in-an-environment situation and to all the forces that are right now interacting within it.

Conclusion

We have examined and observed the various theories of motivation. We have also realized that no single theory can be taken as final. Every theory has some plus points and some lacunae. But it will be better for us to take the theories as complementary rather than contradictory. Let us wait for the day when all these divergent views will be come under one umbrella or a new theory will emerge which will compensate all the deficiencies of these theories. Let us compare it to an elephant. Somebody has seen its ear, another legs, still another the tail. Let us wait for a superman who will see the elephant as a whole and give a conclusive decision.

CLINICAL APPLICATION

In recent days, the concept of primordial prevention has drawn attention to the prevention of chronic diseases. The word primordial means basic and connected with an early stage of development. In primordial prevention, efforts are directed towards discouraging children or young adults from adopting harmful life styles like over-eating, smoking, non-adherence to physical exercise, etc. This prevention is aimed at development of risk factors that are yet to appear. For example, obesity, hypertension, diabetes have their origin in childhood, because this is the time when life styles are formed. The main interventions in primordial prevention are through health education at individual and community level.

We find two kinds of eating disorders that have come to our notice in recent days:
1. The first kind is a type of self-starvation that is very often found among young girls or woman who want to be slim. For this they adopt self-

starvation which leads to various physical disorders like gastritis, renal failure and even death.

2. The second kind is bulimia, in which an individual continually eats huge quantities of food. By this, they trigger obesity and its concomitant variations like diabetes and hypertension. Motivate your patient in the following manner so as enable to control obesity. Bulimia is often found among depressed and anxiety prone people, to whom you should pay attention.

Again, no individual is immune from sexual impulses or drives. A normal person has to bear with it or sublimates for a higher state of living. Some individuals can neither bear it nor sublimate it. They cannot even find the right partner for its fulfillment. They feel shy or they feel they are going to be rejected. For them sex is attractive as well as frightening. This is a type of approach-avoidance conflict that will be dealt in the 19th Chapter of "Conflict". These individuals may attempt with a much lower age group in the form of rape. He may also go for homosexuality by finding a partner who has a similar drive or motivation. He may also go for bestiality i.e., fulfilling the sexual gratification with animals. These deviations are the danger signals not only for the concerned individual only but also for the society. Such individuals should be demotivated from such acts. Moreover, medicines like *Lycopodium*, *Lachesis*, *Conium*, etc. can do wonders for the patient. These or alike medicines give strength to the patients to bear with it or helps in sublimation.

Sometimes parents of a child may complain about their child's behavioral disorder. Before prescribing medicines and other measures it would be better for you to peep into the matter in depth. See whether the child is motivated (without actively being aware of it) in doing so, so that he receives more attention from others. Such instances are specially found in families, where someone else is being paid more attention. Here you have to take the help of motivation. You may also direct the parents of the victim to pay more attention and take due care of him.

Motivation principles help the patient to over-come learned helplessness. Learned helplessness means the depressed patient is convinced that he is out of control and his disease cannot be cured (*Calcarea carb.*). He feels that nothing can done for him and he has to bear with the malady. By this he does not have any motivation even to try.

Now let us discuss the motivational basis of addictive behavior (along with biological basis). Literally, alcoholism means the condition of being an alcoholic. Alcoholism is a condition in which heavy drinking interferes with an individual's ability to function effectively in dealing with other people and in working. This costs job, health and even family. We can help alcoholic individuals through motivation along with medicines like *Acidicum sulph., Quercus glandium spiritus, Sulphur, Syphilinum*, etc.

From a psychological point of view, two things play a major role:

a. First, the process of learning; the individual witnesses the fun or celebration of alcohol in a gathering or society which induces the perception of (its so called) positive feelings. This motivates him to have a taste of alcohol.

b. Second, alcohol itself can provide a powerful reinforcement. It is a depressant drug that acts on the central nervous system to bring feelings of relaxation and reduction of anxiety. Moreover, alcohol very quickly curtails tension and stress.

(**Note:** From a biological point, alcoholic individuals may have a special physiological flaw that results in a craving for alcohol. Some biological differences between alcoholics and non-alcoholics have been recognized.)

As a homeopath, we can take the best advantage of motivation through Homoeopathic Health Education. Health education has basically three aspects:

a. Submission of information to the individuals.
b. Motivating the individuals.
c. Guiding the individuals into action.

You can impart health education to your patients with special focus on motivation to various primordial disorders. Here one example has been delineated as to how to help your patient lose weight. The following motivational techniques may be adopted for him:

1. Motivate him to fix his time and place of eating. By this practice he will prevent various gastric disorders and at the same time extra calories from snacks.

2. Motivate him to eat slowly and with awareness: By this maximum pleasure from the least amount of food can be gained with deep satisfaction, and his hangover for a particular food can be prevented. He should be further motivated not read or watch television while eating.

3. Motivate him to guard himself against fatty and rich-tasting (of course rich calorie) foods. The look, smell and taste of such food will be a motivational force for his stimulation of appetite.

4. Motivate him to eat among the company of moderate eaters. Presence of such people will make him liable to eat more moderately.
5. Motivate him to take the help of visual illusions of using small serving plates with heaped food items. By this a small amount of food looks more than the same amount on a large plate.
6. Motivate him to take regular physical exercise. Physical exercise expends the undesirable energy along with reducing the appetite.

Chapter 16

APTITUDE*

DEFINITION

Santosh is an asthmatic and took B.H.M.S. course last year. Now, he is excelling in each branch of B.H.M.S. course. Krishna also took B.H.M.S. course last year along with Santosh. But Krishna is not doing well from the very beginning. Krishna's previous career including the recent roll number, which is selected on merit basis, is in upper hand to that of Santosh. Such examples are present in large numbers in our society. In many spheres of day to day life we come across people who excel over others under similar conditions and circumstances and become proficient proving, themselves superior to their peers in various given fields. Such people possess certain specific quality or aptitude along with normal intelligence, which helps them to achieve success in the specific occupation of activities.

The dictionary meaning of aptitude is *potential to acquire skill:* A natural tendency to do something well, especially one that can be further developed.

Aptitude may be defined as a specific ability or specific capacity which helps an individual to acquire the required degree of proficiency in a specific field.

According to James Drever, aptitude is an individual's natural capacity with the help of which he is able to acquire some special ability or skill.

Mueller maintains, Aptitude can be defined as the capacity to achieve along special lines. It is a special tendency, bent, fitness or aptness due to a

---

* "The author suggests the CCH authority to change it to 'ATTITUDE'; which will be more useful for the profession."

special neural or muscular organization possessed by the individual, which sets him apart as being superior to average in performance in that trait or activity.

According to Traxler, aptitude is a condition, a quality or a set of qualities in an individual which is indicative of the probable extent to which he will be able to acquire, under suitable training, some knowledge, skill or composite of knowledge, understanding and skill, such as an ability to contribute to art or music, mechanical ability, mathematical ability or ability to read and speak a foreign language, etc.

From above we can conclude that:

a. Aptitude implies the capacity or proficiency in a suitable environment.
b. Aptitude refers to the present condition that may be indicative of the individual's future possibilities or potentialities.
c. Aptitude may be hereditary (say for a singer, the good musical voice) or acquired (for the same singer) coming in contact as in association with a group of musicians (may be father or uncle or alike person, who is a proficient musician).
d. Aptitude solves specific problems. An asthmatic patient may develop interest and subsequent development of aptitude to take a course in homeopathy with success (as above, the example of Santosh).
e. Aptitude also includes the individual's preparedness and suitability for a given field or profession.

Basic Assumptions about Aptitude

Aptitude has three basic assumptions:

1. An individual's potentials are not equally strong in relation to adoption of aptitude. This means one person can not have equal aptitudes for everything. A person may possess good musical aptitude, but it does not mean he would also possess good mechanical aptitude. Rather, the reverse may be true i.e., he might possess poor mechanical aptitude.
2. There exist individual differences in relation to aptitude. All individuals are not gifted with the same input of aptitude nor do they develop equally.
3. Differences among individuals and within individuals are fairly stable or constant. This means, the patterns of aptitude hardly (or little) change.

An individual who is definitely superior in certain aptitudes at the age of 8, will as a rule be above average in that kind of aptitude at the age of say 18 or 28.

Some Clarification of Related Terminologies of Aptitude

Very often aptitude is used as a synonym of ability, achievement, intelligence, interest, etc. Let us analyse these terms for a better comprehension so that we can understand what 'aptitude' means precisely.

Jolly is now seven years old and has an aptitude for swimming, but now he is not able to swim. This implies that Jolly is likely to be a successful swimmer provided he is trained in the right direction, by a right guide through right means. Aptitude is a present condition in relation to future. Ability concerns with present. An ability is the sum total of what an individual has acquired plus what he is capable of acquiring. People differ from each other in their abilities. For example, some public speakers can hold the audience spell bound, while others cannot. Some people are excellent in carpentry while others cannot run a saw. Aptitude is a narrower term as compared to abilities.

Here we should also examine three aspects of ability, which may compete with the meaning of aptitude:

a. Skill means ability to perform a given test with ease and precision.
b. Proficiency, degree of ability already acquired.
c. Capacity, maximum potential ability.

Achievement implies past and indicates what an individual has learned or acquired. Aptitude test measures an individual on which his future achievements may be forecasted.

Again, very often people equate intelligence to aptitude, which is not right. Intelligence tests refer to general mental ability of an individual whereas aptitude test involves specific abilities like motor, mechanical, artistic, etc. or intellectual tasks like an aptitude for painting, for machine operation, etc. Aptitude also refers to specific aspects of intelligence like aptitude for reasoning, word fluency, spatial perception, etc. The test of aptitude is carried out keeping in view a given field, whereas the intelligence tests are carried out in a variety of fields.

Aptitude is also taken as a synonym of interest. Of course, we need interest and aptitude for success in a given field. But both should not be taken as one and the same. For example, you may be interested in cricket but you might not have the aptitude for cricket. That is the reason so many people may be interested in dancing but they do not have an aptitude for it. They simply enjoy the dance. A selection or guidance programme must be an accompaniment for the given activity of an individual.

APTITUDE TESTS

Aptitude tests are available for many fields including arts, sciences, professions and highly skilled vocations. These tests are developed to help individuals learn prior to entering a particular job. These tests help us evaluate the candidates suitability in a given field. It has already been mentioned that interest is one of the important factors in an aptitude test but not everything. Simple interest may not make someone suitable for a given field. Hence, aptitude tests are of immense value for the candidate and organisation to save wastage of time, quality and quantity product.

We can divide aptitude testing under two heads:

A.   General aptitude tests.
B.   Specialised aptitude tests.

A. General Aptitude Tests

In recent days, organisations prefer generalised tests for measuring specific aptitudes called multiple aptitude test batteries to assess the suitability of a person for different professions on the basis of scores in the concerned aptitude tests in the battery. For example:

a.   General aptitude test battery (GATB).
b.   Differentiate aptitude test (DAT).

a. General Aptitude Test Battery

GATB encompass following twelve tests with nine factors:

i.   Intelligence.
ii.   Verbal aptitude.
iii. Numerical aptitude.
iv.   Manual dexterity (2 tests).

v. Form perception (2 tests).
vi. Motor co-ordination.
vii. Form dexterity (2 tests).
viii. Spatial aptitude.
ix. Clerical perception.

GATB was developed by the Employment Service Bureau of USA in the year 1947. Now its later versions are used.

b. Differentiate Aptitude Test

DAT encompasses the following eight tests:
i. Numerical aptitude.
ii. Verbal reasoning.
iii. Abstract reasoning.
iv. Space relation.
v. Mechanical reasoning.
vi. Clerical speed and accuracy.
vii. Language usage I.
viii. Language usage II.

In India, identical aptitude tests are carried out by Union Public Service Commissions, LICs, etc.

B. Specialised Aptitude Tests

These aptitude tests are devised to measure the aptitudes of an individual in a given (i.e. specific) field or activity. Followings are important specific aptitude tests:

a. **Professional Aptitude Tests:** Such types of tests are carried out to determine the suitability of a candidate in a specified professional course like business management, medicine, law, teaching, etc. Important aptitude tests are: American Council of education (ACE), Scholastic Aptitude Test (SAT) developed in U.S.A., Tale Legal Aptitude Tests, Ferguson and Stoddard's Law Aptitude examination, Moss Scholastic Aptitude Test for medical students, etc. Do we not need such tests in homeopathy? We need it definitely. See below.
b. **Scholastic Aptitude Tests.**

c. **Musical Aptitude Tests:** Such types of tests are conducted to discover the musical talent. It is concerned with discrimination of pitch and intensity, determination of time interval and timbre, judgement of rhythm total memory, etc. The whole test is called Seashore measure musical talents test.

d. **Mechanical Aptitude Tests:** The aim of this test is to test the abilities and capacities of an individual for assessing the chances of success in mechanical pursuits. Important mechanical aptitudes carried out are: Minnesota mechanical assembly test, Minnesota spatial relation tests and Bennet tests of mechanical comprehension. These various tests also include test for perception and intellectual, motor ability, etc.

e. **Art Judgement Tests.**

SCORING IN APTITUDE TESTS

Tests like the ones narrated above, have been conducted by the government, as well as private sectors to select candidates through various aptitude tests to fulfil their goals and needs. These results are expressed in terms of average for different occupations. Sometimes these norms are expressed in a way that permits scores to be translated into letters like the marks given in schools A, B, C, D, etc.

Some sectors express these results in terms of intelligence quotient (I.Q.).

$$I.Q. = \frac{M.A.}{C.A.}$$

(*M.A. stands for Mental Age and C.A. for Chronological Age.*)

The percentage can be calculated multiplying the above result by 100.

UTILITY OF APTITUDE TESTS

Utility of aptitude tests is manifold, the following two being most important:

A. Selection of Suitable Candidates

We always want everything to be the best. So also all organisations from where production or management is expected also plan to recruit the best talent for their optimum utility. Government needs suitable candidates for handling the administration and allied services. Hence aptitude tests reasonably enable the organisation or government to decide on the right candidate for a given purpose. People having no aptitude for a given pursuit will prove a disaster for the organisation. Aptitude tests convincingly anticipate the future potentiality of a person for a given prospective. Hence, aptitude tests are the backbone of all kind of guidance services and selection procedures as they are useful for predicting the suitability of a person for specific job chart.

B. Training for an aspirant

Regular practice of aptitude tests also helps an aspirant candidate to qualify for the given job by modulating himself through aptitude training.

NEED OF INTRODUCTION OF APTITUDE TESTS IN HOMEOPATHY

We have to admit that homeopathy is passing through a crucial phase. It has already lost itself in the U.S.A. and U.K. We may blame polypharmacy, practice of low potency and other factors for its downfall. But those reasons are fractional. The fact is entrance of people lacking the aptitude for homeopathy being the main reason for the downfall. Even now in India, most students possess an indifferent attitude towards homeopathy. They enter after failure in medical entrance tests or having no other option, i.e., out of compulsion. Moreover, they do not understand the real spirit of homeopathy and squander time. That is very bad.

Homeopathy is a wonderful science. Its veracity and potentiality can only be realized by diving in its depth, which is not possible for everybody. Hence the need of aptitude test for homeopathy is a must. Through this we can extend our wings. Let only a limited number of people be trained in the true sense. We need aptitude tests also for research and education. Substandard teachers, who possess an antagonistic attitude towards homeopathy, must be thrown out of the institution.

Three Steps of Creating Aptitude Tests for Homeopathic Profession (or Mission): A Suggestion

Step I

First we have to analyse our profession by various studies keeping three factors: Research, Treatment Education and administration as priority. We have to be very practical in evaluating the field study. The harsh realities have to be accepted. False optimistic notions should not encroach our mind.

Step II

Secondly, we have to develop standardized methods of administration and scoring. Aptitudes of various facets should be ascertained through the given tests, otherwise the results will not be reliable.

Step III

The third step is to analyse the results for evaluation. By this we can successfully guage whether the given tests have worked or not. If the tests work well, the tests will be considered suitable.

■

Chapter 17

ATTENTION AND DISTRACTION

We are living in an environment which is full of a variety of stimuli. Our sense organs are always bombarded in a lesser or greater intensity by these stimuli say, the sound of a fan, noise of vehicles, rays of sun, colors of dresses, warm or cold atmosphere, fragrance of flowers, etc. However, these stimuli do not affect us equally. Despite so many stimuli in the environment, only specific stimuli are selected by us. This tendency of selection related to a motivational process is called attention. Attention is considered a power, capacity or faculty of mind, which can be turned on or off at will. But this notion is misconceived. Contrary to common belief, attention is not a power or capacity or faculty. It is a selective process, an act, a function. Hence psychologists urge to use 'attending' (verb) instead of 'attention' (noun). Thus attending (not attention) is the perceptual processing of chosen inputs for inclusion in our conscious awareness at a given time.

DEFINITION

From above, we come to know that attention is a condition of preparedness for a particular stimulus in the environment to where we are exposed. This can be treated as a definition also. Anyhow, let us examine some more definitions by some experts:

Attention is the concentration of consciousness upon one subject rather than upon another (*Dumville, D.E.*, 1938).

Attention is being keenly alive to some specific factor in our environment. It is a preparatory adjustment for response (*Morgan, J.B. and Gilliland,* 1942).

Attention is the process of getting an object of thought clearly before the mind (*Ross, J.S.*, 1951).

Attention can be defined as the focusing of perception that leads to a greater awareness of a limited number of stimuli (*Roediger et al, 1987*).

Attention can be defined as a process which compels the individual to select some particular stimulus according to his interest and attitude of the multiplicity of stimuli present in the environment (*Sharma, R.N.,1967*).

After examining the above definitions along with some other definitions the following version is synthesized, which seems to be comprehensive:

Attention can be defined as an individual's perceptual process of selected input guided by his interest and attitude for its inclusion in his conscious experience.

Moreover, the following lines highlight vividly the definition:

CHARACTERISTICS OF ATTENTION

Attention has the following characteristics:

1. Attention is essentially a process, and not a product. Attention is not a faculty or power. It is also not static. Hence some psychologists suggest using the word 'attending' instead of 'attention'.
2. Attention involves the receptor adjustment to stimuli for its reception. For example, receptor adjustment to visual sensation is made when we attend a football or cricket match on TV. Similarly, receptor adjustment is also made for hearing when we attend a mobile call.
3. Attention is characterized by a set of adjustments:
    a. Postural adjustment.
    b. Muscular adjustment.
    c. Neural adjustment.

    Postural receptors, muscular and neural adjustments make the individual ready to respond to some stimuli in a particular manner. This is called the set towards the action. Set is a motivating condition influencing the direction of response. Set is related in determining the velocity of reaction. Athletes have to with postural, muscular and neural adjustment while running on the track with the sound of a whistle, here the whistle initiates this set of action.
4. It helps making us aware or conscious of our environment.

5. This awareness or consciousness is selective.
6. At any one time, we can concentrate or focus our consciousness on one particular object only.
7. The concentration or focus provided by the process of attention helps us in clearly understanding the perceived object or phenomenon.
8. In the chain of stimulus-response behavior it works as a mediator. Stimuli which are given proper attention yield better response. Therefore, for providing an appropriate response, one has to give proper attention to the stimulus to reach the stage of preparedness of alertness (mental as well as physical) which may be required.
9. Attention is not merely a cognitive function but is essentially determined by emotional and conative factors of interest, attitude and striving.
10. Sensory information is filtered in the process of attention. An individual cannot process all the information in his sensory channels, so it filters out, or checks irrelevant information.

EFFECTS OF ATTENTION

Attention makes us more alert and prepared. By this the mental power is enhanced and we adopt ourselves in a better way for future assignments of a similar nature. We may learn lessons in a better way by paying attention. We can also receive and remember something in an easy manner by paying attention. Attention provides us potency and skill to continue the task of cognitive functioning despite the presence of distractions like noise and music. Mental awareness is developed by attention. Attention also helps in bringing about mental preparation. Thus, attention also helps in developing concentration by focusing one's attention on a given topic. In fact attention is a must for intellectual people like doctors, teachers, philosophers, etc. greater the attention, better the achievements in life. Attention acts as a reinforcement of sensory processes and assists in better organization of perception for clarity. You may be a scientist or a yogi, you still need to develop attention. Lack of attention may jeopardize our observation about a person or an object. Here it is the attention that pays the rich dividends in our goal. Frequent fixation of attention lubricates us in meeting various difficult problems in life. In a nutshell, attention is one of the important factors in our life that is needed to go and get success.

TYPES OF ATTENTION

Many psychologists have classified 'attention' in various ways. The classification of 'attention' presented below is a synthetic compilation, which is presented for an easy perusal.

I. Volitional or voluntary:
   i. Implicit.
   ii. Explicit.
II. Non-volitional or non-voluntary:
   i. Enforced.
   ii. Spontaneous.
III. Habitual attention.

I. Volitional Attention

When we execute our will to an attention, it is called volitional or voluntary attention. We make a conscious or deliberate effort on paying attention. Very often with this type of attention we focus ourselves for a goal. We have a clear cut goal and we become attentive of its accomplishment. In volitional attention, attention is willingly directed to an object. Suppose you are going to appear for 1st B.H.M.S. examination. Now, you direct your attention towards serious study and your specific aim of passing the examination is needed. Similarly attention paid during solving a mathematical quiz or equation, examining a patient in OPD, etc. can be categorized under volitional attention.

i. Implicit Volitional Attention

In implicit volitional attention, a single act of volition is required to bring about attention. Once the author assigned his son Sambit, who was seven years old to carry out an addition. Sambit did not listen him and continued to enjoy some cartoon programme on TV. Then the author warned him to finish the addition fast. Sambit finished the addition instantly. Here the single exhortation of the author brought his son's attention towards the mathematical sum of addition. Here his son Sambit executed a single act of will which can be termed as implicit volitional attention.

ii. Explicit Volitional Attention

This is obtained by repeated acts of will. Now Sambit is preparing for his annual examination of class one. He has to struggle hard to continue being attentive. The annual examination demands Sambit's strong will to stand first in class. The repeated effort of paying attention against heavy odds and distractions is called explicit volitional attention.

II. Non-volitional Attention

In this type, attention is directed by the individual's desire or motivation. It may even go against it. Sometimes it blocks the goal sought for. For example, you are waiting to catch a bus and just when the bus arrives, your favorite film song starts playing at a nearby hotel. Then for a moment you get disturbed and cannot decide what to do: to listen to the song or to leave it. This type of paying attention is categorized under non-volitional attention.

i. Non-volitional Enforced Attention

When the attention is aroused by instinct it is called enforced attention. Sometimes, you feel the sexual urge that comes out of instinct. Paying attention to such instinct comes under non-volitional enforced attention.

ii. Spontaneous Non-volitional Attention

It is aroused by sentiments. It is the outcome of well developed sentiments. We give spontaneous attention towards the object or person around which our sentiment is well knit. Suppose your brother or somebody else who is dear to you was severely beaten by somebody and he enters into your room bleeding. Suddenly your attention is drawn and such drawing of attention comes under this category with the emotion underneath.

III. Habitual Attention

Along with the above two types, a third attention called habitual attention is postulated. In fact, it is the developed form of explicit voluntary type of attention. Some objects in environment draw our attention since a long time. We pay attention to these things or duties out of habit and past experience. We attend them not out of pressure or compulsion, but out of routine. When we get up in the morning, we wash our faces, brush our teeth, attend the call of nature, etc. In a family, mother cooks for members of the family. She attends to cooking out of habit. Similarly, examples can be multiplied: The gardener attends the plants, the betel leaf chewer goes to the betel leaf shop, etc. All these come under habitual attention.

In habitual attention, the person is permanently set for reception of certain stimuli. Let us take an example of watching TV at home. The elderly are attracted towards spiritual programmes, the young couple towards thrillers and the kids are attracted by cartoon programmes.

When a family visits a book exhibition (or even a book shop) the elderly purchase books related to yoga or meditation, the husband may purchase a magazine on sports because he is interested in sports. Similarly, the wife may a purchase book on cooking, she being interested in it. The child may pick up a cartoon book. Infact, habitual attention is guided by aspiration, motives, drives, interest, attitudes, prejudice, etc.

DETERMINANTS (CONDITIONS) OF ATTENTION

Now it has become crystal clear from above that attention is a selective act of mind. The condition may be of two types:

I. External or objective type of attention.
II. Internal or subjective type of attention.

An external stimulus is related to the environment like visual, auditory, olfactory, tactile, etc. There exist innumerable stimuli, but an individual can not go through all the stimuli simultaneously because the stimuli differ in intensity and frequency. Some stimuli are stronger, while others are weaker (and some even imperceptible). Usually the stronger stimuli draw our attention. The factors making these stimuli stronger than others are called external determinants of attention. These are also called objective conditions due to their objective aspect.

Apart from the external or environmental aspect, mental state, cultural background and heredity also play part in attention. These internal governing factors are termed internal determinants. These factors are subjective in nature and hence are often subjective conditions.

I. External Determinants of Attention

1. Nature of Stimulus

There exist various types of stimuli like visual, auditory, gustatory, olfactory or tactile. Experiments have revealed that an individual is more susceptible to drawing attention to form, color and sound. For example:

a. Photographs of humans draw our attention more than that of an animal.
b. Photograph of a beautiful woman draws our attention more than that of a man.
c. Our attention is drawn more to colorful pictures then to its counterpart of black and white. Today best classical Bollywood and Hollywood films of black and white nature are not appreciated by the modern generation.
d. It has also been observed that bright color advertisements draw our attention more than that of a dull color.
e. Similarly, or melodious voice acts like a magnet in drawing our attention paralyzing other voices or noises.

2. Dimension of stimulus

The dimension of stimulus also plays an important role in determining our attention. We have to understand it under two headings:

a. A colossus figure naturally draws our attention. Even while moving on the roadways, big advertisements (colorful of course) draw our attention in comparison to advertisements of smaller size or dimension. We are also susceptible to three dimensional figures than that of two dimensional figures.
b. A small lively picture of an advertisement having a big plain background also holds our attention in a better way.

3. Position of Stimulus

The position of the stimuli also has a decisive role in attracting our attention. It has been observed that the advertisements given on front page or on the upper part of the newspaper draw our attention instantly. Similarly, when a teacher teaches, he gets better attention from the students sitting in front in comparison to students.

4. Change of Stimulus

a. In comparison with unchanged stimuli, changed stimuli (in near past) has more possibility of attracting attention. The modes of change also influence the process of attention. If there is a change absolutely opposite to the present stimulus, it will definitely attract more attention.
b. While studying one does not hear the sound of the clock or electric fan but if either of them suddenly stops, one cannot fail to attend to it.

c. The effect of the change goes on diminishing with the passage of time.
d. Whenever stimuli are changed together and one is left unchanged, the effect of change is not noticeable
e. If changes go on in the changed stimuli, the process of attention is rather permanent and strong.

Man becomes used to regular changes and does not pay much attention to them. But if irregular changes or any sudden change occurs in contrast to regular changes, it draws our attention in a better form.

5. Power of Stimulus

Powerful stimuli have a better edge in comparison to weaker stimuli. Intense stimuli immediately attract our attention. We have learned from aphorism 26 in *Organon of Medicine* that a weaker dynamic affection is over-shadowed by a stronger one. Infact, high sound, excessive pressure and intense pain immediately draws our attention.

6. Disparity of Stimulus

The disparity or contrast of stimuli also acts as a key factor in determining attention. For example, the presence of a woman among men, a man among women, and an old man among children invariably attracts our attention. Such examples can be multiplied in relation to dress code or uncommon amongst a common. A small light in a dark place immediately draws attention.

7. Segregation of Stimulus

A student sitting alone in some corner of the room or in isolation immediately draws the attention of the teacher in an academic institution. The teacher may even enquire about the student. Similarly, a man sitting in some corner of a hotel or club also attracts the attention of an audience.

8. Repetition of Stimulus

We are well aware of the fact that repetition is an important determinant of attention. More the repetition, better the fixation in attention. During our childhood, we were taught lessons by rote. Similarly, a teacher tries to put stress in important matters by repetition, so that the pupils can not forget the same.

9. Duration of Stimulus

Stimulus having more duration will attract more attention. Therefore, a good teacher takes a relatively long time in teaching crucial facts in class.

A word of note: An attempt has been made above regarding the external determinants of attention in general. There may be exceptions in a given situation. For example, you may listen to your name being called by a voice of lower intensity in the market place despite the presence of a horn of a motor car. as you are interested in yourself. This comes under internal determinants of attention. Similarly, frequent repetition of a given stimulus may induce an indifferent reception. Also, duration beyond the threshold can repel the attention and may make an individual bored. Its outcome may be the opposite of the expected one. As a matter of fact, attention does not occur at the mercy of any single external factor but on several internal factors as well.

10. Transformation of Stimulus

We cannot hold our attention for a long time on a particular object. Even in an interesting class or spiritual discourse, our mind comes and goes. Hence, a change of stimulus affects an individual's attention. Even during examinations, when you are glued to your study material, your attention is immediately drawn towards a discord that might be occurring outside your study room. Advertising agencies frequently change their strategy for a given product for this reason. Even the product makes a nominal or trivial change and presents itself in a different manner so that the sale of the product may be promoted further.

Similarly, moving stimuli attract us more in comparison to static stimuli. At night, a static stimulus may attract us, but the moving stimulus attracts us more. We pay more attention to moving stimuli. In a seminar or in a workshop, a static presentation cannot compete in drawing the attention of the audience in comparison to a movie presentation.

II. Internal Determinants of Attention

1. Interest

Interest is one of the prime internal determinants of attention. We can divide interest as *innate* and *acquired*. Both have their importance in their respective fields, but it has been observed that innate tendency attracts more attention for fulfillment. If you are interested in music then it is quite obvious that a newly organized music troop will draw your attention. Similarly the yoga camp advertisement may draw the attention of a diabetic patient as he is interested in getting rid of diabetes.

2. Basic Drives

The basic drives of instincts of an individual play an important role in relation to attention. Our basic drives are hunger, thirst, sex, etc. Hence when we see delicious food or drink, our attention is drawn towards those items. Similarly, a beautiful woman or a handsome man may pull our attention. That is the reason why sex appeal has been so exploited by advertising agencies. They are so expert in their operation that they even use a sex symbol or women in an advertisement which seems to be totally out of context.

3. Emotion

Emotion constitutes vital determinants of attention. Let us take an example of your neighbor boy. When he is summoned by the police, you immediately react and comment that the boy might have been involved in crime, otherwise why should the police summon him. In a similar situation, if your younger brother is involved, you cry that he is innocent and is being harassed by the police. You will also say that your brother is absolutely innocent and the action of police is vindictive. The fact is that we attend to even the smallest fault of a person we do not like, whereas we do not attend to the worst offense committed by the person we love. It is the magic of love that makes the world look beautiful to lovers. All these scenarios are concerned with emotion.

4. Attitude of Mind

Our attention also depends upon our mental attitude. If you are an author, the books will be the sole object of your attention. Similarly, various types of diseases draw the attention of a doctor; beauty deficiencies in women will draw the attention of a beautician even if they are on a holiday tour.

5. Aim and Ambition

Every man has some immediate and some ultimate aims. Currently I am engrossed in writing this book and my immediate aim is to finish this book with good compilation. Hence, now books on psychology will draw my attention. Naturally, libraries, journals on psychology, various book stores, etc. will also draw my attention.

6. Peculiar and Meaningful Events

Nobody likes to dwell on meaningless and ordinary talks. Peculiar and meaningful things attract our attention to a greater degree. When you listen to the news of a dog biting a man, it may not appeal to you and you may not attend to it. But when you listen that a man has bitten a dog, you exclaim, "What?" This peculiar situation draws your attention. It is obvious that striking, singular, peculiar symptoms attract our attention in the clinic and it is on these peculiarities that we base our prescription.

7. Habit

Habit is also counted as an important internal determinant of attention. What do you do the moment you get up from bed? You ask for a cup of tea. Is it not. It is the habit of tea that draws your immediate attention (although you know that bed tea may be injurious to your health). Your time table also draws your attention for a given subject that has been put into habit. It is the habit of an alcoholic that draws his frequent attention to alcohol. Anyhow, in most cases your attention is drawn to a positive atmosphere instead of a negative atmosphere. We usually attend to necessary and desirable objects instead of unnecessary and undesirable objects.

8. Disposition and Temperament

Both are important determinants of attention. You might have come in contact with various people from various walks of life. You might have also noticed that a criminal's attention is drawn towards crime and he may interact with you on crime and criminal talks. A doctor's attention is drawn towards your health and sickness. He may point out your constitution or diathesis or even your nosological disease. Also, a patient's attention is focused to a doctor or books on health in a book shop. Similarly, attention of a spiritual or sex-dwelling man will be drawn towards his respective object. Let us assume that a group of doctors, engineers, geologists, beauticians and carpenters from various parts of India entered a reserved compartment of a train without knowing one another for a fixed destination. Within a few minutes you will find that specific groups will be organized and dwell on a discussion on their profession and interest.

9. Past Experience

Basically we are the product of our past experience. Hence, past experience plays a key determinant of attention. As such we prefer to immerse in past experiences of success (of course to a much less extent in failures), which gives us a pleasant feeling. Moreover, a person's helping deed draws immediate attention and desire to help him, whereas we may reject a lucrative offer from an ungrateful person who has harmed us.

10. Motives and Social Motives

Recognition is a fundamental goal for all of us. We want ourselves and our work to be recognized. Hence our attention is drawn towards social motives like helping others, joining an organization so that we can carry out philanthropic work. We try to accomplish deeds of bravery and valor by saving others. We also attend to our duties because of social motives. Our education and training have a wide influence on attention. Our family, school, college, social structure, organization, etc. of which we are a part, also have an impact on our attention.

DISTRACTION

Distraction means something that diverts attention. Distraction may be defined as interference, division in the process of attention by a stimulus. Distraction can be divided into:

a. **Continuous Distraction:** As the caption suggests, it is the continuous distraction that interferes with attention. For example, continuous use of a microphone during a celebration or festive occasion interferes with your preparation for an examination. However, experts claim that adjustment soon takes place with such type of distractions.

b. **Continual Distraction**: Contrary to above, the distraction is irregular being interspersed with intervals like phone calls that may distract your attention, while you are practicing yoga.

c. **Internal Distraction**: Distraction, in relation to emotional upset, bereavement, fear, health deterioration, etc. comes under internal distraction.

d. **External Distraction**: Varieties of music, noise, inadequate ventilation or light, etc. come under such type of distraction.

How to Get Rid of Distractions

1. Internal distractions need medicines especially homeopathic medicines like *Anacardium, Natrium mur., Acidum phos., Kalium phos.*, etc. along with psychotherapy.
2. When someone becomes active in a given work, distraction proves impotent.
3. Distraction should be disregarded.

4. One can also accept distraction as a part of work. The author in his student carrier used to read lessons while listening to a transistor.

CLINICAL APPLICATION

1. A deficit in attention is one of the clinical conditions that we have to encounter in our clinic. A mild form may not draw our attention but severe form is an indication of schizophrenia. Schizophrenics require the capacity to perceive and respond to situations objectively.
2. Lodging of undue and undesirable factors like bereavement, anxiety, etc. may be at the background of an individual in causing a deficit in attention. In this state, the individual becomes forgetful and cannot follow a job that calls for sustained attention such as reading, teaching or other allied duties. These patients must be taken into trust by the physician and the reality must be explored so that the corresponding medicines may be prescribed.
3. In clinical life you will find chiefly, three types of patients in whom attention is related:
    a. Hypochondriac patients pay much attention to their vague ailments.
    b. Another set of patients do not pay attention to their ailments, even though may be organic in nature.
    c. Hysterical patients present symptoms like loss of sensation in skin, lack of vision or hearing, which do not comply with the corresponding pathological state.

    As a physician you have to play a crucial role in understanding such phenomena as mentioned above in an appropriate way. For the first two conditions, our Master has devoted some instructions in *Organon of Medicine*. Moreover, we are well equipped with medicines like *Ignatia*, *Natrium mur.*, etc. (see repertory) in treating hysterical patients.
4. Attention deficit in children is very often overlooked as normal by us. In this state, the child cannot accomplish an assignment that was initiated due to lack of sustained attention. You should be careful to discover the accompanied morbid problem of conduct disorder or specific learning disability, so that you can help the patient in a better way through homeopathy or other alternatives.
5. Deficit attention is also found in states like delirium (i.e., clouding of consciousness) and hallucinations, where the patient becomes confused,

disoriented (i.e., not knowing the present time or place), etc. In such states suitable measures must be resorted to.

6. Deficit attention is also found in diseases like encephalitis, sleeping sickness, or pressure of a tumor in the brain, etc. These are the conditions related to the brain stem. You must diagnose them at the earliest so as to enable the patient to help in a superior way.

In our armament we are well equipped with medicines like *Aethusa, Anacardium, Medorrhinum, Kalium phos.,* etc. in treating diseases like deficit attention. Of course, the selection of simillimum is carried out after the formation of totality of symptoms, chiefly guided by the constitution (including the miasmatic condition).

Chapter 18

PSYCHOLOGY OF ANXIETY AND ANXIETY DISORDERS

The present age can be designated as the age of anxiety. Disintegration of the joint family leading to isolation, ever growing avariceness, cut throat competition, adoption of foreign culture of disintegrated morality, regular consumption of fast (junk) food, sedentary life style, lack of trust amongst us, non-acceptance of reality and falling in baseless imagination lead us to anxiety. Hence, the phenomenon of anxiety has become a matter of grave concern for us.

Literary portrait of anxiety is submitted below for your appreciation:

"Harassed by headlines, tortured by taxes, tormented by the telephone, laughing and weeping as the sales charts of businessman, wakeful when he should sleep, drowsy when he should be awake, worrying about his blood pressure and nursing his duodenal ulcer, he has 2,500 million neighbours in this world, yet he is alone. And the loneliness is eating him up. He has tranquilizers in one pocket and pep pill in the other. Drugs to dispel nightmares and drugs to *slip into* 'Alice in Wonderland'. He is in search of soul which he has lost in this industrial era."

(Neki in Dutta, 1967)

Let us carry out our the present study under the following heads for an easy comprehension.

A. Anxiety.
B. Normal anxiety.
C. Anxiety neurosis.
D. Anxiety disorders.

A. ANXIETY

Anxiety may be defined as a painful emotional experience with cognitive, somatic, emotional and behavior involvement giving rise to over concern leading to panic or severe fear, which may be real or imaginary and may be related to present, past, future.

The cognitive involvement of anxiety leads to anticipate a diffused and certain danger.

Somatically involvement sets up the organism –

1. to meet threat, by means of emergency responses like increase in blood pressure and heart rate, perspiration, inhibition of functions of immune and digestive system and
2. express itself externally as pale skin, tremor, pupilary dilation etc.

The emotional involvement results in –

1. a sense of dread or panic and
2. physical expressions like nausea, vomiting, diarrhea, chills etc.

Behavioral involvement entails both voluntary and involuntary behaviors like –

1. carrying on a fight or
2. opting for a flight.

Anxiety serves as a vital survival function; it is a warning system that is activated whenever a person perceives a danger or threat. In anxiety, the symptoms are caused by a rush of adrenaline and other chemicals that get the body ready to make a quick getaway from danger.

B. NORMAL ANXIETY

Nobody is immune from anxiety. Everyone encounters feelings of anxiety from time to time. Anxiety can be explained as a sense of uneasiness, nervousness, worry, fear or dread of what's about to happen?

Feelings of anxiety, which rest on the person and the circumstance, can be mild, moderate or severe. An individual can experience a mild anxiety in the form of uneasiness or nervousness or an intense anxiety in the form of fear, dread, or panic.

Again, it's natural for an individual to go through a state of anxiety under a new, unfamiliar, or challenging situation. For example; facing an important interview, a test or a major class presentation can trigger normal anxiety in us. Such situations can cause us to feel 'threatened' and not actually a threat to our safety. Of course these can cause us to feel "threatened" by possible embarrassment, worrying about making a blunder, faltering over words, being accepted or rejected, losing self-importance etc. We can also experience physical sensations like throbbing of heart, sweaty hands, or a nervous stomach, which can be a part of normal anxiety, which subsides unconsciously within a reasonable amount of time. Very often an anxiety can be a boon to us. It can make us alert, watchful, and ready to meet the ensuring problems in a efficient manner.

C. ANXIETY NEUROSIS

This term was coined by Freud. In recent days it is superseded by ICD 10 (International Classification of Disease, version 10) to 'Generalized Anxiety Disorder' (see below under 'Anxiety Disorders'). Moreover, patient (rather the client) must not be injured mentally by the label 'neurotic'.

D. ANXIETY DISORDERS

We have already appreciated the positive aspects of anxiety. It helps us handle a tense situation competently in a working place, study harder for an examination, and keep focus on an important oration or talk. But when anxiety becomes excessive, irrational, and too strong, it interferes with our normal functioning and makes us dread in undertaking a routine task. It causes us to feel paralyzed or tongue-tied and we cannot do what we need. It robs away our efficiency and integrity in discharging ordinary ordeals. This excessive, intense, incessant and irrational anxiety articulated in terms of fear, nervousness, worry or dread is called anxiety disorder. Anxiety disorders cause us to feel preoccupied, distracted, tense, and always on alert.

Anxiety disorders can take many shapes. It can make us so uneasy around people that we avoid them, we isolate ourselves from social gatherings and even we miss prospective friendships. It may fill us with various obsessive thoughts or incomprehensible dread of carrying out ordinary activities. Anyhow, we find various types of anxiety disorders, out of which following five types are very important in our day to day state of affairs.

I.   Generalized anxiety disorder (GAD).
II. Obsessive-compulsive disorder (OCD).
III. Panic disorder (PD).

IV. Post-Traumatic stress disorder (PTSD).
V. Phobic disorders (*Social phobia being most common*).

I. Generalized Anxiety Disorder (GAD)

We have already talked about normal anxiety. Worrying, more or less is a common affair for all of us. Becoming worry is not always bad. Many a time, worry helps us plan for future, make us sure that we are prepared for the interview or presenting a topic for a seminar etc. May the process of worry be never a pleasant drive but without it nothing seems to walk off smoothly. But what will happen if we cannot produce a positive result for us? And most importantly what is the usefulness of that worry; if we cannot stop it. Rather, we know that it is doing us no good and possibly making everyone unhappy else around us. These features characterize Generalized Anxiety Disorder (GAD).

Generalized anxiety disorder or GAD is characterized by excessive, exaggerated anxiety and worry at everyday life events. Patients who are suffering from generalized anxiety disorder always tend to expect a catastrophe or a disaster form oblivion. Sometimes, just the thought of getting through the day produces anxiety in them. They can't stop worrying about health, money, family, work or working place. Their worries are frequently found to be unrealistic. Moreover, their anxieties are out of proportion to the situation. Their day to day life becomes a constant state of worry, fear and dread. Ultimately, over anxiety interferes with their daily functioning, work, social activities and relationships. They suffer from insomnia, startle easily, can't relax, and have difficult in concentration. They also suffer from irritability, headache, nausea, fatigue, tremor, muscle tension, pain at various parts of body, difficulty swallowing, twitching; sweating, dyspnoea, hot flushes etc.

Anyhow GAD is diagnosed when a person

a. Suffers from an anxiety, which is incessant, excessive, unrealistic, and finds difficult to control the anxiety about a variety of everyday problems for at least 6 months (The DSM-IV criteria) *DSM and IV stands for Diagnostic and statistical Manual of Mental Disorder and 4th edition respectively.*)

b. having at least three of the following troubles:
- Restlessness
- Easily tired

- Difficult concentration
- Irritability
- Muscle tension
- Insomnia

Causes of GAD

The exact cause of GAD is not known, but following 4 factors come out to contribute to its development.

1. *Genetics:* It has a role for the development of GAD as it tends to run in families.
2. *Neurotransmitters:* Various studies have revealed that GAD is associated with abnormal levels of certain neurotransmitters in the brain.

   Neurotransmitters are the special chemical messengers, which carry information from nerve cell to nerve cell. Alteration in the level neurotranmitters interferes in carrying messages between cells and thus brain cannot function properly and pave the way to the generation of anxiety.
3. *Emotion:* Mental trauma, stressful events, loss of love or job, death of loved ones; divorce etc. may lead to GAD.
4. *Substance and other narcotis:* The use of and withdrawal from addictive substances, including alcohol, caffeine and nicotine, etc. aggravate anxiety.

II. Obsessive-compulsive Disorder (OCD)

Obsessive-compulsive disorder (OCD) is an anxiety disorder characterized by an individual's obsessive, distressing, intrusive thoughts and related compulsions (tasks or "rituals") which endeavors to diffuse the obsessions. Let us bifurcate the word and go for the definition as fixed by *DSM-IV diagnostic criteria.*

Obsessions may be defined as:

1. recurrent and persistent thoughts, impulses, or images that are experienced by an individual at some time during the disturbance, which are invasive and inappropriate and they cause marked anxiety or distress,

2. whereas the corresponding thoughts, impulses, or images are not simply excessive worries about actual life problems,
3. moreover, the individual attempts to ignore or suppress such thoughts, impulses, or images, or to neutralize them with some other thoughts or actions,
4. and the individual recognizes that the obsessive thoughts, impulses, or images are a product of his or her own mind, and are not based on reality.

Examples of some OCD obsessions:

1. germs or dirt
2. illness or injury (involving the individual or somebody else)
3. across unlucky numbers and day (say 13 or 9 or day like Friday or Saturday)
4. things being perfect or just right in a certain way (i.e. fastidious approach)
5. committing a mistakes or not being sure of it.
6. doing or thinking something negative.

Compulsions may be defined as:

1. repetitive behaviors or mental acts that the individual feels driven to perform in response to an obsession,
2. whereas the behaviors or mental acts are clearly excessive in nature and directed to preventing or reducing distress (or some dreaded event or situation) but the behaviors or mental acts are not linked in a pragmatic way with what they are intended to prevent the said distress (or the dread event or situation).

Example of some OCD compulsions:

- A lady may wash hands every now and them
- A student may count 15 shops on the way before reaching the college
- An individual may, touch every light pole between home and the railway station
- An adolescent may touch everybody's right (or left) shoulder in a clinic or school
- Everyday a student gives gentle stroke to every classmates who sit on benches in the classroom

- A person may check things over and over such as bolting the doors, checking to locks, etc.
- An individual may do things for a certain number of times (moving to and fro for seven times before going to office)
- A lady may arrange and rearrange things in a very particular or neat way
- An employee may ask the same question repeatedly to everybody inside the office
- A person may always move from left to right and right to left constantly while walking on a stair case till he reaches his destination.

An individual is said to be suffering from OCD provided he had obsessions with or without a compulsion as mentioned above. Again the individual must realize that his obsessions or compulsions are unreasonable or out of proportion. Secondly the obsessions or compulsions must take up more than one hour per day, cause distress leading to an impairment in social and occupational life or functioning at working place. Anyhow here you should remember that depression mimics with OCD frequently.

Some symptoms of OCD follow as:

- Repeated hand washing
- Incessant coughing to clean up the throat, although there does not exist any pathology inside the throat
- Fear of going to be crazy
- The individual fears as if he was going to be transformed and he also feels as if he has no control over the transformation
- Sexual obsessions or unwanted sexual thoughts; fears as if we going to be homosexual or fear of becoming a pedophile
- Repetitive useless drills of doing something
- Some OCD sufferers adopt a particular counting system say grouping objects in odd/even numbered groups, etc.
- An obsession with numbers: some sufferers are obsessed with even numbers (or odd numbers) and loathe odd numbers (or even numbers). Odd numbers (or even numbers) cause them a great deal of anxiety and often make the person uncomfortable and irritable
- Feeling like they are needed to have an exact routine, with minor details

- Unreasonable mysophobia: A fear of contamination such as saliva, blood, sweat, tears, vomit, or mucus, or excretions such as urine or feces
- Some OCD individuals do not use soap for the spread of contamination
- The sufferer may play with a doll or a teddy bear in a funny way: Twisting the head like a circle, then twisting it all the way back exactly in the opposite direction
- He may repeat this exercise incessantly without having any aim

Above mentioned symptoms are mere some examples of OCD. But the list is not exhaustive. Simply having some of the symptoms as mentioned above do not point to an absolute diagnosis of OCD. Hence a formal diagnosis should be performed by a mental health professional like a psychologist or a psychiatrist.

Cause of OCD

The exact cause of OCD is not known

In 14-16th century it was believed to be caused by devils and hence exorcism was in vogue.

Some scientists attribute OCD to psychological and neurological origin.

Some other scientist blame Group A streptococcal infection as the contributing factor.

III. Panic Disorder

Panic disorder is characterized by sudden attacks of terror, worry about having an attack, about what it means, or changing the way one behaves because of the panic attacks for no less than a month. Panic attacks are break up and strong periods of fear or feelings of trouble which peak within 10 minutes; but some of the symptoms may last longer. Panic disorder must accompany at least four of the following symptoms:

- Throbbing of heart
- Tremor
- Dyspnea
- Dizziness

- Fear of dying
- Perspiring
- Sense of choking
- Pain in chest
- Nausea or other stomach upset
- Derealization; a feeling of being detached from the world
- Cannot think; feels as if the mind has gone blank
- Sensation of Numbness or tingling
- Chills or hot flashes

Panic attacks usually generate a sense of hollowness, a fear of imminent doom, or a fear of losing control. People, who are suffering from this, claim that they are going to die or having a heart attack or loosing control over their mind. They may express that their mind is going blank or that they somehow do not feel real. They feel as if they were looking themselves form outside of themselves. They can't predict when or where an attack will ensure, and between episodes many worry intensely and dread the next attack. Panic attacks can occur at any time, even during sleep.

Panic disorders are divided into

i. Panic disorder with agarophobia
ii. Panic disorder without agarophobia

i. Panic disorder with agoraphobia

Sometimes panic disorder occurs only once in a life time in many people and they are lucky but in most cases, the course runs longer, even a life time. When the condition progresses far away, the individuals become afraid of open spaces and they are said to be suffering from *Panic disorder with agarophobia*. The term agoraphobia was coined by Westphil in 1871. In the original Greek it refers to the fear of market place (i.e. agora) or a busy, bustling area.

Individuals suffering form PDA experience severe unexpected panic attacks. The suffering individuals feel as if they were going to die or they are losing control over their mind. As they are not in a position to predict the time of attack, they develop agoraphobia, fear and avoidance of situation in which they would feel unsafe. Generally such patients avoid shopping, driving, marketing and journeying (by bus, car, train, aero plane, etc.). They also stay away from visiting theaters, cinema halls, restaurants, crowds, elevators etc. They do not like to leave home by apprehending the attack to PD and need company. They cannot stay all alone there.

Treatment

Panic disorder is one of the most treatable of all the anxiety disorders early detection of PD has better prospectus. The physician's work becomes hard when the patient had additional sufferings like depression, drug abuse, alcoholism etc. Here adoption of judicious treatment a per the totality of symptoms plus Cognitive psychotherapy counts much.

IV. Stress Disorder or Post-traumatic Stress Disorder (PTSD)

It results after an exposure of an individual towards a terrifying affliction which incriminates physical harm or the threat of physical harm. The individual who develop PTSD may have been harmed or may have witnessed a harmful event that happened to a loved one or a stranger. It can develop form exposure to either death or near-death circumstances such as fires, floods, earthquakes, shootings, bus or car accidents, train wrecks, plane crashes, bombings, wars, street violence like stabbing, shelling etc. It also include variety of traumatic incidents such as rape, mugging, torture, being kidnapped or held captive, child abuse or children exposed to horror or pornographic images or acts. The blanketed traumatic event is re-experienced in thoughts and dreams. Common behaviors those are attributed in this respect follow as:

1. The afflicted individual may re-experience the trauma in the awaking state a flashback or during sleep as a nightmare.

    (*An individual having a flashback in this respect may lose contact with reality and believes that the traumatic incident is happening all over again*)

2. He cannot concentrate in any action or thought.
3. he avoids day to day activities, places, or people associated with the sparking off event.
4. He very badly suffers from insomnia.
5. He may become hyper vigilant i.e. may take extraordinary caution in watching the surroundings.
6. He feels a general sense of depression and irritability.

7. He becomes emotionally numb (especially with nears and dears).
8. He may also develop derealization (i.e. feeling of detachment) and anhedonia (i.e. loss of pleasure or interest in previously enjoyable activities)

People suffering from PTSD avoid situations that remind them of the original incident. Their symptoms aggravate on the anniversaries of the incident, when they vividly feel the mishap that occurred to them. Symptoms of PTSD seem to be worse if the event is deliberately initiated by another person, as in a mugging or a kidnapping. Even observing such scenes in a TV channel, may it be real or fictitious, can trigger the sufferings.

The course of the illness of PTSD varies individual to individual. Some people recover within 6 months, while others have symptoms that last much longer. Women are more susceptible to PTSD than men.

All traumatized individuals do not necessarily develop full-blown (or even minor) PTSD. Symptoms usually begin within 3 months. Of the incident but occasionally emerge years afterwards. *The symptoms must last more than a month to be considered as PTSD.*

Note: Common symptoms like chest pain, dysponea, palpitation of heart, reeling of head fainting and weakness generally should be attributed to anxiety and hence demands careful evaluation for PTSD.

Cause of PTSD

Research evidences reveal that PTSD runs in families. Common concomitants of PTSD are depression, substance abuse, or other anxiety disorder.

Treatment

Anyhow Homoeopathy has a wonderful role to play in the treatment of cases of PTSD.

V. Phobic Disorders

Phobic disorders are related to a strong, Persistent and irrational fear of a specific object, activity, or situation that causes to avoid the corresponding object, activity or situation. The person recognizes the fear as excessive and irrational but cannot control the anxiety associated with it.

Phobic disorders differ from generalized anxiety disorders and panic disorders since there is a specific stimulus or situation that elicits a strong fear response. An individual suffering from a phobia of cockroach might feel so frightened by a cockroach that he or she would try to fly out of a running bus or train to get rid of it.

People with such phobias have overwhelming imaginations. They vividly foresee terrifying consequences coming across with such feared objects as knives, bridges, blood, enclosed places (claustrophobia), heights (acrophobia), animals, insects, snakes, etc.

We have already had a glimpse about these fears under 'Anxiety and Fear'. Among dozens of various phobic disorders, social phobia is the commonest and is very pertinent to our study.

Social Phobia (Social Anxiety Disorder)

Suppose you are going to participate in a University debate or for a seminar deliberation for the first time; you are likely to become nervous, feel self-conscious, fill in shy in front of the audience, which are natural. You can also have the feelings of palpitation of heart, sweaty palms, tremor etc. But after some moment you conquer all these troubles in a usual way and successfully present the deliberation before the audience.

In day to day life most people like you manage to get through these moments of anxiety when they need to. But for some, the anxiety that goes from bad to worse with the feelings of shyness or self-consciousness without remission. They feel too nervous to give answers in class, fail to make an eye contact with classmates on the hallway, avoid chatting with others at the lunch table etc. Now we can say that they are suffering from Social Phobia or Social Anxiety Disorder. In social phobia the person dreads of being criticized or humiliated. Performance anxiety is a type of social phobia.

Social Phobia (social anxiety disorder) is defined as an intense, persistent, and perpetual fear of being judged, criticized and evaluated by other people. Physical symptoms that often accompany it include blushing, profuse sweating, trembling, nausea, and difficulty in talking. Although the individuals recognize their fear as irrational, they are filled with the fear of judgement in social situations. They worry for days or weeks before the dreaded situation. Their fear grows, expands and makes them avoid the work and working place.

Even if they manage to tackle their fear, they become extremely uncomfortable throughout the meet, and worry for hours afterwards about how they were judged for.

Social phobia can be related to a particular situation such as chatting with people or eating or drinking in front of others or even writing on a blackboard in front of the students and teachers. The phobia can also be generalized as social phobia, where the individual encounters anxiety around everybody except among the members of the family.

It is very unfortunate that persons suffering from with social anxiety are misdiagnosed almost 90% of the time, because social anxiety is not well understood by common man or even by physicians, psychiatrists or psychologists. People suffering from social phobia are frequently misdiagnosed for "schizophrenic", "manic-depressive", "clinically depressed", "panic disordered", and "personality disordered" etc.

The social phobia may lead the sufferers to resort to substance abuse. It also paralyzes their academic and social activities. Generally, they do not do well in study and other allied activities. Afterwards they have additional occupational difficulties in the working place. They do not enjoy their life or job. Ultimately this phobia induces depression and suicidal ideation.

Causes of Social Phobia

Genetic factors, other anxiety disorders, substance abuse (when used as self medication for anxiety) etc. are blamed for the cause of social phobia

How can social anxiety be treated?

Social anxiety does not come and go like some other physical and psychological problems. This problem usually lasts till the last breathe of the sufferer. Yet, It can be successfully treated with certain kinds of psychotherapy or Homoeopathic medications.

Among various methods, cognitive-behavioral therapy seems to be the best. Cognitive-behavioral methods can produce long-lasting, sometimes permanent relief from the social anxiety. It acts for the following facts

   a. The sufferer recognizes that his thoughts and feelings are somewhat exaggerated and irrational
   b. He also knows that although he is watched and judged by others, he is not really or critically judged or evaluated by them.

ANXIETY DISORDERS: TREATMENT IN GENERAL

First Treat the Underlying Causes of Anxiety Disorder

We have already discussed about various causes of anxiety disorders. But we should also know that anxiety disorders can be sequels of various underlying illness. These illnesses must be ruled out before we confirm the patient to be suffering from anxiety disorders in real sense. *Anyhow, the treatment must be aimed at totality of symptoms as mentioned in Organon of Medicines, Chronic diseases and authenticated Homoeopathic Philosophy.* The underlying illness may be one or more than one among the followings:

1. *Endocrine Disorders*

   Conditions like hyperthyroidism, hypo-parathyroidism, Cushing's syndrome, hypoglycemia, post-menopausal syndrome, etc.

2. *Neurological Conditions*

   Injury to the head, cerebral vascular insufficiency (i.e. TIA), Huntington's chorea, epilepsy, degenerative disorder of nervous system, multiple sclerosis, Alzheimer's disease, infection of central nervous system, etc.

3. *Cardiac Diseases*

   Angina, arrhythmias, mitral valve prolapse.

4. *Pulmonary Diseases*

   Chronic obstructive pulmonary disease (COPD).

5. *Toxic Disorders*

   Lead, mercury, manganese, organo-phosphate insecticides.

6. *Non-psychotropic Medications*

   Insulin, corticosteroids, isoproteronol, levodopa, dopamine hydrochloride, terbutaline sulfate, ephedrine, pseudo-ephedrine, indomethacin, nicotine, ginseng root, monosodium glutamate (used in noodles and other fast foods).

7. *Psychotropic Medications*

   MAO-inhibitors benzodiazepines, etc.

8. *Other Drugs*

   Caffeine, nicotine, cocaine, amphetamines, alcohol or their withdrawal etc.

   The treatment adopted should be of multimodal approach.

I. Psychotherapy

Generally psychotherapy is indicated where occurs personality disorder.

Anyhow we must not forget the directions of Hahnemann's Organon, Aphorism 210-230.

II. Various Behavior Therapies

These include:

a. Cognitive-behavioral therapy of various types is effective for panic disorder. The response rate after acute treatment is comparable to that achieved with tri-cyclic drugs or benzodiazepines. Many different techniques are incorporated into standard cognitive-behavioral packages for panic disorder, including breathe retraining, de-conditioning, cognitive restructuring, exposure, and psycho-education. Cognitive behavioral Therapy is highly effective for social phobia and obsessive-compulsive disorder.
b. Psychoanalysis has a very limited role
c. Catharsis may prove to useful.
d. Other behavior therapies like Bio-feedback and Hyper ventilation control.

III. Crude Drugs

Drugs like Benzodiazepine, Alprazolam and Buspirone are given in allopathy without any significant improvement. With such treatment the anxiety disorder can only be palliated or suppressed.

IV. Relaxation Technique

Patients suffering from mild to moderate degree can be undergoing with relaxation technique, which may prove much beneficial. This includes Jacobson's Progressive Relaxation Technique.

V. Yoga

Yoga is extremely helpful for anxiety disorder. Various Asans or postures, Meditation along with Pranayam are found to be very useful. Pranayam techniques like Vastrika, *Kapalbhati, Anulom & Vilom, etc.* have become household name in India due to its effective result in various mental disorders like anxiety, depression etc.

VI. Homeopathic Treatment

Anxiety Neurosis or anxiety disorders comes under purviews of "Mental diseases". Dr. Hahnemann, the father of Homoeopathy has given all the directions in "Organon of Medicine". This needs special focus on treatment of Psoric miasm and psycho therapy. Repertories and therapeutic books may be consulted for the treatment.

Diet

Sometimes an individual suffering from Anxiety Disorders may be allergic to certain food items. Naturally, he should be advised to avoid those items, which acts as a maintaining or an exciting factor. Again the sufferer must be advised to avoid foods those are hard to digest as consumption of such foods may trigger an adrenaline response to induce muscle tension.

Next, the sufferer must be advised:

a. to avoid white flour products, refined sugar, soft drinks, sweet snacks and desserts, sweetened fruit juice or artificially carbonated water drinks etc.
b. to include more whole fruit in his diet as often as possible.
c. to take fresh or lightly cooked (but not boiled) vegetables.
d. to consume the whole grain food instead of refined food.
e. to drink more mineral water, which would improve the equilibrium of trace minerals.
f. to refrain from the use of tobacco and caffeine as such substances can aggravate the anxiety disorder.

Exercise & Life Style

A regular exercise program must be charted out and advised the sufferer to follow it. Because the chemicals released in the body during exercise have a positive and soothing effect on mood and a person's sense of well-being. Exercises like brisk walking, jogging, cycling, swimming, playing tennis for 20-30 minutes a day may prove a boon to the sufferer. Next, Rest & sleep are very much required for the sufferer and deprivation of these may lead to imbalance the emotional wholeness of the sufferer. Over, the sufferer must avoid stress from his personal life by getting rid of unnecessary activities, and affording time to enjoy a hobby or relaxing more in a congenial atmosphere.

Health Education

Health education has a great role to play in the treatment of anxiety disorders. The patient should be educated about his anxieties so that he can treat himself at home without our assistance. The education may prove very helpful for anxiety attacks of short duration where the cause can be traced. The patient's stress may be relieved by such actions as these:

a. Closing the eyes and projecting that the patient himself successfully facing and conquering the specific fear.
b. Adoption catharsis technique like talking with a compassionate person.
c. Watching healthy TV Programmes (i.e. avoiding pornogrpahic, exciting and horror events etc.). Spiritual discourses may prove immense help.
d. May be allowed to take a long, warm bath provided that suits the individual.
e. Allowed him to take rest in a soothing dark room.

Special Comments From the Author: *anxiety disorders are the creation of modern civilization. Non-acceptance of life as it is the prime cause of generation of anxiety disorders in an individual. A labour who works hard under the Sun from ten to six is less likely to suffer from anxiety disorders. He does not have much ambition and hence suffers from less anxiety disorders. He earns for today and live for today and that's all. Remember a flower cannot be compared with a mass of stone. A flower may live for a day but emits fragrance whereas the mass of stone is likely to stay for hundred years without emitting and fragrance. Hence a flower should not be compared to a mass of stone or vice versa. Hence acceptance as we are the prime key to get rid of anxiety disorders. These are the teachings of our religions irrespective of name. Hence enter in the cut throat competition, try hard to get to the top, but do not get panicked if you fail in your mission. Failure Life is part of life and we have to accept it. Accept yourself and know yourself; that is enough.*

SOME MORE NOTES ON ANXIETY

Types of Anxiety

1. Circumstantial Anxiety

Very often a person may feel anxious in a given circumstance. For example, a college lecturer may feel anxious in an examination hall, where most of the students adopt malpractice. Similarly, an administrator may feel a sense of anxiety while the laborers go on strike.

2. Free Floating Anxiety

It is a constitutional problem. The individual always remains in a state of anxiety. When an individual becomes a part of psychic make-up of the individual; in such instances, an individual will worry about things that have happened and that have not happened. Mostly such anxieties are of imagination. This is called free floating anxiety. Floating anxiety does not denote any specific anxiety.

3. Conscious Anxiety

The individual is aware of *the* cause of anxiety. Moreover, the individual is fully aware that he is anxious.

4. Unconscious Anxiety

Sometimes an individual constantly feels anxiety without knowing its origin or cause. This state of anxiety is ascribed to unconscious anxiety. It is an advanced form of anxiety. The manifestation of this type of anxiety may be attributed to physiological level. Diseases like migraine and urticaria may be related to its manifestation.

5. Irrational Anxiety

Anxiety may be connected to general stimuli of a particular thought or object like fear of death, cancer, etc. When anxiety is attached to specific objects in this manner, it is usually called phobia or irrational anxiety.

Note: All 5 types of Anxiety mentioned above, belongs to old classification. In recent days, we follow ICD-10 Classification as delineated under Anxiety Disorders.

ANXIETY AND FEAR

It is customary in psychology to distinguish between anxiety and fear because both are used as synonyms for each other and the two words are more or less interchangeably used.

Fear is characterised by having a specific, identifiable, 'fear provoking' factor. Anxiety is said to be diffuse and this factor cannot be identified.

Examples of some major phobias:

1. Agoraphobia - Fear of open places.
2. Acrophobia - Fear of high places.
3. Algophobia - Fear of pains.
4. Anthrophobia - Fear of men.
5. Aquophobia - Fear of water.
6. Claustrophobia - Fear of closed places.
7. Hematophobia - Fear of blood.
8. Nyctophobia - Fear of darkness.
9. Xenophobia - Fear of strangers.
10. Mysophobia - Fear of germs.

Phobias can be classified into two:

a. Neurotic phobia.
b. Traumatic phobia.

A *neurotic phobia* may be initiated from a specific object say dog, which may be extended to a generalised form say four legged animals. *Traumatic phobia* is initiated from a traumatic experience which may remain for a long time or life time. Suppose you met with an accident while boating during a study tour, this trauma may remain as a state of phobia for a long time or life time. Next time you will be afraid of boating due to this traumatic phobia.

THEORIES OF ANXIETY

There exist many theories regarding the genesis of anxiety, out of which the following are important ones.

1. Freud's Psycho-analytical Theory of Anxiety

At the beginning, Freud postulated anxiety as a primary physiological response to non-fulfilment of sexual gratification. This deduction was based primarily on his study of patients suffering from anxiety neurosis and neurasthenia. Freud observed with these patients that the genesis of anxiety episodes are closely linked with loss of partner (even a pregnant state), coitus interruptus or masturbation where the sexual gratification is impeded. He also postulated that internal factors like guilt feelings due to non-fulfilment of sex may lead to causation of anxiety.

Later, coming across innumerable patients, he changed his early postulation. He asserted that anxiety is more likely a specific state of unpleasure which worked as a signal of warning. He further clarified that anxiety is generated from the very moment of birth like, being an infant, left alone in darkness, presence of strangers in place of mother, etc.

Psycho-analysis further emphasises that realistic anxiety arises out of perception of real dangers of the ego in the external world. It acts as an early warning signal to make the individual cautious to protect himself from the dangers coming from the environment. To be more precise, psycho-analysis offers the following explanation for the genesis of anxiety disorder.

The Id always wants pleasure without bothering about its outcome. At the same society cannot always allow it for individual's Id. Hence there generates conflict within the individual. The conflict occurs due to individual's instinctive urges of Id and traditional restrictions imposed by the society. Now if the individual go for the satisfaction of his instinctive desires, then he may become an anti-social, who has to defy the society and its standardized norms. If the individual obeys the norms of the society and represses his instinctive desires, then these repressions may ultimately lead to anxiety neurosis. Anxiety disorders are the outcome of the interaction of three forces : The instinct of unconsciousness mind, Ego, & Super Ego (see Chapter VII, Freud and Psychoanalysis)

2. Neo-Freudian Theory of Anxiety

Neo-Freudians maintain that when a child takes birth, he gradually attaches himself to his parents or family. Accordingly, he gets adjusted and leads a usual life devoid of anxiety. When he emerges into the society and undergoes the interaction of social custom, tradition and other norms, he feels a threat and thus genesis of anxiety occurs. Secondly, the child may become aggressive due to non-fulfilment of a given desire or other similar reasons. This aggressive behavior of a child is not accepted by parents. The child learns to control the expression of its aggression by developing defence mechanisms like repression and denial (see Freud). Sometimes even this repression and denial also get threatened. This threatened state creates anxiety in a child. Induction of such a state is called anxiety, which usually leads to neurotic behavior.

3. Personality Theory

Anxiety is not an isolated or single phenomenon. It also has some concomitants. The concomitant may be expressed in terms of subservient (i.e., always doing what other people want him to do), compliant (i.e., willing to do what other people want him to do) self-controlled, restrained and timid (shy and easily frightened) by nature. Such characteristics of the individual compel the individual to repress emotions like hostility, aggression and anguish.

PHYSIOLOGICAL EXPRESSION OF ANXIETY

The physiological manifestation of anxiety can be grouped under:

1. Directly perceptible physiological action:
    a. Shortness of breath.
    b. Rapid or skipped heart beat.
    c. Sensation of tightness over head.
    d. Sensation of lump in throat.
    e. In extreme cases, diarrhea, vomiting, fainting.
    f. Frequent urination.
    g. Insomnia.
    h. Fatigue.
2. Imperceptible physiological action.

    The above symptoms are under the control of autonomic nervous system. It has got a mechanism which enables the body to mobilize itself more effectively to deal with the threatened danger. In this condition, adrenalin plays a crucial role. It compels the organism either to fly or to fight. The action of adrenalin causes the liver to release glucose into the blood stream so that muscles can avail quick energy.

SYMPTOMS OF ANXIETY

1. Gloomy forebodings.
2. Feeling of insecurity.
3. General excitement.
4. Fatigue.
5. Gastrointestinal disturbances.
6. Depression.
7. Cardiac disorder.
8. Emotional disturbances.

9. Feeling of inferiority.
10. Headache.
11. Indecision, intolerance.
12. Panic state.
13. Strange fears.
14. Giddiness.
15. General interest.
16. Neurosis and psychosis.
17. Crime and suicidal tendency.

Chapter 19

CONFLICT

The concept of conflict is not new to homeopathy. It has been scattered throughout our literature. Let us glance at such an example from Roger Morrison's *Desktop Guide*, where he brilliantly narrates the concept of conflict in *Lilium tigrinum*:

> *'Lilium tigrinum is mainly a woman's remedy especially suited for hysterical, intense and rage-filled patients. There is often a deep conflict inside the patient between a strong sexual nature and an equally strong moral side. This conflict or any other strong inner conflict produces a type of frustration which is expressed mainly through anger. We can say that Lilium tigrinum is the most irritable of all remedies. The patient will take offence no matter how kindly she is treated. At other times, the patient alternates between great kindliness and sincerity and this angry, nasty state. The Lilium tigrinum patient can also have great sexual excitement, even to the point of nymphomania. When she crosses a certain barrier she becomes very sexual and cannot restrain these feelings. However, equally deep moral or religious feelings return and she feels great remorse and subsequent depression. Thus from Materia Medica we find "religious despair alternates with sexual excitement" or "lasciviousness alternating with anger".*

(Roger Morrison, 1993)

Human life is not like reel life or a drama where a set of sequences will occur one after another. One has to face several impediments in his real life. Human conflict comprises of both want to reject the same thing (*Staphysagria, Bryonia, Chamomilla,* etc.) and to love and hate the same person (*Ignatia*). Whatever a person does to accomplish one of these motives, it goes against or impedes the other. There is no way out. The more satisfaction he gets from one phase of a thing, the greater the frustration from the other phase. Sometimes there are not just two but several motives, each one of which prevents the remaining ones.

In day to day life, we are always encircled by many motives; some hidden and some obvious. Many of them are active at a given period and with diverse indication of goals. The conflict is initiated when two motives clash; the satisfaction of either of the two leads to frustration or blocking of the other. Interestingly, selection of one motive may not be satisfactory as the motive might have different ways to get close to the goal and the conflict arises at the signal where the paths to the goal depart. An individual may eventually attain the goal; still he has to make a choice that leads to a conflict.

TYPES OF CONFLICTS

According to field theory of behavior, conflict has been classified under the following four categories

1. Approach – Approach Conflict

In this conflict a person gets two desirable but mutually exclusive goals or options and he has to choose either of the two. In this situation it is not easy to select either of them. Both the options are equally attractive and have their own merits. The individual is torn between these two options.

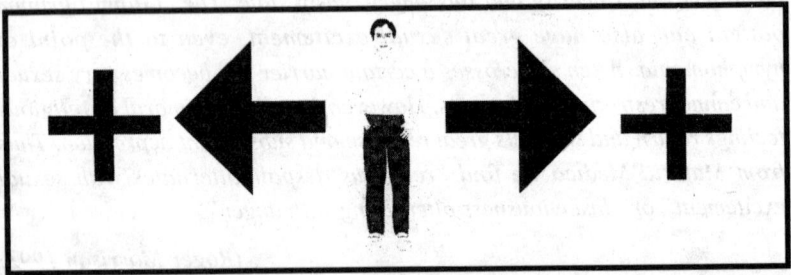

Let us take the example of Shyam Sundar. Recently, he qualified in All India PG Entrance Examination and when he was about to join in the PG course, he got a call letter from the Government to join as a homeopathic medical officer. Now Shyam is in a state of conflict regarding what to do and what not to do. If he joins as medical officer, he cannot pursue PG, which is important for the future. Even his career will come to a standstill by opting for this choice. On the other hand, if he opts for the PG course, then he has to loose the government job as a homeopathic medical officer, which will get him bread and butter throughout his life. This is a typical approach to approach conflict. Here there exist two equally alluring goals having equal chance of appeal and one has to opt to either of the two.

In this type of conflict, ultimately one will lead the other and the return to indecision is not possible.

2. Avoidance – Avoidance Conflict

This is the opposite of the above state. Here an individual gets two unattractive options, both the incentives are negative and none of them is acceptable to an individual. In this type of conflict, the individual develops a strong tendency to escape the dilemma by doing something else.

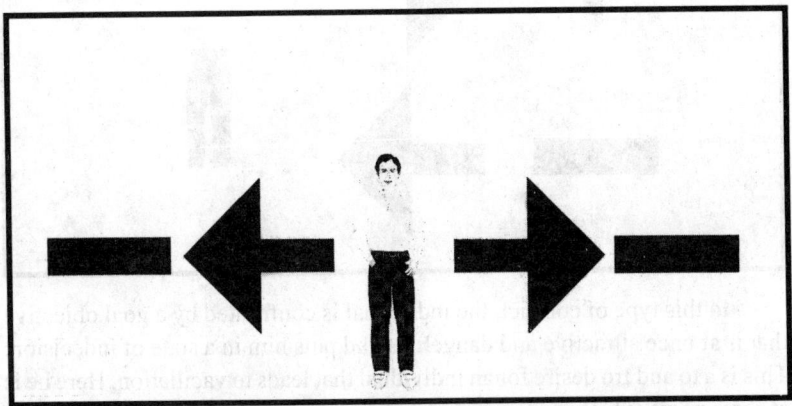

Last night at about 9 p.m., I told my son Osho Sambit, to take his dinner or else go to bed. In response, he started playing with his food with a spoon. He started making excuses by saying that the curry is peppery, that much spice has been added to it, etc. He also asked for frequent supply of water stating that he is thirsty, etc. Now, he is in two negative states. He did not want to eat his dinner and at the same time he was not interested to go to bed either. He was waiting to watch a cartoon show on TV at that time.

In this type of conflict, the food becomes more repugnant when it is on the spoon than when it is on the plate, but the thought of going to bed keeps the child on the table so that he can watch the cartoon show on TV that lies nearby.

3. Approach – Avoidance Conflict

Anacardium orientalis portrays a perfect type of approach – avoidance conflict. Of course, Anacardium is more indicated for pathological conditions. In approach – avoidance conflict, the incentive is at once desirable and not desirable, both positive and negative. The attitude is ambivalent. Let us take an example of a recent diabetic patient who is roaming in the market. While roaming, he desires sweets by looking at a sweets show case. Now he is in conflict: the sweets are delicious making his mouth water, while and at the same time he avoids it as it may raise his blood sugar.

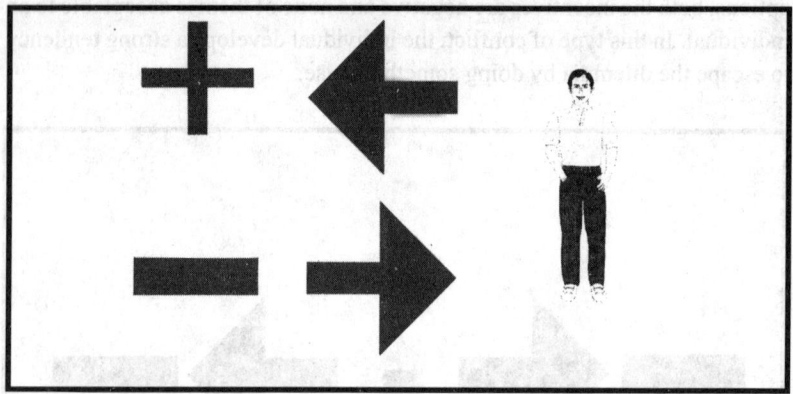

In this type of conflict, the individual is confronted by a goal objective that is at once attractive and dangerous and puts him in a state of indecision. This is a to and fro desire for an individual that leads to vacillation. Here he is at some point, which is near enough to the goal that warns him to be aware of the danger but distant enough to be safe from it.

4. Double Approach – Avoidance Conflict

Very often approach – avoidance conflicts are often combined in a complex pattern. Let us take an example of a family where such a conflict can occur for the son. The father wants his son to be a good football player. The mother wants her son to be a good dancer (or musician). The son wants to be a good cricketer. Now, if the son prefers to play football, the mother will be displeased. If he joins a dance (or music) class and goes for practice, his father will be displeased. If he pursues the career of his choice i.e., cricket both the parents will be displeased. This type of conflict is called double approach-avoidance conflict.

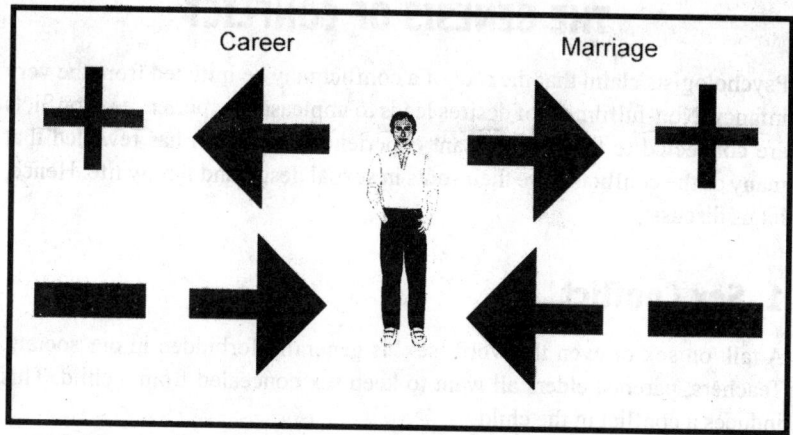

In our society the third type of conflict i.e., approach – avoidance conflicts are very common and have become a part and parcel of our life. It cannot be resolved so easily. First, when we were children, we were depending on others every now and then. Gradually we are trained to stand on our own legs. So when a difficult situation rises we want to take the help of somebody else and at the same time we try our level best to avoid others and want to bring about a solution by ourselves. Second, when we were at school, we were taught to love our fellow beings and at the same time when we do not stand first in our class, our parents and teachers scold for us not coming so. In later life, this also creates conflict. Again we love our freedom. When we want to enjoy something say sex, then the norms of society prevent. Moreover, the law of society also prevent so. Such things put us in a state of conflict. A male having an ugly wife cannot go for a second marriage whereas his impulses urge him to go for an alternative.

THE PRINCIPLES OF CONFLICT

The careful research carried out by various psychologists reveals the following principles of conflict:

a. The tendency to approach a positive incentive is stronger, when the subject is nearer to it.

b. The tendency to repel from a negative incentive is stronger the nearer the subject is to it.

c. Avoidance gradient is steeper than the approach gradient.

d. The gradient of approach or avoidance is guided by the drive upon which it is based.

THE GENESIS OF CONFLICT

Psychologists claim that the root of a conflict may be initiated from the very infancy. Non-fulfilment of desires leads to unpleasant experiences. Conflicts are connected to these unpleasant experiences. Research has revealed that many of the conflicts have their roots in sexual desire and family life. Hence, let us discuss:

1. Sex Conflict

A talk on sex or even the word 'sex' is generally forbidden in our society. Teachers, parents, elders all want to keep sex concealed from a child. This induces a conflict in the child.

Again, during adolescence, boys and girls become inquisitive to know about each other. They also want to have sexual indulgence. This is not permitted in society. They are taught morals and ethics in relation to sex. In such a situation, when the sexual urge appears fiercely during adolescence, his sexual instincts are condemned by the statement that sex is immoral and sinful. This situation gives rise to the genesis of sexual conflict.

A similar situation is imposed upon adolescents, regarding masturbation. In our society, masturbation is being condemned with great hatredness. Usually, masturbation in moderation is not harmful; rather it is a safe outlet for gratification of sex in today's world. However, adolescents are taught that by practicing masturbation he or she will become insane or develop other mental illnesses. This situation creates a state of conflict in an individual.

2. Family Conflict

Man is a social animal. He lives in a society. The society is built on the basis of family and home. In a family, an individual has to interact with different people, which gives rise to different behavior. Hence, if the child is not given proper treatment in the family, the child will suffer from conflicts. There is another contributing factor for the genesis of conflict – it is competition. An individual cannot become successful in every sphere of life. In competition, we compare one another. This comparison also generates conflict in an individual in a family. We have to admit that everybody cannot become a Gandhi or Nehru or Vivekananda. We have to remember that a flower like, jasmine or rose has a smaller life span. Despite their shorter life span, they emit a fragrance, whereas a stone has more durability i.e., a longer life but without any fragrance. Hence a child or individual must be accepted as they are without any comparison so that he does not suffer from conflict.

3. Miscellaneous Conflicts

Various failures lead an individual to a state of frustration. Frustration is the precursor of conflict. Similarly, in order to obtain respect from others, may lead one to conflict. The role of competition also becomes a part and parcel of modern conflict. Even winning a heart or imposing supremacy on others may cause conflict.

Chapter 20

FRUSTRATION

As our civilization and culture advances, our needs also increase. We believe that widening of need will make us more comfortable and respectable. To become respectable and comfortable we extended our desires beyond the sky without maintaining the equilibrium between our desire and achievement. This gap gives rise to frustration.

DEFINITION

It is a state of emotional stress that is characterized by confusion, annoyance and anger. It occurs whenever goal-seeking behavior is interfered with. In other words frustration is the result which takes birth when one's path or right of entry to a goal is blocked. A goal may be blocked because an obstruction has been set up to prevent access, as when a roadblock prevents a vehicle from going to its destination. On the other hand, a goal may be unreachable

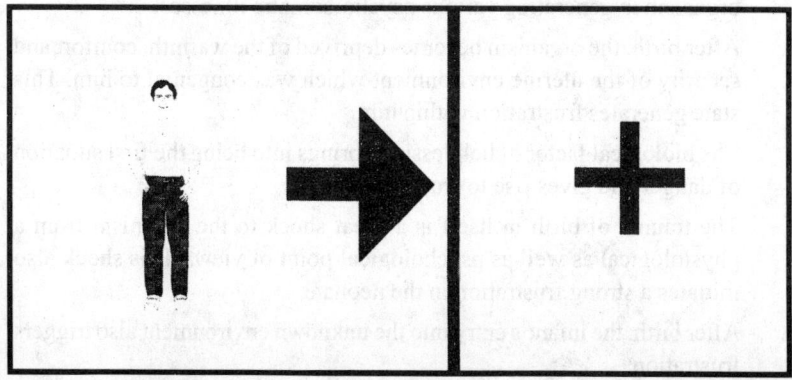

Frustration

because one lacks the resource to advance it, as when the vehicle is out of diesel or fuel. The person is aware of his inability to satisfy his drives and is let down as he cannot reach the goals he has set for himself. So he feels helpless and suffers from injured pride.

PHYSIOLOGICAL EXPRESSION

Frustration is initiated inside and expressed outside. It is almost impossible for an ordinary person to push it inside. Frustration expresses itself through postural tension. The greater the frustration, greater its expression in rigidity, stiffness and tension. In postural tension, changes in respiration, galvanic skin responses, increased pulse rate, increased in muscular tension, and changes in E.C.G. are known to occur.

EVOLUTION AND GENESIS OF FRUSTRATION

Psychologists claim that frustration starts from the very birth of an organism. The organism, before birth is in a state of tranquility. So, when he takes birth, his tranquility is disturbed and becomes frustrated. Accordingly, anxiety is a sequelae to frustration.

1. The neonate brings frustration with birth. The organism, before birth remained in a state of relative calm and tranquility. Some psychologists postulate that frustration is even generated during the period of conception. This statement seems very controversial. However, from the homeopathic point of view, we cannot underestimate it. Mother's frustration during the period of conception definitely reflects on the organism in generating various psycho-somatic illnesses.

2. After birth, the organism becomes deprived of the warmth, comfort and security of the uterine environment which was congenial to him. This state generates frustration within him.

3. The biological factor of helplessness brings into being the first situation of danger and gives rise to frustration.

4. The trauma of birth in itself is a great shock to the organism from a physiological as well as psychological point of view. This shock also initiates a strong frustration in the neonate.

5. After birth, the infant's entry into the unknown environment also triggers frustration.

6. The newborn is quite incapable of having a defense mechanism for his protection.

7. Separation from mother as a unit, and adjustment with the current environment also causes frustration.
8. Again, on the very first day of arrival on this earth, the organism feels the first pangs of hunger. He expresses this by crying. If may evoke a favorable or an unfavorable response from the mother. If the mother responds by slapping or expressing the anger, the vicious cycle of frustration continues.
9. Frustration also develops due to bottle feeding. A bottle cannot substitute the breast, the mother's milk, the flavor, its taste and the warmth.
10. When breast milk is cut off, due to some reason or the other, the infant has to again suffer from frustration. Breast was the first and sole object of love for him and when he departs from it, there occurs severe frustration. This frustration affects the developmental of personality to a great extent.
11. During growing years, growth and development occurs. This also creates frustration. Developmental stages like oral, anal and phallic stages creates tremendous frustration (see Freud and Psycho-analysis, Chapter VII).
12. We must remember that a mother is also a human being, full of fraility and weakness. Hence her erratic behavior may cause frustration in a child, who is helpless and quite dependant on her. Her answer with a slap, which is very common in an illiterate family or in rural areas, not only creates a sense of frustration but also leads towards psychogenic shock.
13. The attitude and behavior of parents including that of attendants plays a tremendous role in creation of frustration.
14. Lack of attention produces instant frustration as he feels nobody cares him.
15. Pampering makes him look forward to more and more, which may not be given to the child. This also generates frustration.
16. In recent years, divorce, family discords, non-comprising nature, etc. have grown in phenomenal proportion in India. The child wants affection and appreciation of both of the parents. He becomes a sandwich in the discord. He becomes a sacrificial animal at the altar of conflict. The whole process instills tremendous frustration in the child. Sometimes, this frustration leads to schizophrenia or puts one on the path of crime in search of a security leading to another labyrinth of frustration.

17. In school and college careers, he has to face tremendous competition which leads to frustration.
18. In later years, when he tries to understand the world, he discovers that people are mean, untrustworthy, deceitful and highly selfish. He feels that the empathy, the righteousness, the truthfulness are misused by the devils of society. These create frustration leading to schizophrenia.
19. During adulthood, he has to face other situations like disappointment of love, search for a career or job, adjustment in society, etc., which also generates frustration.
20. Some other causes of frustration can be stated:
    - Faulty upbringing of child
    - Rigid attitude of parents
    - Strict norms of society and religion
    - Rigid and inflexible thinking
    - Unhappy and pathological home environment
    - Over-protection and too much care
    - Negligence of the child
    - Uncared attitude of the parents
    - Deep breach between level of ambition and height of achievement
    - Over-estimation of one's abilities, etc.

SOURCES OF FRUSTRATION

There exist a number of sources of frustration, out of which the salient ones are given below:

I. Obstacle in the Physical Environment

Factors like accident, fire, war, death of near and dear ones, famine, cyclone, etc. come under this category of frustration.

II. Obstacle in Social Environment

The norms and values of society act as a barrier and generate frustration in an individual. For example, sexual gratification or even masturbation is being condemned in society. This creates severe frustration as well as a conflict in an individual. An individual also has to struggle in society for status, establishment, job, home, etc. Any dissatisfaction in these goals leads to frustration.

III. Personal Deficiency

The individual has a low economic status, lack of intellectual ability and skill, short stature, ugly look and other physical deficiencies, disappointment in love, failure in marital life, low education, etc. These points also generate frustration in an individual.

IV. Miscellaneous

- Conflict between opposing and incompatible motives
- A bright child is likely to be frustrated when he learns lessons from an institution which is meant for average students
- A young homeopath posted in a village can also feel frustrated
- When teachers and parents impose their ideas and thoughts upon a child rather than considering what he wants to do, the child suffers from frustration
- When there is great ambition without achievement
- Aspiration for independence is thwarted by economic dependency
- Many frustrations owe their origin to a conflicting motive when a young man is compelled to do something which is not agreeable to his conscience

REACTION TO FRUSTRATION

Frustration is not an isolated phenomenon. It has an array of concomitants.

Frustration very often leads to restlessness and tension. The restlessness may be expressed through whispering, sighing, complaint and unhappiness. An increase in tension levels or excitement also occurs, when adults are blocked or thwarted. They may express frustration through a blow or may remain in a state of tremor with clenched fists. Adults may also bite a nail, may start smoking or chewing gum as an outlet for their restlessness and tension. Children also show reactions like thumb sucking, nail biting, etc. in relation to frustration.

Very often, tension and restless movements are added by a feeling of anger. Anger leads an organism to launch destruction and hostile attack. When the desire of a child is blocked by negation, the child expresses itself through knocking, kicking, breaking, destroying or throwing something. Very often, aggression is expressed directly against the sources of frustration.

I. Aggression

As mentioned above, the type of hostile, injurious or destructive behavior or outlook caused by frustration is called aggression.

The expression of aggression may be of two types:

1. Direct aggression.
2. Displaced aggression.

1. Direct Aggression

Very often, aggression is expressed directly against the very sources of frustration. When a toy belonging to a child is taken by another child, the former child is likely attack to the latter for regaining the toy.

2. Displaced Aggression

Sometimes, it may so happen that frustration may be caused by:

a. A source, which is vague or intangible.
b. A source which is too powerful to meet.

In such conditions, the frustrated individual cannot express the aggression satisfactorily against the corresponding source, then the aggression is displaced somewhere else.

A child may break something when chided by his father. Here he cannot attack his father. Hence he resorts to breaking a nearby object as an outlet. There is a beautiful joke. When a boss scolds a subordinate staff, the staff shows his aggression over his wife at home. The wife displaces this aggression over their innocent child and the child breaks the toys as a reaction. In fact, such incidents can be observed in day to day life.

From above, it is clear that when the circumstances block direct attack, the sources of frustration, aggression is displaced. Displaced aggression is against an innocent person or object rather than the actual cause of the frustration. A child pulls the tail of his cat in case he cannot pull on with his playmates.

The practice of "scape-goating" is an example of displaced aggression. An innocent individual may be targeted or blamed for one's trouble and becomes an object of aggression.

Miller and Bugelski (1948), p. 436, cites an example of scape-goating, as follows:

"An experiment with boys at a summer camp shows the relationship between frustration and scape-goating. The boys were required to participate in a lengthy and boring testing session which ran overtime so that they missed their weekly outing to the local movie. A survey measuring attitudes towards Japanese and Mexicans given before and after the testing session showed a significant increase in unfriendly feelings. The boys displaced their anger verbally towards remote people rather than expressing it directly towards the administrators of the test."

II. Apathy

One of the factors complicating the study of human behavior is the tendency for different individuals to respond to similar situations in a variety of ways. Thus, although a common response to frustration is active aggression, another response is its opposite – apathy, indifference, withdrawal. We do not know why one person reacts with aggression and another with apathy to the same situation, but it seems likely that learning is an important factor; reactions to frustration can be learned in much the same manner as other behaviors. Children who strike out angrily when frustrated and find that their needs are then satisfied (either through their own efforts or because a parent rushes to placate them) will probably resort to the same behavior the next time their motives are thwarted. Children whose aggression outbursts are never successful, who find they have no power to satisfy their need by means of their own actions, may well resort to apathy and withdrawal when confronted with a frustrating situation.

(Hilgard et al, 1975)

Learned Helplessness

Studies with animals have demonstrated a reaction that has been called "learned helplessness". A dog placed in a shuttle box (an apparatus with two compartments separated by a barrier) quickly learns to jump to the opposite compartment to escape an electric shock delivered to its feet through a grid on the floor. If a light is turned on a few seconds before the grid is electrified, the dog can learn to avoid the shock entirely by jumping to the safe compartment on signal. However, if the dog has previously been placed in a situation where shocks are unavoidable and inescapable – where nothing it does terminates the shock – then it has great difficulty in learning the avoidance response when appropriate. The animal simply sits and takes the shock, even though an easy jump to the opposite compartment would eliminate the discomfort. Some dogs never learn, even if the experimenter demonstrates the proper procedure by carrying them over the barrier. The dogs had previously learned that they were helpless to avoid the shock, and this *learned helplessness was very difficult to overcome*

Experiences of Prisoners of War

Studies of inmates in concentration or prisoner-of-war camps indicate that many prisoners develop attitudes of detachment and extreme indifference in the face of continual deprivation, torture and threats of death. In fact, apathy may be a "normal" reaction to frustrating conditions of long duration from which there is no hope of escape. Interviews with American servicemen released from prison camps after the Korean war showed that almost all experienced, at some time during their imprisonment, a period characterized by listlessness, indifference to the immediate situation, and total lack of emotion. Since these men could respond appropriately when spoken to, and since their speech and behavior did not suggest psychosis, the reaction has been described as apathy. The most severe of such "apathy reactions" frequently resulted in death. Two remedies seemed capable of saving the man close to death; getting him on his feet and doing something, no matter how trivial, and getting him interested in some current or future problem. Usually the efforts and support of a friend helped the individual to snap out of a state of apathy.

(Strassman et al in Hilgard, 1975)

III. Fantasy

In general, we may cope with various types of frustration by adoption. It is common sense that all the frustration cannot be successfully met. Very often, the problem becomes too great. The problem becomes so great that we feel as if a multitude of demons are sitting on our head. We feel that those demons will tear us into pieces. We feel a sense of incapacity to meet the situation. Hence the organism has to make some alternatives. The organism searches for an escape to enter into the world of fantasy. The organism finds this measure a solid solution for the current problem. But this solution is not a realistic one. Let us take an example from student hostels. The students are prevented from sex. Hence frustration become inevitable. They adopt a life of fantasy. Sometimes they carry the photograph of their beloved inside their wallet purse. Very often they look it for a long time and enter into a world of fantasy as a substitute for love and romance. This situation can also be observed from the pin-up of girls in soldier's barracks. They accept fantasy as real.

Guetzkow and Bownar (1946) carried out experiments and showed that a starving man lost interest in women and instead of having their pin-up on the wall, pictures of prepared food were cut from magazines and put there.

Once, the author was invited to treat a case of malarial fever in a girls hostel of a reputed college. There, he saw pin-ups of famous actors on the room walls. He happened to find a student's diary by chance, where the picture of a famous film star was decorated with artificial flowers. These are example of fantasies. When the gap between source of frustration and its achievement is great, fantasy is adopted.

Very often, these fantasies are self limiting and short lived. The world is too big and challenges us for worse and renewed problems. Hence, the organism has to enter the realities from the world of fantasy. The lady who worshipped the film star has to enter the world of marriage after few years and refrain himself from star worship. We must know that if this dimension becomes severe and continuous, the person may become schizophrenic in the long run.

IV. Stereotypy

One of the consequences of frustration may take the shape of stereotype behavior. In this type, the subject tends to exhibit repetitive, fixated behavior. Generally, an individual attempts to meet the blocked goal by finding out a new direction with a flexible attitude. When repeated frustrations confuse and perplex a person, some flexibility appears to be lost and the person will foolishly make the same effort again and again though experience proved to be in vain.

V. Regression

Regression means reversion to an earlier state: A return to an earlier or less developed condition or way of behaving. In psychology reversion is defined as a return to more primitive modes of behavior i.e., return to a less maturer state or reversion to an earlier less adaptive emotional or mental level, often involving the appearance of forms of behavior associated with childhood. There are two interpretations of regression.

First, in the midst of insecurity the individual attempts to return to a period of past, which seems to be secured. This is called retrogressive behavior, a return to behavior once fitted into the situation. Here the older child wants the love and affection that was given during his childhood. So he adopts the corresponding behavior of a younger age.

Second, interpretation of regression is that the childish behavior following frustration is simply a primitive kind of behavior (not actually a return to earlier behavior) like fist-fight. Here he may adopt actions like fist-fighting although he belongs to a civilised society. This is called primitivation.

VI. Withdrawal

Sometimes an individual may not able to solve a problem. Despite repeated efforts he may fail. The individual gives up everything and resorts to withdrawal. He escapes from the situation psychologically or physically. These instances are found amongst frustrated lovers.

VII. Rationalization

When an individual gets frustrated, he sometimes does not want to accept it before others. Hence, he adopts rationalization. This is clouding over frustration. By this, he saves his self-respect and is able to avoid criticism at the hands of others. When a boy fails in getting his love, he tells others that he has no time for affairs or he may say that it is the career that matters more to him than love. The main theme of this rationalization is that the reasons for failure are all concocted and the greater the number of arguments produced, the more evident is that person's hollowness.

VIII. Anxiety

The biggest and immediate contribution of frustration is anxiety. This is a common reaction to frustration. All the details have been dealt in the Chapter 'Psychology of Anxiety and Anxiety Disorders'.

FRUSTRATION : ITS ROLE IN DEVELOPMENT OF PERSONALITY

The world is not so green as the poets depict through their narration. Frustration is a way of life. It starts with the womb and ends with the tomb. Hence, the role of frustration in the development of a personality cannot be underestimated. Frustration experienced in infancy and childhood becomes an important determinant in the development of personality in the future. We have read various stages of development of personality in the Chapter of 'Freud'. Various frustrations generated due to habits of feeding, elimination, toilet training, nurturing, etc. determine the development of a personality. The child who is frustrated with feeding develops the habit of biting others. Sustained frustration leads to various maladaptive behaviors. Sexual frustration may lead to commitment of rape, sodomy, lesbianism, bestiality and homosexual acts. Extreme and rigorous discipline leads to aggressiveness and antisocial activities. Freud comments that frustration is the most immediate, most easily discernable and most comprehensively exciting cause of neurotic illness. Frustration may lead to self-devaluation and an inferiority complex.

CLINICAL APPLICATION

In clinical practice, we may not take care of minor frustrations. But when it interferes with the very life of the patient as a concomitant variation like depression, anxiety, etc., then we must provide a plausible solution.

We have to adopt two methods for meeting frustration:

A. Coping with frustration in a general way i.e., without medicine.
B. Coping with frustration the homeopathic way.

A. Coping with Frustration : The Non-Medicated way

The very definition of frustration states that there is a barrier that is present and this restricts an individual's action. We can divide the barriers under two heads:

1. *Internal barriers* like weakness, lack of will power, lack of skill, low intelligence, etc.
2. *External barriers* include our relationships like father, mother, friends, etc. This also includes geographical distribution, weather, time, etc.

One or more than one of the above factors block the goal and lead to a state of frustration or unsatisfied motive. Hence we need to deal with the barrier and readjust with the situation. Hence, the frustrated individual resorts to a course of action. It may so happen that he may be able to discover a way of meeting the barrier. If not so, a substitute action is resorted to. Even if the solution cannot be found, the individual withdraws from the situation or worse, he enters the world of fantasy in which there is no barrier to encounter.

1. should take an effort to encounter the barrier,
2. undertakes an exploratory behavior and probably discovers a solution to it.

B. Homeopathic Way

We have to translate frustration into our language and it should also be related to other mental rubrics of mind. The following alike rubrics may be examined for frustration:

Abandoned or forsaken feeling, anxiety, childish behavior, confusion, depression, gloomy (morose), helplessness, hypochondriasis, irritability, lamenting, love disappointments from, feelings of pity, of self-rage, feeling fury, screaming, shrieking, shouting, etc.

■

Chapter 21

DIMENSIONS OF DEVELOPMENTAL PSYCHOLOGY

Life begins with the very fertilization of the ovum (from female) with the destined unit of semen (from male). This fertilization forms a zygote. A simple and single zygote is a dynamic organism which undergoes various changes and ultimately expresses itself into a human being due to its potentiality to grow, because one of the chief unique points of living organisms is their ability to grow and develop. Hence, *developmental psychology may be defined as a systematic study of the changing events embodying all aspects of an organism from fertilization to death.* Growth and development of an organism is guided by the interaction of various factors like genetic endowment, endocrine function, life style (and rearing), socio-economic conditions, geographical distribution, etc.

I. NATURE OF GROWTH AND DEVELOPMENT

In day to day life, terminologies like growth and development are exchanged and treated as synonymous. Psychologists also use these terms together as synonyms in practice because the process of growth and development are inter-related, inter-dependent and cannot be separated easily. Again, growth and development are the collective result of heredity and environment. Moreover, development as a matter of fact is achieved through growth. Despite such resemblance and integration, there exist many salient differentiation points between these two terminologies, some of which are presented below:

Growth means an increase in size, height, weight, length, etc., which can be measured in terms of centimetres and kilograms, whereas development means functional or physiological maturation, which cannot be measured through such measurement. Development indicates attainment of mental, emotional and social abilities. Mental abilities stand for acquisition of skills, emotional abilities include development of right attitudes, and social abilities mean fitness to family and society. Growth refers to changes in the particular or regional aspects of the body while development refers to the organism as a whole.

Another difference between growth and development is that growth does not continue throughout life. Human beings grow up to a certain age, say upto twenty to twenty five years of age (peak being at adolescence). Development, on the other hand, progresses throughout one's life. In other words we can say growth stops at maturity while development continues throughout life. Growth involves changes in body proportions, stature and weight while development characterizes changes in an organism from its origin to its extinction. Development is a progressive series of orderly changes that tends towards the goal of maturity. Growth and development go side by side. Growth without development is meaningless. For example, when the body grows in structure, it also develops in function. But sometimes the reversal may be observed; for example, sometimes a child may grow fat with lack of any functional progress or development, which cannot be categorised as normal.

II. PRINCIPLES OF GROWTH AND DEVELOPMENT

1. Principle of Continuity

Development is a non-stop process and follows the principle of continuity Life begins from the very moment of fertilization development continues till death. But the intensity of growth is marked till the attainment of maturity. Later, growth becomes too sluggish and it is a never ending process. The changes continue and display themselves in the characteristics of the personality. Gradual development of both physical and mental activities continues till its maximum possible extent.

2. Principle of Uniformity of Pattern

Development follows a pattern. Development occurs in an orderly manner and follows a certain sequence. Thus, infancy, early childhood, late childhood, adolescence and maturity, adulthood, etc. are the series of developments that take place in an individual. A uniformity in the pattern of development is also observed in relation to physical, mental, psycho-social and cognitive abilities, which are spread throughout various developmental stages of an individual's life.

3. Principle of Development From General to Specific Response

Development proceeds from general to specific responses. The responses or the reactions of a child are of general nature to start with at birth. First he reacts to the situations and external stimuli with his body as a whole. Gradually, he learns to have specific responses, say by pointing a finger to a dangling toy. This is not only true of his physical responses only, but also of his intellectual and emotional responses. The responses of a child which are of general nature first, gradually become more and more specific.

4. Principle of Lack of Uniformity in the Developmental Rate

Different aspects of growth develop at different rates. Though development is a continuous process, the rate of growth is not uniform for various aspects of growth and development. Thus, there are periods of accelerated growth and periods of decelerated growth in an individual's life. During the first three years of infancy, the rate of growth is rapid, and then the rate of growth slows down. The growth is again accelerated around the adolescent stage. Similarly, neither all parts of the body grow at the same rate, nor do all aspects of mental growth progress equally.

5. Principle of Interrelation

Most traits maintain a correlation in the process of growth and development. Normally, it has been observed that the child, whose intellectual development is above average, is also superior in so many other aspects of life like health, sociability, special aptitudes, etc. Similarly, the mental development of an individual is closely associated to his physical growth.

6. Principle of Interaction

Development is a product of interaction of the organism and environment. Neither heredity alone nor the environment alone is responsible for the development of an individual. Both the factors are accountable for growth and development. Of course, it is not possible to estimate precisely in what proportion heredity and environment share the contribution of an individual's growth and development.

7. Principle of Individual Difference

There exist wide individual differences in the growth pattern. Individuals differ from each other in their pattern and rate of growth. The differences may not be perceived from a physical point of view, but the differences from intellectual and personality point of view can be marked in individuals. The individual differences are caused by differences in hereditary endowment and environmental influences. Of course, the individual differences in rates of development are found to remain constant. It has been observed that children who are slow in learning during early childhood usually remain so throughout their life. Similarly, it has also been observed generally that a bright child will be so from his early childhood till the end of life provided his health status remains in good condition.

From a homeopathic point of view, if the miasmatic cleavages are well dealt with their corresponding anti-miasmatic medicines, then the child can bloom with the best possibility of development.

8. Growth is Both Quantitative and Qualitative

Physical growth can be termed as quantitative growth which has been illustrated above. Along with these, qualitative aspects of growth called personality also develop. That means the child's physical, mental, emotional and personality growths proceed simultaneously. All this growth and development is inseparable.

9. Principle of Predictability

Development is predictable. The rate of development of each child is fairly constant, that is, a slow learner will ever remain so, and a superior child is so from the very beginning. Thus, it is possible to predict at an early age the range within which the development of maturity of a child is likely to fall; though the prediction cannot be made accurately.

10. Principle of Orderly Sequence

Development follows an orderly sequence in an individual, out of which following are the main trends:

a. Cephalocaudal

Development proceeds in the direction of longitudinal axis i.e., head to foot.

This is the reason why the child gains control over his head followed by arms and then legs. (Can you recall Hering's Law of Cure?)

b. Proximo-distal Tendencies

Development from the near to distant parts i.e., centre to periphery. This explains why in the beginning, the child gains control over the large fundamental muscle of the arm and the hand followed by gradual control over the smaller muscles of the fingers. (Can you connect this to Hering's law of Cure?)

c. Locomotion

The sequence of locomotion can be confirmed from the fact that infants belonging to various religions, castes, creeds, geographical distributions show uniformity, creeping, crawling, walking, etc.

11. Principle of Spiral Versus Linear Advancement

Although we have talked so much of growth and development, we have to remember that the development in a child is:

a. Not linear.
b. Not straight.

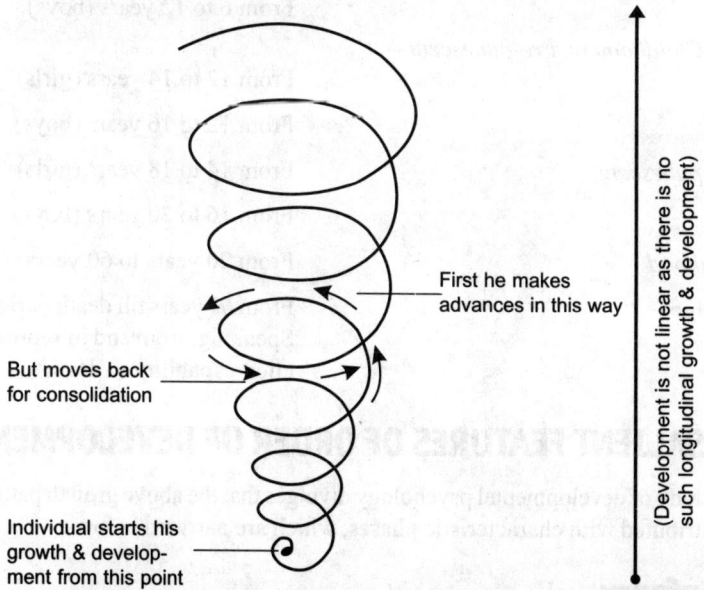

Spiral Pattern of Movement in Development (as Opposed to Linear).

c. Does not take place at a steady pace.

Moreover, after the development to a certain stage, there comes a period of consolidation when development becomes imperceptible. Then again, development proceeds and moves forward in a spiral pattern.

III. STAGES OF GROWTH AND DEVELOPMENT

Prenatal

Ovum - 0 to 14 days.
Embryo - 14 days to 12 or 14 weeks.
Fetus - 12 to 14 weeks to birth.

Postnatal

Newborn -	Birth to 4 weeks of life.
Infancy -	From birth to 2nd year of life.
Toddler -	From 1 to 3 years of life.
Early Childhood (Pre-school going) –	From 3 years to 6 years.
Middle Childhood (School going) –	From 6 years to 10 years (girls). From 6 to 12 years (boys).
Late Childhood or Pre-pubescent –	From 12 to 14 years (girls). From 12 to 16 years (boys).
Post-pubescent –	From 14 to 18 years (girls). From 16 to 20 years (boys).
Adulthood –	From 20 years to 60 years.
Old Age –	From 61 years till death (strictly Speaking, from end of reproduction capability to death).

IV. SALIENT FEATURES OF ORDER OF DEVELOPMENT

The study of developmental psychology divulges that the above growth pattern is distributed with characteristic phases, which are narrated below :

1. Infancy

Infancy is the smallest period in the life of an individual. During this short span he tries to acclimatise and accommodate with the environment. He also learns to suck and swallow milk from mother.

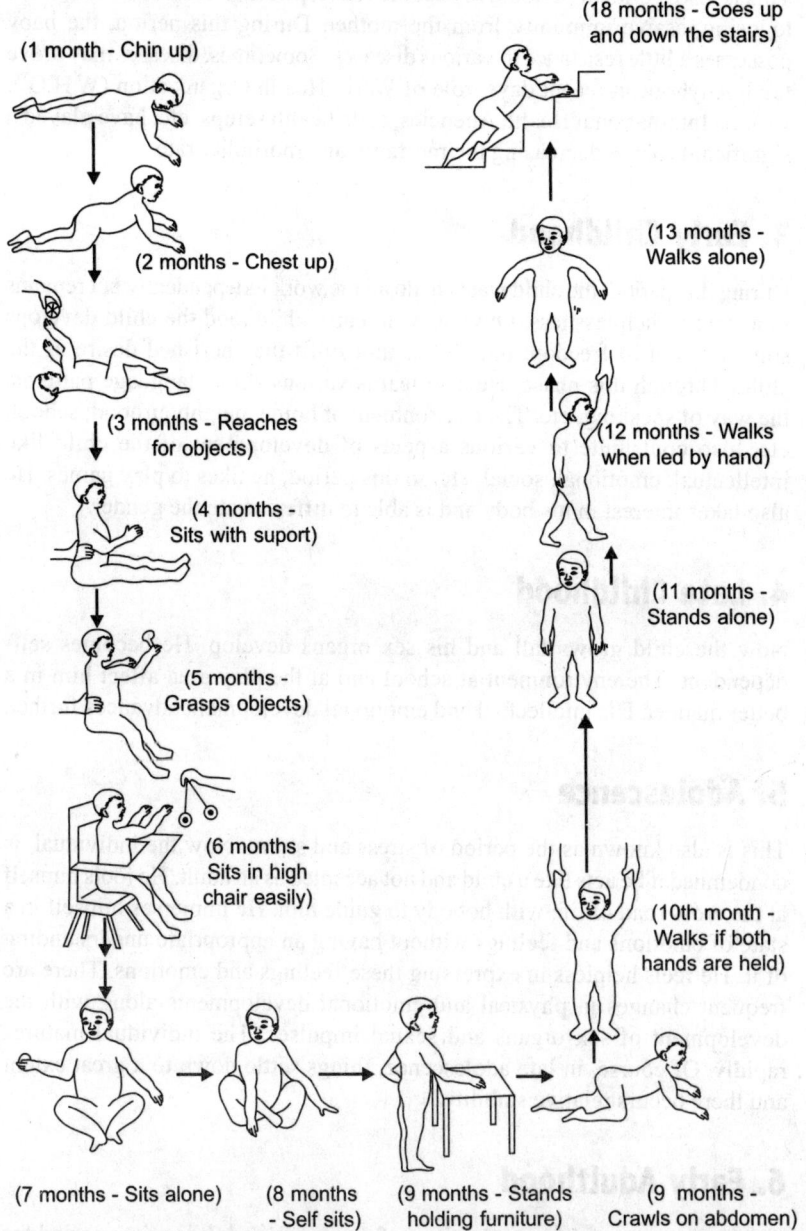

Development of Posture and Locomotion in the Infant.

2. Babyhood

This is also a critical period. He becomes susceptible to various diseases due to losing passive immunity from the mother. During this period, the baby possesses a little resistance to various diseases. Sometimes, diseases may prove fatal. Anyhow, in recent days, role of World Health Organization (W.H.O.), various International Health Agencies, state health setups, etc. have played a significant role in decreasing the mortality and morbidity rate.

3. Early Childhood

During this period, the child wants to do all the work independently but remains in a state of helplessness. Obviously, in early childhood the child develops some amount of freedom but that cannot fulfil the cherished desire of the child. Through this phase, He also learns various skills, language patterns, the way of speaking, etc. The environment of home, neighbourhood, school, etc. also contribute to various aspects of development of the child like intellectual, emotional, social, etc. In this period, he likes to play games. He also takes interest in his body and is able to differentiate the gender.

4. Late Childhood

Now the child grows tall and his sex organs develop. He becomes self-dependent. The environment at school and at the play area affect him in a better manner. His intellectual and emotional development advances further.

5. Adolescence

This is also known as the period of stress and storm. Now the individual is condemned if he acts like a child and not accepted as an adult. He fools himself at the cross road of life with nobody to guide him. He immerses himself in a state of emotions and feelings without having an appropriate understanding of it. He feels helpless in expressing these feelings and emotions. There are frequent changes in physical and emotional developments along with the development of sex organs and sexual impulses. The individual matures rapidly. Of course, in late adolescence, things settle down to a great extent and there occurs relative stability.

6. Early Adulthood

In this stage, power of reproduction is fully developed. It is prime period for an individual to establish himself in society. The individual seeks success, establishment and recognition.

7. Middle age

The age group from 40-60 is called middle age. This is a period of transition to old age. This is the age of achievement. The professional and family responsibilities become enormous. In case of females, there occur significant changes in personality due to appearance of menopause.

8. Old age

This is the ultimate stage in man's development. Here the development comes to a halt. Infact, this is a period of decline and degeneration. During this period the interest in sex declines and the interest in religion increases. Generally in old age people feel themselves useless. But it is the period when an old man can guide the new generation with his experience for betterment.

V. FACTORS AFFECTING GROWTH AND DEVELOPMENT

Human growth and development is a very complex phenomenon. It is affected by a number of factors. These factors include internal factors, external factors and miscellaneous factors.

Internal factors belong to the conditions within the body. These include intelligence, sex, glands of internal secretion, racial difference, cultural background of the child, etc.

The *external factors* include sunlight, season, fresh air, climate, ventilation, food and nutrition, etc.

Other miscellaneous factors that govern growth and development are heredity, environment, learning and maturation, etc.

1. Internal Factors

a. Intelligence

Low grade intelligence is associated with retardation, slow learning and poor performance. On the other hand, high grade intelligence is associated with acceleration, quick learning and excellent performance.

b. Endocrine Glands

Secretions from endocrine glands play an important role in human growth and development.

For example, hyperactivity of the pituitary glands gives rise to a giant appearance to different parts of the body. The hypo activity of the same gland results in a dwarf size appearance. The deficiency of sex glands cause delay in puberty. The over-activity of these glands produces early sexual maturity. Other glands such as parathyroid and thyroid glands also affect growth and development in an important manner.

c. Gender

At birth, boys are slightly bigger in size than girls. When the process of growth sets in after birth, girls exhibit rapid growth and attain a full size earlier than boys.

2. External Factors

A large amount of physical growth depends partly upon environmental factors like sunlight, fresh air, conditions of climate and partly upon food and nutrition.

Psychologists attribute seasons of the year as another external factor that influences growth. Accordingly, utmost gain in weight takes place between October and December and the least amount of weight gain takes place between April and June.

3. Miscellaneous Factors

a. Heredity and Environment

An individual is the product of his heredity and environment. Potentialities of development (and not gained skills, knowledge and attitudes), are handed down from parents to their off-springs. The prospective development of a full personality is controlled by genetic endowment, favorable environment and specific training. Unfavorable environment or lack of training may result in an under developed or a weaker personality.

b. Maturation and Learning

Development is the result of maturation and learning.

Maturation means development of traits potentially present in an individual because of his hereditary endowment from his parents and other ancestors. This maturation is the inner growth process unaffected by training.

Learning implies exercise, training and experience on the part of an individual. Learning may result from practice, which in due course, may bring about a change in the individual's behavior, or it may result from training. Training is an indicator of a selected, well directed and goal oriented type of activity.

Maturation and learning are closely inter-related, and one influences the other. Learning develops the trait potentiality present in an individual to the highest extent possible. Thus, even though factors like learning and environment have a great influence on growth and development, maturation supplies the raw material for learning and decides to a large extent the more general patterns of the behavior of an individual.

VI. ASPECTS OF DEVELOPMENT

The following are the major aspects of human growth and development:

1. Physical growth and motor development.
2. Intellectual development.
3. Emotional development.
4. Social development.
5. Moral development.

Physical growth refers to the progressive development of the various parts of the body and their capacity to function properly.

Intellectual development includes abilities like attending, perceiving, observing, remembering, imagining, thinking, solving problems and growth in intelligence, language, etc.

Emotional development refers to distinct emotional experience, specific to the particular stage of development.

Social development is "the progressive improvement, through directed activity, for the individual in comprehension of the social heritage and the formation of flexible conduct patterns of reasonable conformity with this heritage."

Moral development means learning social or moral values which include lessons about honesty, kindness, charity, service, obedience and the like.

1. Physical and Motor Development

One of the chief characteristics of a living organism is its ability to grow. Physical growth is the progressive development of the various parts of the body and their capacity to function. Physical growth is determined by a variety of factors, some of which are not yet understood. We have already discussed about these factors under internal, external and miscellaneous factors.

The initial changes immediately after birth, include the expansion of the lungs and certain changes in the circulation of blood. The growth of the brain during the first year is very rapid. The bones start growing in length and thickness. Milk-teeth start erupting within the sixth to the eighth month. By two and a half years, all twenty teeth of the first set erupt. These teeth start falling off after six years and teeth of the permanent set start erupting. The last tooth of the permanent set normally erupts by the 25th year. About the age of 13 years, the individual starts attaining sexual maturity. This age is called the *age of puberty*. During puberty, girls start menstruating and like the boys show secondary sexual characters. Complete growth is attained by the age of 16 years in girls 20 years in boys.

2. Intellectual Development

a. Meaning of Intellectual Development

Intellectual or mental development is an important aspect of growth, which embraces the various mental abilities. Mental development includes such abilities as attending, perceiving, observing, remembering, imagining, thinking, solving problems, learning languages, growth of intelligence, etc. These abilities grow and mature with age. Inspite of a general pattern of mental development, each individual grows and develops in his own unique manner.

The various mental abilities are inter-related, inter-dependant and develop as a whole. Moreover, mental development is a continuous process. The factors that affect mental development include maturation, learning and education. Mental development is a function of the brain and nervous system.

b. Phases and Aspects of Intellectual Development

Under this, we will discuss various developments that take place in an individual.

i. Formation of Perceptions

Since birth an individual is exposed to various types of stimuli. These stimuli are responded to in the form of sensations and these sensations are perceived. Sensations and perceptions therefore form a significant aspect of mental development. Sensations act upon the individual through the sense organs and give a meaning to it through perceptions. Perceptions are concrete and objective. For example, one can perceive a book or TV or computer, which is concrete and objective.

In the beginning, the infant's sensation and perception remains hazy about the environment. Gradually his sensation of taste, color, sound, touch, etc. gets related with various concrete objects. Gradually he is able to discriminate between objects, people or events through sensations and perceptions. The child's perceptions are also resolved by his needs and interests. As the child grows older, his sensations and perceptions are customized by his beliefs, estimations and ideals. Thus, his knowledge grows to complexities and leads to abstract concepts. Formation of perceptions is a major factor in the mental development of a child.

ii. Formation of Concept

Mental development takes place through the increase of knowledge. During the initial stage, perceptions give an individual the basis of knowledge. But the real knowledge evolves when the perceptions are converted into concepts, or are generalized. Concepts are the outcome of an individual's perceptual experiences. A concept is the generalized meaning that is attached to an object. We arrive at concepts of things, persons and qualities as a result of our perceptual experience, our ability to compare the common qualities, and to generalize the same.

For example:

Concept of things

Desk chair, ballpoint pen, computer, etc.

Concept of persons

Father, mother, brother, sister, friend, etc.

Concept of quality

Honesty and truthfulness, benevolence, etc.

The child's concepts increase with perceptions and experiences along with comparison of relationships between old and new circumstances. Among various concepts, self-concept and social-concepts of inter-personal relations greatly influence the child's thinking and behavior. The child's social concepts are influenced by the nature of inter-personal relationships at home, relationship in the neighbourhood, in the play ground and other social activities. Therefore, concept formation, is one of the most important aspects of mental development.

iii. Development of Language

Language is a powerful force in the mental development of a child. Infact, mental development pre-supposes a good command over language. Our mind develops through thinking, and thinking is impossible without language. Thus, language development is one of the crucial factors that is required in mental development. The process of concept formation is helped by the development of language. Infact, language development and mental development go side by side. Learning a language involves listening, speaking, reading and writing. Language is a tool of both thinking and communication. It is the basic tool for social communication and personality development. Hence, language is one of the most crucial factors that have been attributed for mental development.

iv. Growth in Thinking

Thinking is a potent mean for mental development. Thinking along with language encompasses various strategic involvement of objects and situations around the individual, which gives rise to logical development of various conclusions. Hence, thinking and reasoning are potent vehicles for the mental development of an individual.

v. Development of Intelligence

Development of intelligence is the most important characteristic of mental development. The growth of intelligence is related to other aspects of the individual like, health status, physical growth, language, personality, emotion, etc. along with his environment.

Intelligence has heightened growth during the period of infancy and it is marked. Moderate growth occurs during childhood and slow growth during adolescence and the latter periods. Of course, there are individual variations. Some individuals show a rapid increase in certain areas of intelligence, whereas others indicate a rapid increase in other areas of abilities. From homeopathic point of view the role of miasm needs re-experiment with these areas.

In addition to this, intelligence seems to grow on up to a certain age, and then it ceases. Psychologists set the age of 16 to 20 as the peak period of mental growth. The various conditions or factors which affect intellectual development or the growth of intelligence are the intellectual atmosphere at home, the socio-economic status, geographical distribution, health and disease condition etc. But the fact remains that growth of intelligence or intellectual development is a significant factor in the mental development of the individuals.

3. Emotional Development

See next chapter (along with 'Emotion', Chapter 10)

4. Social Development

Practically, no one can live in a state of complete or even partial isolation. A human being cannot lead a secluded life. Perhaps that is the reason a killer or murderer is jailed and kept in isolation. After all, human beings are essentially social beings. In modern life, man has come to feel the necessity of human relationships more than ever before. It is by living in society that man develops human qualities for the evolvement of a civilized society. An infant takes birth in a social milieu, but he is unaware of the social aspects of life. It is the society and social environment that rear, shape and adjust him into a total individual in their framework. As the child grows up, he develops not only in physical, mental, emotional spheres but also in the spheres of social behavior that becomes a part of society.

a. Social Development: What is it?

Social development implies the process of adapting the biological individual into a human person. In social development, an individual learns the standards, values and traditions of group standard. He becomes imbued with oneness in social structure making an acceptable rapport and cooperation. It is the accomplishments of maturity in social relationships. During the process of social development, an individual gives a positive response to tastes, attitudes and behavioral patterns of society. Social development presupposes that growth must be progressive with a flexible pattern of reasonable compliance to social heritage.

b. Other Aspects of Social Development

Social development is inter-related and interwoven with other aspects of development like physical, mental, emotional, intellectual, etc. It is an individual's interaction of physical constitution, mental make up, emotional disposition, maturity, etc. with corresponding aspects of other individuals, either to promote or to dissuade the desirable social attitudes and behaviors at any stage of development.

Socialization is another aspect of social development where an individual learns about the society and its customs, traditions, language, morals, ways of living, thinking and other allied norms. Every individual takes birth in a family. A family is also a unit of social group. As a member of a family, an individual has to learn a language, modes of behaving with siblings, parents and other members of the group. As he grows up, he has to acquire certain modes of behavior and existing social attitudes of the society.

Socialization is the process by which an individual learns the behaviors, the values, and the expectations of the social structure. Socialization enables him to play various social roles along with social learning and allied developmental tasks along with shading his own personality in society. Next, in social development, the individual increasingly amplifies, intensifies and strengthens his social field so that he becomes an integral part of society where his views and activities are also accepted and shared.

Some of the important characteristics of socialization are given below:

a. A desire of belongingness and to be socially accepted by an individual.
b. An individual's interest and ability to take interest in others.

An individual's interest to share, co-operate, to work as a member of group, to develop friendship and acquaintance, to develop social perception etc.

The most important aspect of social development is the attainment of social maturity. A socially mature individual is capable of exhibiting desirable social traits in a given age level, i.e., a socially mature child of 8 years must exhibit social traits that are prevalent amongst most of the 8 years olds in a given society. Anyhow, a socially mature individual (especially an adult) must be able to:

- make judgments and decisions
- arrive at logical conclusions
- take appropriate action in resolving problems and critical issues
- fit himself to his fellowmen and new circumstances
- adjust his fellowmen and situations to himself, etc.

c. Factors Affecting Social Development

i. Home Environment

Home is the first agency of socialization for an individual from where all social virtues and qualities develop. Family is the starting point from where the social structure begins. It is the family where the child gets an opening of social life. It is in the family that the child learns different behavioral patterns like eating, sleeping, toilet training, etc. He also learns language and the mode of expression at home. A happy, content and well-knit family helps in advancing social adjustments of the individual members. A good family instills 'the feeling of 'we' instead of 'feeling of I'. It is a general note that charity begins at home. The principle of intra family cooperation later extends to inter-family and inter-social cooperation and mutual aid.

Another aspect from home environment should be undertaken, i.e., love and affection provided by the family to a child. Love and affection are the basic psychological needs of a child. It boosts the feeling of security and self-confidence in a child. Rearing in love and affection gives him the needed courage to enter into social relationships outside the family. If the child acquires love and affection from home, it is quite natural that he will also look forward to love and affection from others also. This interaction will develop a social harmony and amicability in a social set up. As a result, there develops a positive attitude towards life and society. In fact, the famous saying 'to spare the rod is to spoil the child' is absolutely wrong. Even the love of a teacher works like a reinforcement.

ii. Socio-economic Status

The socio-economic status is also an important issue in the process of socialisation. Higher socio-economic conditions make the child interact in a higher and wider circle of society, which teaches him various etiquettes, manners and other socially accepted behaviors in a natural way. By associating with a range of people and wide social circle, the child develops a solid foundation of socialization. It has been observed that children belonging to a high economic group become extroverted having an integrated and positive personality for the enrichment of socialization. On the other hand, children born in poor families or broken homes frequently experience difficulty in proper social adjustment. It has also been observed that criminals and anti-social people are generally associated with low socio-economic conditions.

iii. Social Interaction

Social interaction through various social organizations widens the field of child's social connections and increases his social perception. He learns and absorbs the qualities of leadership, cooperation and endurance. The narcissistic or self-love attitude of the child is transformed to philanthropic and benevolent actions through social interaction.

iv. Friends and Groups

When the child grows up, he starts playing and participating in small groups outside home which widens his social contacts. Gradually he is influenced by friends and playgroups through social relationships, who exert effective influence on his social life. During the interaction, friends and playmates admire child's certain traits and disapprove others. The traits appreciated by the friends are further adopted in a social process by the child. The rightness of the trait does not matter much to the child. If his immoral deeds are appreciated by his playmates, then the child may even adopt those immoral qualities. At this crucial juncture of life of the child the role of parents becomes crucial. They should be careful and take special steps to prevent the child going astray.

v. Role of School

School is another potent organization for the social development of the child. School is a prescribed agency of education and it makes attempts for "a systematic socialization of the younger generation". School acts as a complementary social institution to home. In the school, the child comes in contact with a large number of students through which he experiences different kinds of social experiences. In addition to these, school programmes and activities help him to build a communication among their friends, classmates, peers, etc. The guidance from teachers also determines to a large extent the development of social skills and attitudes. Schools also teach some of the basic social attitudes, moral lessons, principles of good conduct, etc., which helps in blooming of social qualities in a child. The school also socializes the child by teaching cultural elements of the society in which the school functions. School also helps the child to gains skills essential for fitness in the society through group activities like games and projects.

vi. Community and Religion

Community and religion definitely contribute and modify the process of socialization. Both material and non-material resources of the community help in socializing the individual.

Religion has long been regarded as a primary social institution. It certainly exerts a special influence on a child for socialization. It is unfortunate that we talk of religion but not of religiousness. If the child is taught of religiousness, then a wonderful society in this universe can be evolved. Moreover, by this the current parochial trend of fighting for a religion can be curbed. Religiousness can help in shaping the social attitude of the individual in a far superior way.

vii. Other Factors

Other factors like heredity, age, language, personal property, health status along with agencies like government and private sectors, also play a substantial role in socialization for an individual.

5. Moral Development

The word 'moral' and all its derivations come from Middle French (via Latin) moralis, and 'Mos' which means manner, custom and habit. It is concerned with the principles of right and wrong in behavior. It also implies ethical judgment sanctioned or operative on one's conscience. In the present context, the word 'moral' refers to personality traits of an individual that synchronizes with the inner nature of the individual and ideals approved by the society. Moral development is one of the important processes of development of an individual. Moral lessons are related to service, sincerity, truthfulness, honesty, kindness, compassion, charity, obedience, respect, etc. Morality also encompasses relations between children and their peers, between children and adults, between men and women, etc. Moreover, rules of games and sports also come under the purview of the morality.

a. Factors Affecting Moral Development

i. Family Set Up

Family plays a crucial role in a child's moral development. The various behaviors those are observed by the child in a family set up become ideal for him. The child is neither moral nor immoral in himself. He develops moral behavior as a reaction of having reward or punishment, praise or condemnation from the family. His first initiation into the mysteries of the good and the bad is determined through his parent's acceptance or rejection of his various actions. The actions, which are approved by the parents, are regarded as good and those rejected by them are regarded as bad. It is the family where the foundations of a child's moral development are laid down.

ii. Play Companions

When the child is exposed to his external environment like neighborhood or school for playing, he comes in contact with his playmates, some of who are senior to him. He is influenced by the notions of good and bad that prevail among his chosen senior companions.

iii. School and Educational Institutions

School and other educational institutions also play a significant role in shaping moral concepts in a child. The child is influenced by the notions of good and bad as a result of his relationship with his school environment such as peers or classmates, senior students, teachers and others. Children accept many things which they observe from the deed and actions of seniors. The child may find some conflicting concepts that have been learnt at home. At this time, the child accepts the new morals and discards or confirms the lessons that he has learnt at home. The teachings of moral science and moral education influence the child to a greater extent. It is very unfortunate that such lessons are not given due importance in the school curriculum, as a result of which the child goes astray when he enters a college. Today, moral lessons remain more in spirit than in its real execution.

iv. Society and Culture

The general social impression also shapes the moral development of an individual. It is this reason why the moral behavior of individuals belonging to cultured societies is noticeably different from that of individuals belonging to uncivilized societies.

v. Age

Age is an important factor in the formation of moral concepts and moral behaviors in an individual. As the individual passes from infancy to adolescence, he becomes more tolerant towards certain ideals which sometimes do not tally with his standard of acceptance of morality. The individual as a child was obeying his seniors unconditionally, but when the individual attains adolescence, he becomes defiant to the seniors and asks questions about the validity and utility of morality. Of course, in the later period of adolescence, he accepts many things which he had rejected earlier.

vi. Gender

Gender is majorly related to moral development of an individual. Generally, girls feel a sense of guilt and shame if their behavior is not within the accepted moral code of society, whereas boys in contrast are usually more aggressive and hence set their own standards of moral behavior.

vii. Cinema, TV and Computer

Cinema, TV and computers in no way influence a child less in modifying moral development. The criminalization and success of immoral people displayed in cinema or TV (or even fighting games loaded in software) must be kept in strict vigil otherwise the child or the adolescent may be inspired by such deeds and go wayward.

viii. Books

Books have a great bearing in moral development of an individual. Good books develop morality in an individual and facilitate the path to be a good citizen. Similarly, bad books may lead a child or adolescent astray. Hence, care must be taken so that the child or adolescent is not exposed to pornographic books or magazines where the immoral and abnormal relations are highlighted. Children should be encouraged to read books on Rama, Krishna, Christ, Nanak, Vivekananda, etc. so that they can practice morality and understand humanity in a better way. Moral developments are complex processes in which the action and interaction of an individual and those surrounding him are of great importance.

VII. NEED OF READING DEVELOPMENTAL PSYCHOLOGY

1. Problems concerning the welfare of a child.
2. Making a legal decision on divorce.
3. Removing children from abusing families.
4. Understanding Sexual behavior.
5. Infant day care.
6. Behavior emotional problem.
7. Early childhood education.
8. Process of child development.
9. Situational influences on children's behavior.
10. Research questions.

11. Role of:
    a. Heredity and environment.
    b. Passive and active nature of the child.
    c. Continuity and discontinuity of developmental changes.
    d. Stability of behavior.
    e. Consistence across situations.

THEORIES OF PERSONALITY DEVELOPMENT

PIAGET'S WORK ON COGNITIVE DEVELOPMENT – A SPECIAL NOTE: Jean Piaget's work on cognitive development in the child is more significant than that done by any other psychologist. Besides distinguishing four major stages in the process, Piaget identifies many sub-stages within the four major ones. Piagetian work on cognitive development shall be discussed under two heads: Key concepts, Four stages of Cognition.

1. Key Concepts

Piaget worked out his four stages on the basis of the following key concepts:

a. Schemes

'Schemes' are patterns of behavior that children exhibit in dealing with objects in space. In case of children, schemes can be simple like the pattern of behavior shown by a child in grasping an object within his reach. It is complex in case of adults. They show it when they try to solve an intricate mathematical problem.

b. Assimilation

Assimilation takes place when the organism uses some object in the environment in the course of its activity. It occurs when the new is drawn into the old behavior pattern and becomes part of the child's inner organisation. For example, when something new is perceived that resembles an old, already familiar object, it is used like the old object. It is, however, necessary that the object or event to be assimilated must fit an existing scheme.

c. Accommodation

Accommodation refers to adjusting the old pattern to account for the new one. Hence, new activities are added to the infant's previously learnt pattern and these are modified to accommodate them.

d. Equilibrium

Piaget says that when the organism fails to handle the new situation with the help of the previously learnt pattern of behavior, some sort of inequilibrium or imbalance is created. However, the individual tries to reduce such imbalance. He does so by focusing his attention on the stimuli that has caused the imbalance. He develops new schemes or adopts old ones until the equilibrium is restored. This process of restoring balance is called equilibrium.

2. Piagetian Four Stages of Cognition

Piaget conceives the following periods of intellectual development:

i. The period of sensori-motor activity.

ii. The pre-operational stage.

iii. The concrete-operational stage.

iv. The period of formal operations.

v. The above stages are discussed in brief in the following paras.

i. The Period of Sensori-Motor Activity

The period of sensori-motor activity covers the period of birth until 18 to 24 months. During this period, the infant's actions are not yet internalized in the form of thoughts. The infant exercises sensori-motor capacities by sucking, handling or by moving objects. He behaves as if objects that have disappeared from view have ceased to exist. "Out of sight, out of mind" might be said to characterize the view of the infant.

For example, Piaget tells us that an infant of five to eight months of age, already old enough to seize a solid object, will lose interest and turn away if a cloth thrown over the object before his hand reaches it. At a slightly older age, he is capable of seeking an object behind a screen. This is the beginning of the notion that objects have permanent exteriors, and that they are there in the world, independent of himself. However, at this stage, the child's intelligence level is equal to that of intelligent animals.

ii. The Pre-operational Stage or the Stage of Pre-concepts or Representations (2 Years to 6 or 7 Years)

This stage coincides with the period of two years until six years or seven years (early childhood) of age. This is the period preparatory to that of concrete operations. As the stage of early childhood sets in, the child begins to make internal symbolic representations and to invent solutions rather than depend on trial and error. This is the beginning of pre-operational stage. Symbolic play with a toy gun as a real gun or a tricycle or a horse illustrates this stage.

Ego-centricism

This stage is marked by ego-centricism. There is natural shift from the sensori-motor stage to logical and social ego-centricity. His own perspective of the world is all that matters for him. He fails to understand another's point of view. He does not understand that someone else has a different point of view for things and objects in space. His attitude is, "I am I and you are you, and how can you be I and I be you?" "The child's own personal perspective," says Watson, "Is absolute, not relative".

Animism

Animism is another characteristic of this stage. Children between four and six years of age, regard everything to be alive unless it is broken or damaged. Children up to seven years of age regard everything that moves to be alive. For children of eight to ten years, everything that moves by itself is alive. Children at the late childhood stage, reserve life for animals and plants or animals alone.

iii. Concrete Operational Stage (7 Years to 12 Years)

As soon as children reach the end of the pre-operational stage, children begin to understand the principle of conservation. Conservation is the ability to recognize the basic attributes of an object such as number or weight, to remain the same even when the appearance of the object is changed. At this stage, ego-centricism is diluted. Now, the child communicates with others, compares others' points of views with his own and takes a decision after some thought. At this stage, spirit of cooperation and competition can be developed.

iv. Stage of Formal Operations (From 12 Years Onwards)

During this stage, the child develops the ability of thinking and reasoning of the objects which are beyond the immediate world. Now the problems are systematically solved. Trial and error gives way to some logic. The child also learns by mistakes.

■

Chapter 22

DEVELOPMENTAL PSYCHOLOGY

There exist different ways of describing human development. However, the most accepted way of describing this method belongs to chronological pattern or age pattern. We can divide this under two heads:

I. Pre-natal development.
II. Post-natal development.

I. PRE-NATAL DEVELOPMENT

Stages of Pre-natal Development

Pre-natal development indicates the development from conception to birth. This stage is divided under three heads:

1. Period of ovum.
2. Period of embryo.
3. Period fetus.

1. Period of Ovum

The period of the ovum starts from the time of fertilization and lasts up to 14 days.

Fertilization takes place in the fallopian tube after the union of sperm and ovum. After fertilization, the zygote divides itself and becomes a morula. The morula reaches the uterine cavity by the 7th day and is fully embedded by the 14th day after ovulation. Then the morula converts to a blastocyst. The blastocyst gives rise to the trophoblast from its outer shell. The troubleshot helps in supplying nutrition to the embryo. Later, the zygote gains access to the maternal blood supply by embedding in the decidua which enables to receive further food and oxygen from the maternal source.

2. Period of Embryo

The period of the embryo continues from the third week to the end of second or third lunar month. In this stage, respiratory system, nervous system, etc., develop. This period is characterised by rapid growth. The embryo becomes susceptible to environmental effects. Most of the birth defects occur in this phase.

3. Period of Fetus

This stage is initiated by the eighth or twelfth week and ends in birth. With the emergence of the first bone cells, the embryo develops into a fetus. The fetus look like a miniature human being. The fetus can move and kick in this phase.

Week Vise Pre-natal Development

Week	Development
1	Fertilization occurs and embryonic period begins.
2	The cell mass differentiates into endoderm and ectoderm.
3	The lady misses the menses. Mesoderm appears.
4	Embryo forms a human-like shape, arm and leg buds appear.
5	Primitive mouth appears.
6	Primitive nose appears.
7	Eyelids start to grow.
8	The organism's gender can be differentiated as there appear ovaries (female) and testes (male).
9	Period of fetus ensues.
10	External genitalia can be discriminated.
20	The approximate weight and length becomes 450 gms and 20 cms respectively.
25	The approximate weight and length further becomes 900 gms and 25 cms respectively.

28 – Eyes become open and fetus turns head down.
38 – Full term.

Factors Affecting Pre-natal Development

1. Maternal Nutrition

The mother needs additional 300 to 500 calories during pregnancy in comparison to the usual calorie intake. Adequate nutrition is highly essential for the health of the expectant mother. Malnutrition may lead to still born babies, low birth weight infant, etc.

2. Rh Incompatibility

This condition may lead to death or permanent injury to the neonate.

3. Maternal Age

Maternal age before 21 and after 27 may have an adverse affect on the neonate due to deficient hormonal activity.

4. Maternal Emotions

Maternal emotions have a tremendous impact on the fetus through glandular changes caused by emotion. Maternal stress may cause an increase in the fetal heart rate and movement, and may also lead to various abnormalities.

5. Vitamin Deficiency

Deficiency of vitamins and minerals can cause a deleterious effect on the neonate.

6. Drugs

Various drugs have been attributed in causing various damages to the fetus. Hence all mothers seek and should also take the advice of a doctor for the use of drugs. Of course, homeopathic medicines are safer alternatives.

7. X-rays

It has an adverse effect on the fetus, even if it is used for diagnostic purposes. It has a damaging effects on the fetus. It is wiser to avoid X-rays as much as possible.

8. Infections and Chronic Diseases

Mothers suffering from various diseases can have a deleterious effects on the fetus. Mothers suffering from:

a. German measles, gives birth to a mentally retarded child.
b. Syphilis, gives birth to a weak and mentally deficient child. Also, the mother may undergo a miscarriage. You, being a homeopathic student should appreciate it in a better way from a miasmatic point of view.
c. Diabetes may induce the child with various respiratory and circulatory diseases.

Such examples can be multiplied.

9. Alcohol and Substance Abuse

Obviously, use of alcohol and allied substances may severely impair the physical and mental development of the newborn.

II. POST-NATAL DEVELOPMENT

As mentioned in the last chapter, we will carry out the study under the following caption:

A. Infancy.
B. Early childhood.
C. Late childhood.
D. Adolescence.

A. Infancy

The word infant has originated from a Latin word meaning 'without language'.

The period between birth to 2 years is called the period of infancy. This period is characterised by rapid growth and development in terms of height, weight, size, etc.

The first four weeks of life is termed as neonatal period, which is a transition period : the transition from intrauterine life to extrauterine life.

1. Physical Growth

The infant is on an average 20" long and weighs around 7 pounds. A male infant weighs on an average 0.2 pounds more than a female infant. Surprisingly, the weight of an infant is doubled in six months.

In the first few weeks of life, the infant has no control over his body, except the ability of turning the head from side to side while lying on the back, which is gained at birth. Gradually, he learns to raise his chin and head while lying on the abdomen.

He starts smiling at the age of about two months. At this age he can also affix his eyesight steadily on the to and fro movement of a dangling toy.

He can also strongly hold any nearby object by this time. By six months of age he can reach out and grasp the dangling toy. At this age, a baby is able to sit with a slight support.

Between 9 to 18 months, the baby rapidly learns:

- to creep,
- to stand with support,
- to climb stairs,
- to walk and,
- is constantly moving about

At the end of two years, there is an increase of strength in arms and legs and he learns to walk.

By the time the infant reaches a height of 28.25 inches, his weight increases to 19.7 pounds. However, averages in height and weight may vary from individual to individual.

Besides changes in height and weight, growth in large muscles affects body proportions.

Changes are also noticeable in respect of cutting teeth. At first there are no teeth. The baby's teeth appear and are followed by different sets.

There are many other changes which are connected with:

- digestion,
- respiration,
- toilet habits, etc.

Changes also occur in:

- nerves and glands, and
- in reproductive organs

The baby's bones are more pliable and the joints are less firm. There is always the risk of infection because of low calorie intake. There is always an extra danger of infection after six months of infant feeding, when the infant lacks passive immunity obtained from the mother.

By two, most infants will go to the toilet when they feel the need; by three, most infants will stay dry all night.

2. Development of Sense Organs

An infant possesses the senses of sight, hearing, smell, taste and touch.

a. Touch is the earliest sense to develop in infants. The infants are highly sensitive to pain.
b. The sense of sight tends to develop in infancy. The infant can blink. He has a fair color perception and can follow a moving light. Still the sense of sight is less developed in comparison to other sensory organs during this phase of life. Their optic nerve and retina are yet to be fully developed.
c. Newborns are sensitive to hearing and turn their head towards sound.
d. Newborns respond to sense of smell. They can know from where a particular smell is coming. Surprisingly, an infant of 6 days old prefers to have mother's breast in comparison to someone else's due to the fact that he can sense the smell of his mother. Infants do not like the smell of rotten egg, fish, strawberry, vanilla, etc.
e. Newborns are also sensitive to taste and love tasty things and avoid non-tasty things.

A Synopsis of Motor Development Observed in Infancy:

Age in Months	Motor Activity
1	Chin high.
2	Raising chest.
3	Gripping and releasing an object.
4	Sitting with some assistance.
5	Sitting on lap and holding objects.
6	Sitting on chair.
7	Playing with toys.
8	Standing with assistance.
9	Self-standing with the help of a wall.
10	Crawling on knees.
11	Raising oneself while holding the wall.
12	Walking with assistance.

13	Starts climbing staircases.
14	Stands without anybody's help.
15	Walks without anybody's help.

3. Intellectual Development

The baby has all the senses and is ready to carry out various mental activities. The baby can think at this stage. Hence, he seeks approval from his parents for the things he likes. He becomes curious during this stage, which is a characteristic of mental development of this period. He makes an attempt to know about his immediate environment. He is also able to distinguish people and things in the environment to which he belongs.

4. Emotional Development

There exist controversies regarding the emotional development in infancy. But it is safe to state that emotions in infancy remain in an undifferentiated and diffused form. The emotional reaction grows to be less diffused and can be differentiated as the baby grows further. Watson, is of the opinion that the three emotions of fear, anger and love identify infants. For example, distress and delight are the two emotional patterns that get differentiated from excitement. Similarly, fear, anger and disgust are differentiated from distress before the age of six months.

5. Social Development

This period is not very important for social development. Anyhow, at the age of one month, the infant notices the adults around him, from where social behavior begins. During this period, the infant begins to respond to the behavior of those elders who supply his needs. At about one year of age, he develops a fairly satisfactory pattern of responses to adults. The following table points out some salient features of infant behavior during the first year:

Infant Responses / Behavior	Age in Months
Returns glances of adults with smiles	1 – 2
Cries when the attendant leaves him	2 – 3
Quietened by caressing	4 – 5
Shows denial response to strangers	5 – 6
Stretches out hands towards the attendant	7 – 8

Seeks attention by movements	9–10
Starts imitating other children	9–10
Organised play activity	10–11
Looks to other child leaving aside the toys	11–12

6. Moral Development

Moral development evolves with toilet training in an infant taught by parents. Hence, child's first experience with 'right', 'wrong', 'good' and 'bad' is perceived from toilet training. The appearance of sense of guilt is developed around the age of two. At the age of three plus, this sense is further heightened by the mere thought of a prohibited act.

B. Early Childhood

The period of early childhood refers to the period from two years to five or six years. This is also an important phase of life. Various physical and psychological changes are observed during this stage. During this period, most of the changes come from maturation and less from learning. This stage is very important for the following two reasons:

First, this is the stage where the child is reared for entering into formal education.

Secondly, during this stage, the child leaves home and enters school, which is a totally new circumstance for him.

Due to the emergence of kindergarten (lower and upper) schools, early pressures are put on the child with new expectations from parents as well as teachers.

1. Physical Development

The following features of physical development during the period of early childhood are noteworthy:

a. This period is discernible by physical growth and motor development, which are very conspicuous.
b. At the age of 3, the average height of the child reaches approximately 90 cms and at the age about 5 or 6 years, the height comes up to 110 cms.
c. At the age of 3, the weight of a boy becomes about 30 pounds and at the age of 5–6 it becomes around 43 pounds.

d. Generally a weight gain of about four or five pounds per year is also noticed during this phase.
e. Girls are slightly shorter in height in comparison to boys in this stage of development.
f. There develops a lot of motor development and muscular coordination. This enables the child to perform various types of essential activities like walking, running, jumping, throwing, etc.
g. Different parts of the body such as head, hands, arms, legs, etc. grow proportionately.
h. The nervous and lymphatic system grow to an appreciable extent.
i. The respiratory and circulatory systems become more capable. The breathe becomes regular, deep and longer.
j. Primary teeth appear at the age of 3. At the attainment of 6 years, these teeth are replaced by permanent teeth.
k. The stamina of the child also improves.
l. The immune system revives in a more efficient manner.
m. There is a marked improvement in the functioning of sensory organs.
n. The child pays instant attention to noise, sound, color and light. He begins to recognize faces and expresses the feelings of pleasure and pain through his facial expressions.
o. The influence of learning may be readily seen in such skills as talking, writing, buttoning clothes, etc.
p. However, they become proficient in climbing, jumping, throwing and catching balls, tricycling and so on by the time they reach the age of four of five. Sex variations in this respect are also noticeable.
q. It is important to note that each child has his own tempo of growth. Some children grow slower during the early years and faster in later years. Boys and girls grow at different rates. It is found that 60 percent of the adult height is reached by girls at 3 ½ years and by boys at 4 ½ years.

2. Intellectual Development

a. There occurs rapid language development during this stage. The child gains increasing ability of expression.
b. The child is able to express himself in a potent manner, which certifies his mental development.
c. The child also gets hold of a variety of sensory and perceptual experiences, which adds a lot towards his mental development.

3. Emotional Development

In this stage, significant emotional developments are conspicuously marked.

a. Significant emotional developments are marked in this stage. Emotions of distress and delight get differentiated from excitement.

b. During early childhood, three important emotions viz. fear, anger, jealousy are developed (for details see the Chapter X).

c. Between the age of 2-4, children become afraid of various animals (especially dogs), darkness, etc. Unfortunately during this period the child cannot differentiate realism from unrealism. In recent days, often fear is induced through horror or violent movies from cinema or TVs. The child takes everything as genuine. Moreover, they feel totally powerless in front of such fears.

Characteristics of Childhood Emotions

a. Children's emotions are:
   - Brief and last for only a few minutes
   - Intense
   - Transitory and changeable, shifts instantly from tears to smiles; from jealousy to affection.
   - Appear frequently

b. Children express their emotions frankly, the way they feel it.

c. Variability is found in the emotional responses of children. One child in fear may run out of the room, another may hide under a chair.

4. Social Development

a. During this stage, the social behavior of the child progresses from the individual aspect to social aspect. He starts sharing his comfort and possessions with other members of the family in volition.

b. He also develops the sense of cooperation in the company of other children who are brought into his life. Now, he considers 'what is mine is mine' but he also starts gaining in understanding that 'what is yours is yours'. At the age of four, he comes to realize that 'what is mine is yours also' and likes to share or exchange his toys and other belongings with his playmates.

c. He also begins to subscribe his affiliation to the social group, to which he belongs. He also takes pride for such an affiliation. He also becomes responsive to the feelings and thoughts of others around him

d. Children of both sexes learn to play together.
e. Some of the important forms of social behavior during this period are negativism, rivalry, quarrelling, teasing with a blend of cooperation and social approval.
f. Four year old children quarrel more in comparison to those of two years of age.
g. Boys fight with their companions more in comparison to their counter part, girls. Girls's quarrel is limited to verbal only.

Early childhood is an important period an individual's life. Habits of social response developed during this period leave a solid foundation for future social activities of life. In this respect, a model nursery school will prove immensely helpful for developing healthy social behavior in a child in his early childhood.

5. Moral Development

a. Children count good and bad only in terms of specific acts approved or disapproved by parents.
b. They start obeying elders, helping co-fellows along with developing the mutual relationship of give and take.
c. Children want that their performances should be accepted and appreciated unconditionally as correct. If their wrong deeds are brought to their notice, this leaves them in a state of worry and unhappiness.
d. Children develop the sense of responsibility during this period. When they are ordered, etc. to go to a grocery or departmental store, they gladly do it with a sense of cooperation. They also adopt this tendency of cooperation and team work in a play ground and at the homes of friends and relatives.
e. They also like to help parents in setting the dining table, making their beds and tidying up their rooms and other domestic chores.
f. Children become interested in God and like to listen to moral stories.

During this period, parents should be vigilant about the child's exposition to environment including TV and cinema shows. In TV serials and cinemas, many immoral acts are generalized and highlighted. They inspire the child to adopt immoral practices. Such shows should be discouraged or abandoned, so that the child can learn the right things to become a successful, healthy and productive citizen.

C. Late Childhood

The period between the age of 6 to 12 is attributed to late childhood. In this stage of later childhood, growth and development becomes slow, steady and uniform in contrast to the period of infancy and early childhood where there was rapid growth and development. During this period, the following developments become conspicuous:

1. Physical Development

The average height of the child at twelve is about 145 cms. He weighs 42- 45 kgs. The child becomes tall and slim. He gains about 3 kgs of weight in 2 to 3 years until the pubertal growth spurt takes place. Girls show a sudden growth called the growth spurt in 10th or 11th year of age, whereas boys put on height at the age of 12 or 13. Maturity occurs about two years earlier among girls than boys.

During this period, muscles become strong. The development of motor skills becomes more specific, by which the children gain better control over their muscles. Development of greater strength and endurance in children is also observed during this stage.

Milk-teeth start falling around the age of 6 and are replaced by permanent teeth within the following 5 years. Bones also become harder during this period.

During this stage of life, resistance and immunity to many diseases is developed.

From the age of 9 or 10, children start playing outdoor games and sports like running, jumping, swimming, cricket, football, etc.

An outline of motor development of children is mentioned below:

Age	Behavior
6	Activities like skipping and throwing improves, but girls do better in this respect.
7	Hopping and jumping becomes improved along with balancing feet. They can hop and jump in squares.
8	Hopping, jumping, throwing becomes more refined. Grip strength also improves.
9	Running and vertical jumping can be performed. Boys surpass girls in this field of activity.

10	Children can estimate and stop the pathways of small balls when thrown from a distance
11	A boy and girl can do standing broad jump of 5 feet and 3 feet respectively.
12	Children can also do standing high jump of 3 feet.

Various illnesses and disorders like upper respiratory tract infection, eczema, scabies, bed wetting, etc. are found during this stage of life. Many start suffering from acne, headache, etc. and transitory emotional upsets occur as they approach puberty.

Important Note: *The motor development gaps between sexes widen after 13. Boys continue to improve while girls stay at the same or even decline in this respect. We must also know that the growth variances are attributed to genetic endowment and environmental influences, which include climatic condition, geographical distribution, socio-economic status, etc.*

2. Intellectual Development

During this period, rapid intellectual development in a child occurs. The child becomes interested in studies. He feels a sense of pride while increasing his knowledge. He relates the studies learnt into his practical life. He now presents himself in a refined manner and expresses himself with an improved version of language. He searches for new friends and peers. He also takes interest in meeting people, and talking and chating with them on various topics. Such interactions become very useful for the intellectual development the child. However, parents must guard their precious child against wrong education and wrong circumstances.

3. Emotional Development

This is the period of stability and control of the emotional aspect of the child. Now, the child is able to cope with various of emotions. He realises the futility of his anger. He also understands that his violent emotions are no more accorded by anyone. But it does not mean that the child becomes free from emotions. The reality is something deeper. At the age of 9 months, the infant, instead of crying out loudly and wholeheartedly shifts to a subdued response as the child gradually becomes aware of social prestige. Hence, his expression remains in latent form which may develop into acting out behavior or depression. He is also adorned with pleasant emotions which he expresses also. He laughs and enjoys being laughed with.

We must remember that the child has emotions like anger, fear, jealousy besides other common emotions.

During this phase, acting out behavior may play a decisive role. Emotional turmoil expressed through misbehavior is called acting out behavior. Acting out behaviors may include fighting, telling a lie, stealing, destroying something or breaking rules. In the long run, culmination of this trend may lead to development of antisocial activities.

During this period, anxiety disorders may also find a place in the child. This is generated due to separation of near and dear ones, say mother or father, to whom the child was very attached. This is found in close-knit, caring families.

Sometimes depression may also be found. If you find 4-5 symptoms from the following list in the child, then the child is said to be under depression:

a. The child feels tired.
b. Looks unhappy.
c. Crying out of rage.
d. Intense feeling of guilt.
e. Complains of physical ailments.
f. Loss of appetite.
g. Suffering from anxiety disorders.
h. Extremely active or inactive.
i. Thinking of suicide or death.

4. Social Development

Exposure to school environment increases the child's prospect for expansion of his social development. Radical changes are observed in the child's social behavior in school.

The period is often called the 'gang age'. The important characteristic of the 'gang age' is that children groups have a proclivity to expand and to become highly organized. Now the child does not like to play only with the children of his neighbourhood. He develops friendship with other students at school. He discovers new peers. He plays with them, builds up and enlarges his circle of friends and enjoys their company. Now he prefers group play instead of individual play. He no longer wants to depend upon a limited environment at home. He wants to be in the wider social world of peers. He does this for social endorsement and recognition. The child organises or becomes a part of organising for realising some of his goals. He ascertains the social norms by becoming a member of the gang. After forming a gang, the children invite other groups (or gangs) for a game or play competition. Each member feels pompous to be the member of the gang. They also arrange meetings themselves at the corner of the street or in dilapidated houses or in playgrounds or alike places. Girls due to restriction meet at the house of a member of the group. The gangs enact drama, go for a picnic or outing, or may play cricket or football. During the process of social adjustment, there may occur frequent quarrels and bickering. Hence, the child also learns how to adjust with society. During this process, envy, jealousy, aggressiveness, etc., also develop. They also develop good qualities like sympathy and benevolence. They also learn getting adjusted to a situation or a company, judgement, loyalty, honesty, obedience, etc. Boys grow more aggressive than girls whereas girls harbor more jealousy and enviousness than boys in matters of companionship.

Social praise and disapproval effect the behavior of children immensely. Hence, it is advised to praise the children for their good acts, and approval should be the norm in rearing a child for making him a better citizen of the country.

Some causes for unsocial activities may be :

- bad health,
- lack of proper diet,
- bad environment,
- adverse home condition,
- disregard of parents,
- low socio-economic status,
- heavy home or school tasks, etc.

5. Moral Development

During late childhood, the child is fairly competent to understand what is right and what is wrong. This moral development is the outcome of environmental influences. The role of home, neighborhood, peer group, school, etc. aids substantial growth in his understanding of morality: The ideas of right and wrong. He also develops positive moral aspects like tolerance, honesty, justice, co-operation, etc.

It has been also observed that gang plays a dominant role in manners, speech and the general behavior of a child. Sometimes their so-called, moralization creates a state of conflict. The so-called morality taught by the 'gang' goes against the lessons learnt in home. The child finds himself in a state of confusion with the moral concepts that have been taught at home, and which are being opposed by his 'gang'. In this stage there is a strong chance that the child may be swept away by the ideas preached by the 'gang'. Moreover, the advice of the 'gang' looks much more alluring to him.

The 'gang' is usually interested in immediate and temporary pleasure. This so-called pleasure lures the child to bypass morality. Abnormal behavior like stealing, lying and bullying may develop among the children at this age. So every parent must be vigilant to understand their offspring, who may go wayward. However, the effect of home always remains dominant especially regarding religion and race.

D. Adolescence

This word means immature, involving, relating or meaning somebody who is immature. This is a 15th century French word that appears via Latin word 'adolescence' which mean 'to grow', 'be nourished'.

The period between childhood adulthood is termed as adolescence. This period of adolescence is characterised by rapid growth and change in nearly all aspects of a child's physical, mental, social and emotional life. It is a very critical period in one's life, as the growth achieved, the experiences gained, and the relationships developed at this stage determine the complete future of an individual. It is the most critical period of human life. This period is called the age of teenagers.

Very often this period is referred as 'period of transition' and 'period of stress and storm'. During adolescence, an individual has to pass through a very crucial phase. At this juncture he is not accepted as an adult and he is condemned or criticized for various immature and child-like activities. Elders exhort that he should not act like a child. They expect the adolescent to behave in a mature and dignified manner as a grown up. At the same time he is not accepted as an adult by the society. He always remains in a state of conflict and suspension.

1. Physical Growth

Physical growth and development achieves its summit during the stage of adolescence. The human body including internal and external organs accomplish its ultimate form and figure during this period. Other aspects of physical growth like size, weight and height are also gained to their utmost during this period.

Let us explore this caption further under:
a. Puberty and menarche.
b. Adolescent growth spurt.
c. Primary and secondary sexual characters.
d. Other associated aspects.

a. Puberty and Menarche

The period of adolescence begins with puberty i.e., sexual maturation. Usually, puberty sets in between the age of 11 to 13. Sometimes the onset may become delayed, say at the age of 15 or 17. In developed countries, like U.S.A., Japan and Western Europe, very often puberty is set at an early age, say at the age of 9 or 10 which is called 'precocious puberty' or 'secular trend' in psychology. This growth trend has been observed since the last century. The secular trend is usually not found in India. However, it is beginning to appear in India amongst the affluent families who maintain a high standard of living. An advanced lifestyle is held responsible for this trend.

In this stage an individual attains sexual maturity. The body of an individual becomes capable of functioning sexually. The attitude and behavior becomes more mature.

In girls, the first menses called menarche, marks the beginning of their puberty. Pubertal changes are initiated at the age of 9 or 10 and is expressed as sexual maturation at the age of 13 or 14. The role of the endocrine system is held responsible for the causation of this sexual maturity. In tropical and sub-tropical countries, girls mature earlier in comparison to those of cold countries.

In boys, onset of semen, pubic hair, a lower voice along with growth of penis and testes occurs. In boys, generally puberty and sexual maturity appear around at the age of 12 and 14 years respectively.

The stage of puberty may be divided into three stages:

i. Pre-pubescent Stage

In this stage, the reproductive organs do not function but secondary sexual characteristics begin to appear.

ii. Pubescent Stage

During this stage, the reproductive organs start functioning. In case of females, the ova and in case of males, the sperms are produced. The secondary sexual characteristics develop further.

iii. Post-pubescent Stage

During this stage, the sex organs are capable of adult functioning and the secondary sex characteristics are well developed.

b. Adolescent Growth Spurt

Growth spurt is one of the foremost characteristics of adolescence. There occurs a sudden shoot in height. Rapid growth is observed twice during a life time; first from birth to six months of age and second during the period of adolescence. This growth spurt usually starts at the age of nine and reaches its peak by twelve. After attaining the age of twelve the growth spurt gradually slows down and almost ceases between fifteen to eighteen years of age. During this growth spurt, girls gain almost 9 cms height in a year and 5 kgs of weight. Hips of girls become wider due to deposition of fat and it develops a round appearance

The growth spurt in boys beings between the age of 11 to 14 and reaches its peak at about 15 years. There after, it slowly declines till the age 20 to 21. Boys grow 10 to 12.5 cms in a year and add 5 to 6 kgs of weight. A boy develops wider shoulders and muscles. His legs become longer in comparison to his trunk. His forearms become longer in contrast to his upper arms and his height.

The sex difference displays a distinct character during this stage of development. At the age of about 15, boys surpass girls in growth spurt.

c. Primary and Secondary Sexual Characters

During adolescence, development of primary and secondary sexual characters occur.

Primary sexual characteristics point to those characteristics of physical organs that are essential for reproduction. In males the testes, penis, prostate, seminal ducts are related to primary sexual characteristics. The first sign of sexual maturity in boys is the arrival of sperms, which may appear in urine or may release in semen while a sleep (especially with amorous dreams).

In girls (rather women), the primary sexual characteristics are connected to the development of ovaries, uterus, fallopian tubes, vagina, etc.

Secondary sexual characteristics pertain to those physiological maturation which are not directly related to reproduction. Such signs include voice changes, appearance of hair in axilla and pubic region, enlargement of breasts, etc. In case of females, the nipples and areola enlarge. The skin also becomes thicker and the sebaceous gland activity increases, which frequently gives rise to acne.

d. Other Associated Aspects

Voice change in boys is a common feature. The voice of boys becomes hoarse and that of girls sweet. The change of voice has a link to the behavior of adolescents.

The capacity for performing physical activities is enhanced in this period.

Boys take more interest in physical activities and usually surpass girls. Adolescents also prefer to engage themselves in athletic activities instead of mental occupations.

There is also an increase in height and weight during adolescence. There are also general changes in proportions of various physical functions. Different parts of the body grow at different rates and reach their maximum development at different times.

2. Intellectual Development

During this period, tremendous intellectual developments occur in adolescents. Intellectual development reaches its climax during this period. Various mental abilities like perception, attention, observation, thinking and reasoning, memory, intelligence, etc. are augmented and sharpened to a greater degree. As a result, the individual becomes interested in aesthetic creativities. He solves problems in an analytical and systematic manner. The ability of observation also grows in depth.

In this period of adolescence, there is an increased ability to generalise facts. He develops generalisation from particulars. Earlier during childhood, he was only concerned with a particular or parochial reasoning. Now he generalises and examines other facets of the problem. For example, if you display a picture of a bike accident on the road to a child, he will immediately hold the truck responsible for the accident while overtaking the bike, whereas an adolescent will analyse it as:

- from where did the truck come,
- whether the bike rider was on the left side or not, i.e., was he obeying road rules,
- whether the bike rider's breaks failed,
- whether another party (say a bull or a child) entered between the bike and the truck,
- whether the truck driver was drunk,
- what was the mental condition of the bike rider,
- what could be the other conditions of the location, etc.

Even in a science laboratory his imagination and concept building functions along with reasoning. During this stage, the adolescent is able to think in terms of abstraction along with generalisation. His depth of understanding develops. Abstract thinking leads to a heightened imagination.

Decision making ability also develops to a greater degree during adolescence. Communicating skills also develop during this period. They like to argue and ask for plausible explanations for an enquiry while interacting with others.

3. Emotional Development

It has already been mentioned that in this period of adolescence, an individual demonstrates signs of development in every sphere of life. Hence it is obvious that the expression of emotion should also go through a transformation.

This period of life is compared to spring. It is exciting, alluring, charming and wonderful, but full of bumps and bizarre path that bridges the gap between childhood and adulthood.

In adolescence, the individual becomes very prestige conscious. He always guards his prestige from injury. He cannot bear any adverse comments or remarks against him. He also becomes sensitive to his appearance and health. A little toothache or colic or a small abscess over the skin may be magnified as if he is suffering from cancer. Sexual instincts reappear in an intensified form. This impulse is new, intense and unknown to him. His reaction to the emotion of love is almost maniacal. He is easily deluded to fall in sex or love without understanding its nature or phenomenon. The individual cannot control himself and is attracted to the opposite sex. He seeks sexual gratification without understanding the ways and means. In this mode of life this aspect must be sublimated in studies. If this sexual instinct is not sublimated, he succumbs to masturbation or homo-sexuality or sexual gratification with the opposite sex. This leads to a sense of guilt and sin against himself which leaves an indelible mark for the development of his personality. Moreover, this may interfere in his married life resulting in various maladjustments and misunderstanding with the spouse.

Sometimes the love of an adolescent is sublimated towards the nation and he becomes patriotic. Then he talks of the nation and gives various solutions for its development. His sensitiveness further extends against the existing corruption and injustice in the society. He raises his voice against these vices and wants to fight them. This state of adolescence seems to be fit for *Causticum*. The *Causticum* patient is highly sympathetic in the sense, his sympathy is related to fight for a case of justice. Anyhow, adolescence is the period of emotional imbalance and is full of strain and stress.

The adolescent finds himself in conflict with himself, and many a times, this conflict extends to his family or society. Frequently, he goes into fits of anger easily and he represses his emotions. The present trend of job insecurity is another cause of emotional disturbance on the part of the adolescent. They are always haunted by the uncertain future which adds fuel to their emotional disturbance. The adolescent also becomes a victim of anxiety, guilt, etc. during this stage. On the outside, he represses his emotions but inside, he magnifies it in his day dreams and imagination. Hence as a homeopath, we have to advise the adolescents for sublimation of these emotions along with providing them with anti-miasmatic (and constitutional) medicines for relief.

4. Social Development

The period of adolescence is characterised by significant changes in social behavior and interaction. At home they are caught in the twilight area – neither a child nor an adult. They want to be treated with high esteem but nobody treats them the way they desire. During this stage, the adolescent becomes highly ambitious and wants to be something. He wants that he should be recognised at home and outside. He wants to be the centre of his surroundings. He also wants that his presence must be felt and no one should neglect him. He craves social status and social prestige.

Now his interest swings from himself to other members of family in an advanced form. His interest also proceeds from the family to the external world so that he and his work can be recognised.

He makes friends with his peers and elders. He serves and derives service from them and thus social interaction is intensified. In every need the individual stands as a service man to society. But he gains maximum satisfaction and comfort in close association with those of his age who appreciate his service.

Appreciation and recognition of his aid, instills a positive sense of security in him.

Gradually he makes strong bonds with his associates, where he gets his appreciation and recognition. On the contrary, he is rejected home being immature. This state induces him to lean towards his associates. This bond becomes so strong that he can even wage a confrontation with his own parents. The individual asserts that his friends are very important people for him and hence they must not be betrayed. This notion very often makes an individual go astray. Many adolescents, after interacting with peers and associates, develop some positive qualities like leadership, fellow feeling and cooperation.

If in the same family two or three children are passing through the adolescence period, they often form a gang among themselves and take decisions in a unified form like close associates as mentioned above.

Adolescence is the period of 'show off' or of affected manners. Freudian psychology clearly claims the awakening of sexual impulse during this period. Now the adolescent becomes interested in the opposite sex. He wants to impress the opposite sex with effective appearances. Boys start maintaining special dress codes and present a smart look to attract the attention of girls. Girls also do the same to attract the attention of boys. They crave praise, appreciation and recognition from boys. Subsequently the adolescent always remains appraising of his or her relationships and manners – the way he looks, talks, or behaves.

Parents play a crucial role in the adolescent's social development. If the adolescent is caught midstream, so are his parents. Parents expect a lot from boys, which may be beyond their ability and capability. This creates a sense of frustration and leads the adolescent wayward. Parents want to dominate, guide and give directions to him and still they expect him to act independently. This induces confusion and uncertainty in the adolescent. Some parents transfer their responsibility to their friends and relatives to advise the boy or girl if something goes wrong. By this act of parents, the adolescent understands the limitation of his parents and considers them impotent. This leads to a vicious circle. The adolescent resorts to revolution and this attitude compels him to miss the warmth of affection and sense of ownness from his parents. The situation may be aggravated further if friends or relatives of parents fail where the peer group succeeds in solving the problem of the adolescent. By this, the adolescent values his gang more than the values his family. Ultimately, the adolescent adheres to habitual disobedience to parents and elders which may lead him to the road of waywardness, thus transforming him into an irresponsible person in society.

Another aspect of this age is hero worship. The adolescent makes someone his ideal. Now-a-days cricket stars are the most common heroes. Among yester generations, film stars were the role models for adolescents. Prior to this, Vivekananda, Mahatma Gandhi, were the heroes along with Rama, Krishna and other Gods. This phenomenon has a definite impact on the future moulding of the personality.

5. Moral Development

Moral development of an adolescent is the effect of internal dictation rather than of peripheral imposition. As a child, he accepted the concepts of right and wrong as preached by his parents or elders around him without asking them any questions. But when he attains adolescence, he questions all moral concepts and demands a plausible answer.

With passing days and growing social interaction, the adolescent finds a number of inconsistencies in the moral concepts of people around him. So he wants to change them. He expects that everyone should follow the code and conduct of morality. He also raises questions on every aspect of morality that does not conform to his own standard of moral code. He even builds his own moral theories as a measure to solve the problems around him. But his theories are more in spirit than in real execution, because his theories on morality are out of tune with the existing circumstances and society. Along with these harsh realities, he finds himself in a baffled position regarding various concepts and hence feels helpless.

An adolescent develops a sense of guilt and shame during this stage. Moreover, he is exposed to surrounding social expectations. These two important factors develop the conscience of an individual. He also takes moral matters into his own hands and sets higher standards of morality. When he cannot realize or fails to practice the standards fixed by him, then he himself suffers from guilt and a troubled conscience. He seeks guidance and vision of a practical and feasible nature from others. The adolescent wants recognition for his good work and does not hesitate to accept any punishment for the wrong deed.

However sometimes, some adolescents become victims of various misdemeanors. Misdemeanor means a misdeed or a deliberate disobedience of rules. Some adolescents become victims of home misdemeanors. They leave home without giving any notice to any member of the family. They may also leave their home for petty tussles. They also defy the family norms. They hang outdoors beyond time. Sometimes, they run away from home or elope with somebody (may be a member of the opposite sex). Some of the adolescent students irritate their teachers, pass direct or indirect comments to them, or harasses classmates (like snatching money, taking pen or compass, important note books, etc.). They also fall prey to smoking, drinking, eve-teasing, etc.

Juvenile delinquency is quite common at the adolescent stage. Juvenile means a boy who has not attained the age 18 years. Delinquency does not merely mean juvenile crime. It embraces all deviations from normal youthful behavior including incorrigible, ungovernable, habitual disobedience and alongwith desertion of their home and mixing with immoral people. They suffer from behavioral problems and indulge in anti-social practices. Delinquency may be assessed from the following:

a. Self injury.
b. Harm to self or others.
c. Assaulting people.
d. Disturbing the crowd.
e. Damage to public property.
f. Misappropriation of property.
g. Theft or burglary.
h. Disobedience to authority.
i. Sexual misconduct.
j. Carrying weapons without proper authority.

Anyhow, in late adolescence, most of the individuals come on the right path. They become gentle and more liberal. They also understand their own and other's limitations and weaknesses. They become morally mature individuals. They understand that they cannot be a law unto themselves. They also understand the laws of society, which they cannot over-rule. So, ultimately they understand, realize and hence practice the common moral codes of society.

6. Health Problems of Adolescence

a. Obesity

In recent days, the advent of over-calorification of food including junk food, minus intake of fibres, lack of exercise, over-gluing to television, computer and internet, etc., has lead to the development of obesity. This situation has serious repercussions in the future. Obesity accentuates diseases like diabetes, hypertension, etc.

b. Alcohol and Substance Abuse

Inspite of stringencies made by Governments, some adolescents want to have a taste of alcohol and ultimately they get addicted to it. First, they start providing company to their elders, who preach pseudo theories and plus points of alcohol and drugs. Later alcohol and drugs within themselves become a great reinforcement to the adolescents. In this way they throw themselves in hell. Some of them choose the way of crime and other anti-social activities.

c. Sexual Transmitted Diseases

During this period, there is a re-awakening of sexual impulses in adolescents. This impels adolescents for doing the sexual act. They do not hesitate in adopting unsafe means for getting sexual gratification. Thus, they suffer from sexually transmitted diseases (STDs) like syphilis, gonorrhea and even AIDS (acquired immune deficiency syndrome).

d. Teenage Pregnancy

As mentioned above, sexual impulse leads both the male and female adolescents for experimentation which sex. Lack of knowledge of contraceptive practices leads to teenage pregnancies in females. It has serious outcomes including death of the expectant mother.

e. Juvenile Delinquency

This has already been discussed.

DEVELOPMENT OF PERSONALITY

As already described, that onset of puberty gives maturation to sexual activities. It is the transitory phase that connects childhood to adulthood. This stage is full of disturbances and very often this stage is called the period of stress and storm.

Immediately before puberty, wide-ranging physiological developments occur. Boys and girls start exhibiting their respective physical signs. Girls start having menstrual cycles and their organs acquire rounded contours. Boys grow beards and moustaches and their voices become heavy. Puberty causes an awareness of the noticeable physiological changes and this state leads to a feeling of adulthood. They also become interested in sex. They want to know all about it, but they have to suffer a set back as the elders do not want to handover knowledge on the subject. Rather, they are denied information on the ground that it is not their age for knowing all this. Elders do so because of the existing social taboos. Lack of sex education makes these adolescents face various problems, out of which some become more intricate. In India, there are less sex restrictions in primitive tribes as compared to the youth of cultured groups. Thus, the transition from adolescence to adulthood becomes easier for the tribal youth than the other youths. Absence of means of satisfying sexual curiosities and a social feeling of immorality induces a guilt conscience and anxiety in the adolescent, which becomes an impediment in the proper development of his personality.

Adolescents also experience an increase in the feeling of independence. The adjustment of adolescence is a problem which differs with culture. Interestingly, the study made by Mead reveals that the disturbance of an adolescent in civilised societies is not found amongst people of some primitive cultures like Samoa. So he submits that disturbances of the adolescent stage are due to those mental conflicts which cause imposition of the norms of civilisation. The author fully agrees with views submitted by Mead from his observation in the village of Kebidi, a remote place in the district of Koraput in Orissa, where he was posted as a homeopathic medical officer. In those areas sex does not give rise to any conflict in an adolescent. Interestingly, in their culture, one is allowed to adopt another's wife with her consent just by giving some money. There is not much discord on the issue. In fact, conflicts generated lead to many social problems like breaking of joint family, lack of sexual fitness, self-dependence, choice of profession, etc. in this age. In this respect, the role of parents, existing educational system, role of teachers should be amended. They treat the adolescent as a child. But the individual wants to prove his assertion. Hence he wages a revolt against it. Of course, in many instances, it soon subsides automatically. Adolescence is a stage in the development of personality and development is an unremitting process in which infancy shapes adolescence and adolescence shapes adulthood.

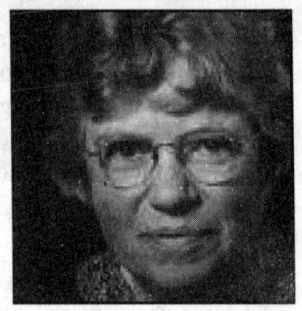

Margaret Mead (1901-1978)

(Along with the above, you must also add Freud's (Chapter 7) Genitalia stage, Erik Erikson's stage V, i.e., identity versus identity confusion (Chapter 8).

Chapter 23

MODEL QUESTIONS

Psychology : An Introduction

1. Delineate the nature and scope of psychology.
2. Narrate the contributions of Wundt and Titchener of experimental psychology.
3. Narrate psychology as the science of consciousness. Describe its plus and minus points.
4. Do you agree that psychology is a science? Justify your statement
5. What are the limitations of psychology as the 'Science of Soul'? Give an acceptable definition of psychology.
6. Discuss different branches of psychology.
7. Write brief notes on the contributions of the following to psychology :
   a. Watson.
   b. Freud.
   c. Jung.
   d. Adler.
   e. Neo-Freudians.
   f. Practical application of psychology.
   g. Organism and environment.

Psychology : Its Relation to Other Sciences

1. Examine the relationship of psychology to sociology, logic and medicine.
2. State the subject matter of psychology. How is it related to biology and medicine?

Schools of Psychology
Trace the historical development of contemporary psychology.

Psychology of Cognition : Sensation and Perception
1. What are the attributes of sensation? Discuss the steps involved in sensation.
2. Describe the structure and function of eye with the help of a diagram.
3. Describe the structure and function of ear.
4. Examine the theories of color vision.
5. Critically examine the various theories of hearing.
6. What is gustatory sensation? Describe the mechanism of taste sensation.
7. Describe the mechanism of olfactory and tactile sensation.
8. Discuss briefly kinesthetic, static and organic senses. Are they useful in human life?
9. Write brief notes on the following :
    a. Cornea.
    b. Iris.
    c. Aqueous humor and vitreous humor.
    d. Lens.
    e. Rods and cones.
    f. Blind spot.
    g. Mechanism of vision.
    h. Dark adaptation.
    i. Purkinjee phenomenon.
    j. Color vision.
    k. Cochlea.
    l. Basilar membrane.
    m. Telephone theory.
    n. Taste buds.
    o. Pain sensation.
    p. The Static sense.

Learning (Scientific Study of Behavior : Pavlov, Skinner, Watson)

1. "Learning is a process which brings about changes in the individual's way of responding as a result of environment". Explain.
2. Explain the importance of maturation in learning.
3. Explain the relationship and difference between learning and maturation.
4. Discuss operant conditioning technique. What are its practical applications in life.
5. What is insightful learning theory? Explain the characteristics of insightful learning.
6. Explain the following:
    a. Generalization in conditioning.
    b. Spontaneous recovery.
    c. Reinforcement in learning.
7. What is reinforcement? Discuss the various schedules of reinforcement.
8. Distinguish between :
    a. Learning and maturation.
    b. Classical and instrumental conditioning.
9. Examine the contributions of the following psychologists to learning psychology:
    a. Pavlov.
    b. Watson.
    c. Skinner.

Freud and Psycho-analysis

1. Explain the importance of unconscious mind.
2. Describe Freud's concept of mind.
3. What do you understand by daily psycho-pathology? Describe its various defense mechanisms.
4. Describe vividly infantile sexuality and psycho-sexual development.
5. Narrate psycho-analysis as an adjuvant therapy to a homeopath.
6. Describe how psychosexual development plays a crucial role in the determination of personality in a human being.

Neo-Freudian Psychodynamics

1. Who are the prominent Neo-Freudians? Describe their contributions to psychology with a thematic approach.

2. Describe Adler's individual psychology in short.
3. Describe Jung's 'Analytical Psychology' in short.
4. Describe Erik Erikson's eight developmental stages.

Psycho-somatic Manifestation of Dreams

5. Describe the process of dreaming and examine the theory of Freud that dreams are wish-fulfillment.
6. Compare and contrast night dreams with day dreams.
7. Discuss the various theories of dream interpretation.

Emotion

1. What is emotion? Examine the importance of physiological factors in emotion.
2. "Emotion is an acute disturbance of the body, psychological in origin involving, behavior, conscious experience and visceral functioning". With reference to the above definition, explain the characteristics of emotion.
3. Differentiate between feeling and emotion.
4. What are the theories of emotion? Which one do you consider the best? Justify your response by subscribing suitable examples.
5. Discuss in brief the different types of common emotions.
6. What is meant by bodily change in emotion? Discuss the various physiological changes for different types of emotional experiences.
7. Write notes on the followings :
   a. Causes and treatment of anger from a homeopathic point of view.
   b. Jealousy and envy.
   c. Sentiment.
   d. Joy and delight.
   e. Role of hypothalamus in emotion.
   f. Opponent process theory of emotion.

Memory

1. What do you understand by remembering? Discuss the various processes of remembering.
2. Examine the contributions of Ebbinghaus to the concept of remembering?

3. What is forgetting? Explore the various factors that contribute to forgetting.
4. Describe the characteristics of a typical forgetting curve? Compare and contrast the forgetting and retention curves with a suitable example.
5. Enumerate and explain the causes of forgetting with special reference to the interference theory of forgetting.
6. Distinguish between memory and retention. What methods do you know for its improvement?
7. Explain the phenomenon of forgetting. Describe five important homeopathic medicines for restoration of memory.
8. What do you understand by retention? Discuss the factors that influence retention.
9. What is short-term memory? How does it differ from long-term memory?
10. Critically explore the various theories of forgetting.
11. Discuss the importance of psycho-analytical causes of forgetting in practical life.
12. What is proactive inhibition? How does it differ from retroactive inhibition?
13. Write brief notes on the following:
    a. Retrograde amnesia.
    b. Theory of Disuse.
    c. Recitation vs Mere learning.
    d. Recall vs Recognition.

Intelligence

1. Define intelligence. Discuss its characteristics.
2. What is the nature of intelligence? How is it measured?
3. Describe any test of intelligence that you have studied.
4. What do you understand by individual and group tests of intelligence? Give examples from each category.
5. Distinguish between verbal and non-verbal tests of intelligence. Under which circumstances are non-verbal intelligence tests carried out?
6. What is mental age? How is it related to I.Q.? Explain how I.Q. is calculated.
7. Discuss the structure of intelligence.

8. What are the various types of intelligence tests? Describe some of them.
9. Explain the various theories of intelligence.
10. Examine the role of heredity and environment in the development of intelligence.

Thinking

1. Define thinking. Describe the chief characteristics of thinking?
2. Explore 'thinking as a problem solving behavior'.
3. What are the steps involved in problem solving? Describe the strategies of problem solving.
4. Narrate the role of set, direction and motive in thinking.
5. What is creative thinking? Discuss the various stages involved in creative thinking.
6. Discuss the relationship of thinking with symbols, language and past experience.
7. What is a concept? Describe some experiments on concept formation.
8. Write brief notes on the following :
    a. Percept.
    b. Language and thought.
    c. Thinking and images.
    d. Incubation.

Personality

1. Define personality. Discuss its nature and characteristics.
2. Give a critical estimate of the classification of personality.
3. What do you understand by 'trait'? Describe some important traits of human personality.
4. Describe that various determinants of personality. Why personality is called a social by-product?
5. Examine the role of home environment and child rearing practices in the development of personality.
6. Discuss briefly the various techniques used to assess personality.
7. What do you understand by psychometric tests of personality? Describe

some paper-pencil tests of personality.
8. What is a projective technique? Discuss the advantages and disadvantages of Rorschach test as a measure of personality.
9. Write brief notes on the following :
   a. Sheldon's classification of personality.
   b. Introversion-Extroversion.
   c. T.A.T.

Motivation

1. What is motive? Discuss the need, drive and incentive relationship.
2. Discuss the different types of motives.
3. Explain the importance of biological motives in human life.
4. What do you understand by personal motives? Critically examine the effect of culture on personal motives.
5. What is socialization of motives? Discuss the need for achievement and need for approval.
6. Critically examine the various theories of motivation.
7. Examine the role of motivation in learning. Illustrate your answer with experimental evidences.
8. All behaviors are motivated: Elucidate.

Aptitudes

1. Should we introduce aptitude tests in our curriculum? If so justify your assumptions with suitable instances.
2. Narrate different types of aptitude tests.

Attention and Distraction

1. Define attention and discuss its process.
2. Narrate the characteristics of attention? How does it differ from perception? Discuss attention as a selective process.
3. Why is attention is called a pre-perceptive attitude? What is the role of mental set in attention?
4. What are the types of attentions? Describe them with illustrations.
5. What are the various determinants of attention? Explain the objective determinants in detail.

6. Examine the role of interest, needs, motives and habit in attention.
7. Discuss the internal and external determinants of attention. Which one of them plays a greater role?
8. Is it possible to do two things at a time? Support your answer with illustrations and experimental evidences.
9. Explain the following:
    a. Involuntary attention.
    b. Attitudes, moods and attention.
    c. Attention as a receptor process.
    d. Span of attention.
    e. Distraction and inattention.
    f. Shifting of attention.
    g. Neural adjustment in attention.
    h. Postural set.
    i. Attention and interest.
    j. Figure and ground.
    k. Habitual attention.
10. What do you understand by distraction? How would you overcome it?

Psychology of Anxiety and Anxiety Disorders

1. What do you understand by anxiety disorder? Can we help a patient suffering from such a disorder with our medicines?
2. Narrate various types of anxiety disorders along with probable homeopathic medicines?
3. Describe various theories of anxiety disorders.

Conflict

1. Define conflict. Elucidate types of conflict in detail.
2. Define conflict and give a note on its genesis.
3. Define conflict and give a not about its principles

Frustration

1. Define frustration and bring forth its evolution and genesis in short.
2. What are the sources of frustration and narrate how an average man is

going to react to it.
3. How is frustration related to the development of personality.
4. In which way are you going to help your patient who is suffering from frustration?

Developmental Psychology

1. Name one major factor for growth and development of the child.
2. What do you mean by growth and development? Delineate the salient differences.
3. Narrate the principles of development.
4. What is meant by physical development? Explore various aspects of physical development.
5. Explain 'Why do we need proper knowledge of the patterns of physical growth and development?'
6. Describe emotional development of a child. Discuss five important remedies in relation to this aspect of child.
7. Justify 'Emotions are the springs of human action'.
8. Define emotion. Explore three common emotional traits.
9. What do you understand by 'socialization'? Discuss its associated factors that determine it.
10. Describe the social development from childhood to adolescence.
11. What is the difference between social development and socialization?
12. Moral development is a complex process: Discuss.
13. What do you understand by moral development? Give an account of the moral development before the onset of adolescence.

■

BIBLIOGRAPHY

1. Abraham Sperling (1990 Reprint, Ed. 1981) *Psychology Made Simple*, Rupa & Co by arrangement with Hehnemann Professional Books, London.
2. Adler, A. (1927) *Practice and Theory of Individual Psychology*, New York : Harcourt Brace & World.
3. Ahuja N. (1996), *A Short Text Book of Psychiatry* (3rd Ed.) New Delhi, Jaypee Brothers Medical Publishers Pvt. Ltd.
4. Arya, S.C. (1991), *Rational Pediatric Practice* (1st Ed.), Bombay, Indian Academy of Pediatrics.
5. Atkinson, J.W. & Birch, D.C. (1978). *An Introduction to Motivation* (2nd Ed.) New York : D.Van Nostrand.
6. Bajpai, S.R. (1993) *Methods of Social Survey and Research* (14th Reprinted), Kanpur, Kitab Ghar.
7. Bandura, A. and Walters, R.H. (1963) *Social Learning and Personality Development*, New York : Holt, Rinehart and Winston.
8. Bandura, A. (1968) *A Social Learning Interpretation of Psychological Dysfunction*. In P. London & D.Rosenhan (Eds), Foundation of Abnormal Psychology. New York : Holt, Rinchart and Winston.
9. Barlow David H & Durand V. Mark, (2000) *Abnormal Psychology* (2nd Ed.), London, International Thomas Publishing, Europe.
10. Baron, Robert A; et al (2003) *Psychology, Delhi,* Pearson Education (Singapore) Pvt, Ltd. 2nd Indian represent.
11. Berk Laure E 1991, *Allyn & Bacon* (A division of Simon and Schuster, inc. 160 Gould Street, Needham Heights, MA 02194 USA.
12. Bhargava, K.B. et al (1994) *A Short Text Book of E.N.T. Diseases for Students and Practitioners* (3rd Ed.), Bombay : Usha Publications.
13. Bhatia, H.R. (1968) *Elements of Educational Psychology* (3rd Ed.), Calcutta: Orient Longmen.
14. Bhatia, K.K., (2002) *Educational Psychology and Techniques of Teaching* (6th Revised and Enlarged Ed.), New Delhi, Kalyani Publishers.
15. Cattell, R.B. (1965) *The Scientific Analysis of Personality*, Penguin, Harmondsworth.
16. Cattell, R.B. (1971) *Abilities : Their Structure, Growth and Action*, Boston : Houghton Mifflin.

17. Chaube, S.P. (2003): *Developmental Psychology* (1st Ed.), Hyderabad, Neelkamal Publishers Pvt. Ltd.
18. Chauhan, S.S. (1984) : *Advanced Educational Psychology,* Sahibabad : Vani Educational Books (A division of Vikash Publishing House Pvt. Ltd.)
19. Dollard, J. & Miller, N.E., *Personality and Psychotherapy,* (1950) New York: McGraw Hill.
20. Dumville, D.E. (1938) *The Fundamentals of Psychology,* 3rd Ed., London: University Tutorial Press, 1938 (p.315).
21. Dutt, N.K. (1963) *Psychological Foundation of Education for Advanced Studies,* Delhi Doaba House.
22. Eysenck, H.J. (1990) *Trait Theories of Personality.* In A.M. Colman (Ed.) *Companion Encyclopedia of Psychology.* Vol. 1, London : Rutledge.
23. Fernald & Fernald, (2001) *Munn's Introduction to Psychology* (5th Ed.), USA. Wm.c. Brown Publishers.
24. Freud, S. *An Outline of Psycho-analysis* (1939), New York, Norton.
25. Freud, S. (1931) *The Interpretation of Dreams* (translated by A.A.Bril), New York, Carlton House
26. Freeman (1971) F.S., *Theory and Practice of Psychological Testing,* Bombay, Oxford & IBH.
27. Garry et al (1986): *Obstetrics Illustrated* (3rd International students Ed.) Edinburgh, Churchill Livingstone.
28. Ghorpade, M.B. *Essentials of Psychology* (3rd Ed.) Bombay, Himalaya Publisher .
29. Gupta, M.C., & Mahajan, B.K. (2003), *Text Book of Preventive and Social Medicine,* (3rd Ed.), New Delhi Jaypee Brothers Medical Publishers Pvt. Ltd.
30. Guyton, A.C., & Hall J.E. (1998) *Text Book of Medical Physiology* (9th Ed.) Hartcourt Brace & Co., Asia PTE Ltd. Philadelphia, PA 19106.
31. Hahnemann, Samuel (5th & 6th Ed), New Delhi, *Organon of Medicine,* B.Jain Publishers.
32. Hall Calvins. Et, al (4th Ed.) 1997 *Theories of Personality,* New York, John Wiley and Sons, Inc.
33. Hurlock, E. B. (2001), *Personality Development* (17th Reprint) New Delhi, Tata McGraw Hill Publishing Co. Ltd.
34. Hurlock E. (2003), *Developmental Psychology- A Life Span Approach* (29th Reprint), New Delhi Tata McGraw Hill Publishing Company Ltd.
35. *Induction Training for Newly Appointed Medical Officers,* State Institute of Health and Family Welfare, Orissa.
36. Kent, J.T., *Lectures on Homoeopathic Philosophy,* B. Jain Publishers, New Delhi.

37. Kohler, W. (1927). *The Mentality of Apes,* New York : Harcourt, Brace & World.
38. Labarba, Richrard C. (1981), *Developmental Psychology* (1st Ed.), London, Academic Press Inc.
39. Lange, C. (1922). *The Emotions.* Baltimore : Williams & Wilkens (Ongoing published 1885).
40. Lefton, L.A. (1985), *Psychology* (3rd Ed.), Allyn & Bacon, Newton, Massachusetts.
41. Mangal, S.K. (1994), Advanced Educational Psychology New Delhi, Prentice Hall of India Private Limited.
42. Maslow, A.H., (1962) *Towards a Psychology of Being,* Princeton, N.J., Van Nostrand.
43. Mehta M., (1998) : *Behavioral Sceince in Medical Practices* (1st Ed.) New Delhi, Jaypee Brothers Medical Publishers Pvt. Ltd.
44. Michael 1993, New York, *Scientific American Books,* Cele Sheila R. Cele.
45. Mohanty, G.B. (1997) *A Text Book of General Psychology* (2nd Revised Reprinted Ed.), Delhi Kalyani Publishers.
46. Mohanty, G.B. (1991) *A Text book of Abnormal Psychology* (2nd Reprinted Ed.) , New Delhi, Kalyani Publishers.
47. Morrison, R. (1993), *Desktop Guide to Keynotes & Confirmatory Symptoms* (1st Ed.) , Mumbai, Homoeopathic Medical Publishers.
48. Morgan, C.T. et al (1993), *Introduction to Psychology* (17th Ed.), New Delhi, Tata McGraw Hill Publishing Company Limited.
49. Munn, Norman L. et al (1972) *Introduction of Psychology* (3rd Ed) New Delhi, Houghton Mifflin Company, Boston, USA.
50. Murphy Gardner (1968) *An Instructor of Psychology* (2nd Reprint India Edition), Harper & Brothers, New York.
51. Murphy R. (1994), *Homoeopathic Medical Repertory* (1st Indian Ed.) New Delhi, B. Jain Publishers.
52. Nandy A., 2001, *Principles of Forensic Medicine* (2nd Reprint Ed.) Calcutta, New Central Book Agency (P) Ltd.
53. Nema, H.V., Nema N. (1998), *Text Book of Ophthalmology* (3rd Ed.), New Delhi, Jaypee Brothers Medical Publishers Pvt. Ltd.
54. Osho Rajneesh, *Unio Mystica* (Vol. I and II) Poona, Rajneesh Foundation.
55. Page, James D. (27th Reprint zero) *Abnormal Psychology,* New Delhi, Tata McGraw Hill Publishing Company Limited.
56. Papalia Diane E. (2004), *Developmental Psychology* (9th Ed.) New York, McGraw Hill Higher Education.

57. Piaget, J. (1932), *The Moral Judgment of the Child.* Routledge and Kegan Paul, London.
58. Park, K. (2005) *Text Book of Preventive & Social Medicine* (18th Ed.) Jabalpur, Benarasi Das Bhanot Publishers.
59. Prince, Morton (1929) *The Unconscious* (2nd Ed.), New York : Macmillan.
60. *Reproductive and Child Health Module for Medical Officer* (P.H.C.), National Institute of Health & Family Welfare, New Delhi, Reprint November, 2002.
61. Ross, J.S., *Groundwork of Educational Psychology,* 2nd Ed., Boston: George G. Harrup & Co., 1951, pp. 170-75.
62. Roediger, H.L., Rushton, J.P. e al., *Psychology,* London: George G. Harrup & Co., 1987, p.161.
63. Samuels Andrews (1985), *Jung a Post Jungians,* Rutledge and Kegan Paul London.
64. Sharma, R.N. (1967), *Educational Psychology,* Meerut: Rastogi Publications, 1967,
65. Sharma Poonam, & Lata G. (1990) *Fundamentals of Child Development & Child Care,* New Delhi, Sterling Publishers Pvt. Ltd.
66. Sharma, Ramnath (1982-83), *Outlines of General Psychology,* Meerut, Kedar Nath Ram Nath.
67. Sheldon, W.H., *The Varieties of Temperament* (1942) : A Psychology of Constitutional Differences, New York, Harper.
68. Skinner, B.F. (1938), *The Behavior of Organisms.* New York : Appleton-Centure-Crofts.
69. Sternberg, R.J. (1984) *Metaphors of Mind : Conceptions of the Nature of Intelligence.* New York : Cambridge University Press.
70. Suhail Shaizad, Bapat Ashwinee (1999), *Developmental Psychology,* New Delhi, Himalaya Publisher.
71. Varma, A.K. & Varma, M. (1989), Allahabad (1st Ed.), Vohra Publishers & Distributors (1st Ed.).
72. Watson, J.B. *Behaviorism,* (1930), London, Kegan Paul.
73. World Health Organization (1983). *Doctor-Patient Interaction and Communication,* Geneva.
74. Vatsayan, *General Psychology* (10th Revised Ed.) Meerut, Kedar Nath, Ram Nagar.
75. Weber, A.L. (1991) *Introduction to Psychology,* (1st Ed.) New York, Harper Collins Publishers.
76. Woodworth, R.S. (1965), *Contemporary Schools of Psychology* (Revised Ed.) London : Methuen.

■